Wid Scalpel and Shillaleh

Wid Scalpel and Shillaleh

The Life of William Hudson Daly

Robert M. Grom

America Through Time®
ADDING COLOR TO AMERICAN HISTORY

To my wife, Carol; children, Adam and Jessica;
and parents, Ann L. and Robert G. Grom

America Through Time is an imprint of Fonthill Media LLC
www.through-time.com
office@through-time.com

Published by Arcadia Publishing by arrangement with Fonthill Media LLC
For all general information, please contact Arcadia Publishing:
Telephone: 843-853-2070
Fax: 843-853-0044
E-mail: sales@arcadiapublishing.com
For customer service and orders:
Toll-Free 1-888-313-2665

www.arcadiapublishing.com

First published 2019

ISBN 978-1-63499-168-1

Typeset in 10pt on 13pt Sabon
Printed and bound in England

Preface

I first learned about William H. Daly while working at the Western Pennsylvania Hospital Foundation during the late 1980s and early 1990s. At the time, I served as executive director of a special project tasked with researching and updating the history of the Western Pennsylvania Hospital (also known as West Penn). A secondary goal of the project was to collect, catalog, preserve, and showcase surviving historical artifacts.

The "Antiquity Project," as it became known, was an endeavor to capture the hospital's history and update it for modern use in education and marketing. In the truest sense, the "Antiquity Project" was an "applied history" venture. Its primary purpose was to use what was learned and gathered to inform and educate patients, visitors, medical staff, and employees.

As the first chartered public hospital in Western Pennsylvania in 1853, West Penn had a long and noble history. The deeper I delved into the institution's history, the more I learned about the many great stories there were to tell. The life of Dr. William H. Daly is among the best.

Acknowledgments

Writing a book is never simple, nor is it typically representative of only the work of the author whose name appears on the cover. This book is a case in point.

First and foremost, I am grateful for the love and support of my wife, Carol, and my children, Adam and Jessica. Together, they have served as my chief editors and primary research assistants. Their critical eyes for teasing out details and their infrequent constructive criticisms were helpful throughout the research and writing process. I am likewise indebted to Wayne Winters, a friend with many years of experience writing and editing educational materials in the insurance industry. His proofreading skills are superb and his editing recommendations invaluable.

There are many other individuals and institutions who were helpful in the process of writing this book. In particular, I wish to recognize Bruce B. Wilson of St. Davids, PA, a relative of William H. Daly, who generously provided a wonderful family photograph for use in the book and rich details of Daly family history I had not previously known; Bill Marshal, Director of Facilities of Allegheny Health Network in Pittsburgh, PA, recently granted me access to old records of West Penn Hospital's Athalia Daly Home; and Brian A. Butko, Director of Publications at the Heinz History Center and Editor of the *Western Pennsylvania History* magazine in Pittsburgh, PA, was helpful in permitting my use of images and materials from an article about William H. Daly I had written many years ago.

I also wish to acknowledge with heartfelt appreciation the assistance I received from many librarians, archivists, and curators across the country. This wonderful group of individuals include Arlene Shaner, Historical Collections Librarian at The New York Academy of Medicine Library in New York, NY; Madeleine Bradford and Karen Wight, Reference Assistants at the Bentley Historical Library in Ann Arbor, MI; Michael Kraus, Curator at Soldiers and Sailors Hall in Pittsburgh, PA; Arlene Balkansky, Reference Specialist in the Newspaper and Current Periodical Reading Room, Library of Congress, Washington, D.C.; John Jackson at Virginia Tech University Libraries Special Collections Department in Blacksburg, VA; Jacklyn Burns at the J. Paul Getty Museum in Los Angeles, CA; Laura R. Brooks, Library Associate in the Archives & Special Collections Department at the University of Pittsburgh in Pittsburgh, PA; Amber L. Dushman, Manager, Records Management & Archives at the American Medical Association in Chicago, IL; Samantha L. Harper, Archivist at the Buffalo Bill Center of the West in Cody, WY; Jeremy Bonfini, Executive Director of the Allegheny County Medical Society in Pittsburgh, PA; Gilbert Pietrzak, staff member in the Pittsburgh Photographic Library at Pittsburgh Carnegie Library's Pennsylvania Department in Pittsburgh, PA; and Mary Jones, Chief Librarian at Heinz History Center in Pittsburgh, PA.

I would also like to gratefully recognize the many images and the great deal of reference material made possible through the resources of the U.S. National Library of Medicine, the Library of Congress, and the U.S. National Archives and Records Administration.

Contents

Introduction

In 1738, Benjamin Franklin wrote in *Poor Richard's Almanac*, "If you wou'd not be forgotten as soon as you are dead and rotten, either write things worth reading or do things worth the writing."[1] A little more than 100 years after Franklin penned his wise aphorism, William Hudson Daly was born in Western Pennsylvania. From his birth in 1842 until his death less than sixty years later in 1901, Daly took Franklin's advice to heart. As a young man, he overcame many challenges, including the loss of his father and, shortly afterward, his mother in 1858. After their deaths, he was forced to move from Pennsylvania to Virginia in 1859, where he found himself with little money and poor prospects. After joining the Confederate Army in Richmond in 1861 and successfully surviving several battles, he was captured at the Battle of Lee's Mill in 1862. Upon swearing an oath to never bear arms against the Union again, he was paroled. Shortly after his parole, and after taking an oath of "true" allegiance to the United States of America, he traded his field gray army uniform for the blue junior officer's frockcoat of the Union Army's medical cadet corps.[2] By the age of twenty, Daly already achieved some "things worth the writing."

His adventures did not end with capture and change of allegiance, nor did he forget the other part of Franklin's dictum about writing things worth reading. Between his brief military confinement in 1862 and his death in 1901, Daly would continue to accomplish extraordinary things worth being written about, and he would go on to author some sixty books, articles, and presentations on a diverse range of subjects. Most of his publications covered medical topics that reflected his interest in medicine and his chosen specialization of rhinology and laryngology; others related to his love of sports hunting and nature. Several of his published medical works were recognized in the United States and Europe as being at the vanguard of medical practice and science as it progressed rapidly in the late nineteenth century.

During the last quarter of the nineteenth century, Daly would move seamlessly between his medical practice, sports hunting, writing, military service, and family. While focused on these primary interests, he also spent considerable time and resources over the years advancing his and his wife Athalia's social standing through the cultivation of professional and business relationships and the arts. Financially, his medical practice grew to be quite lucrative; however, he enjoyed supplementing his income through a broad range of real estate and business investments.

In Pittsburgh, his reputation in medical and social circles was carefully developed and well-honed over the years. He built one of the city's preeminent medical practices, he married well, and he associated with all of the right people. His fame rested initially on his pioneering work in the medical specialties of laryngology and rhinology. Later in his career, it was the imbroglio he caused while serving as Surgeon-in-Chief of the Volunteer Army of Pennsylvania and major and chief surgeon of the U.S. Volunteers under his old friend, General Nelson A. Miles, during the Spanish-American War that brought him national notoriety.

Seemingly never being motivated by politics or public celebrity, his medical training and intellectual curiosity nevertheless entangled him in both during and immediately after the Spanish-American War. If a century had not separated him and Benjamin Franklin, it is likely Daly would have served as a contemporary example of the practical application of Franklin's wisdom.

1

Early Years

William Hudson Daly was born on 11 September 1842, about 40 miles east of Pittsburgh in Blairsville, Indiana County, Pennsylvania. He was the eleventh of thirteen children, with six brothers and six sisters all born over a period of twenty-five years between 1823 and 1848. Of the thirteen children, five died while very young. His parents, Thomas and Mary Maher (Marr) Daly, were married on 18 June 1822 at St. Paul's Catholic Church, Arran Quay, Dublin, Ireland. Seven of their children were born in Ireland; the remainder, including William, were born in the United States.

Emigrating from Ireland around 1838, they first arrived in Philadelphia. In September 1839, William's older brother, Thomas Lafayette, was the first child born in the United States. Between Thomas's birth and William's, two sisters, Mary Jane and Margaret, were born but died early. After William's birth in 1842, two additional children were born. His younger brother, Patrick, died in infancy; his sister, Mary Ellen, the last of the thirteen children of Thomas and Mary Daly, was born in June 1848.[1]

According to the 1850 United States Census, the family of Thomas and Mary Daly lived in the Spring Garden area of Philadelphia, near the Schuylkill River, the Pennsylvania State Penitentiary, and Fairmont Water Works. At the time of the census, Thomas was fifty-two years of age and Mary forty-four. They lived with seven of their eight living children: James, Alice, John, Jane, Agnes, William, and Mary Ellen. Their other son, Thomas Lafayette, aged eleven, had already left home to work on a farm in Wilmington, Delaware. He began work three years earlier at the age of eight.

William's father, Thomas, was a distiller by trade and worked in Philadelphia and the Wilmington, Delaware area for a number of years before relocating to Western Pennsylvania in 1856. Thomas Daly worked for John Gibson, an Irishman who had established a multi-city whiskey business with its headquarters in Philadelphia. Gibson had difficulty obtaining the steady flow of rye and other whiskeys he needed to supply his large number of customers. His answer to the supply problem was to create a distillery in Western Pennsylvania where the best rye grains in the country were grown.

In 1857, Thomas was engaged to superintend the building of the Gibsonton Mills distillery to be known as John Gibson Son's & Co. in Rostraver, Westmoreland County, Pennsylvania, along the Monongahela River. Construction of the original distillery and associated structures began on 40 acres of property surrounded by 300 acres of farmland. The building plan for the distillery included "eight bonded warehouses, a four-story malt house, a distillery millhouse, drying kiln, saw mill, boiler, two carpenter shops, a cooper shop, a blacksmith shop, and an ice house."[2] Recognized for its Monongahela rye and other wheat and malt whiskeys, the distillery soon reportedly became the largest rye distillery in the United States.[3]

Prospects for success looked good for the family as Thomas now had a great job with excellent opportunity for growth since a dramatic expansion of Gibsonton Mills was already envisioned as soon as distilling began in 1857. Things were going so well in fact that William's older brother, Thomas Lafayette, returned from Iowa to assist his father in the construction of the Mills. When the family moved to Western Pennsylvania, Thomas Lafayette, as noted earlier, had remained in the Wilmington, Delaware, area for a period to work on the farm and in the flouring mill of Samuel Anthony. He later moved to Iowa to spend time on a farm with his older brother, James. His return to Western Pennsylvania brought joy to the Daly family household.

The outlook for the family, however, soon changed for the worse. On 07 April 1858, disaster struck with the untimely accidental death of the father when "he was killed by falling through a hatchway of the mills."[4] Not long afterward, Mary Daly passed away as well. Just a few months before his sixteenth birthday, William was faced with the loss of not just his parents, but also the financial wherewithal and family stability he had become accustomed to over the last few years since moving to Western Pennsylvania.

Thomas Lafayette would remain in the area and assume greater responsibility at the distillery. Throughout the remainder of his life, he would continue to progress through higher and more important roles at Gibsonton Mills, eventually becoming its superintendent in July 1873. He held that position for more than a quarter century.

William's life, on the other hand, would soon be further disrupted. Sometime between his parents passing in 1858 and the beginning of the Civil War in April 1861, he made his way to Virginia. Little is known about his life during this period other than the fact that he moved to the Richmond, Virginia, area in 1859. Just one month after the start of the Civil War, with the firing on Fort Sumter in April 1861, William decided to join the Confederate Army. On 14 May 1861, he volunteered for military service. He soon experienced war firsthand. The casualties he encountered very early in the war would forever change both his life and life's work.

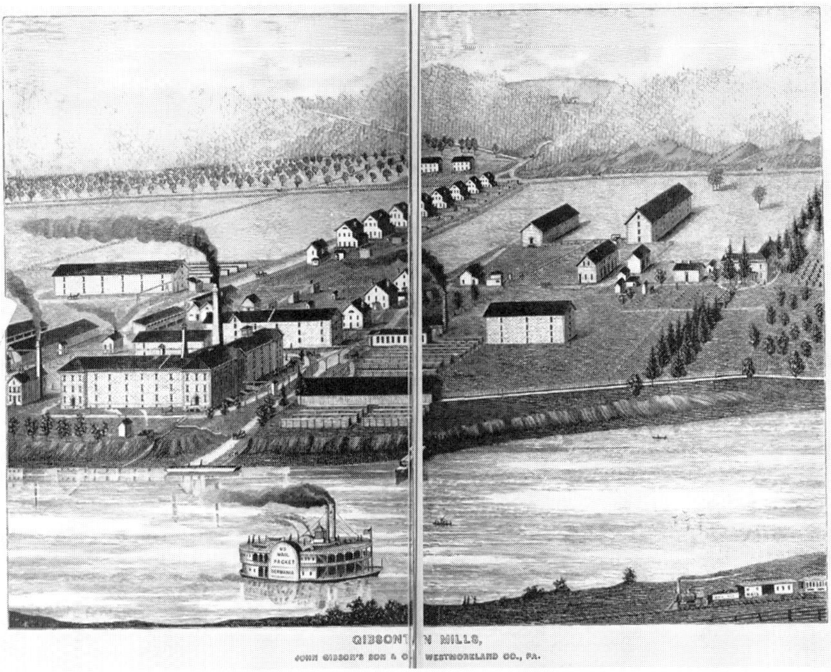

Gibsonton Mills, Westmoreland County, Pennsylvania, *c.* 1882. (*History of the County of Westmoreland, Pennsylvania*)

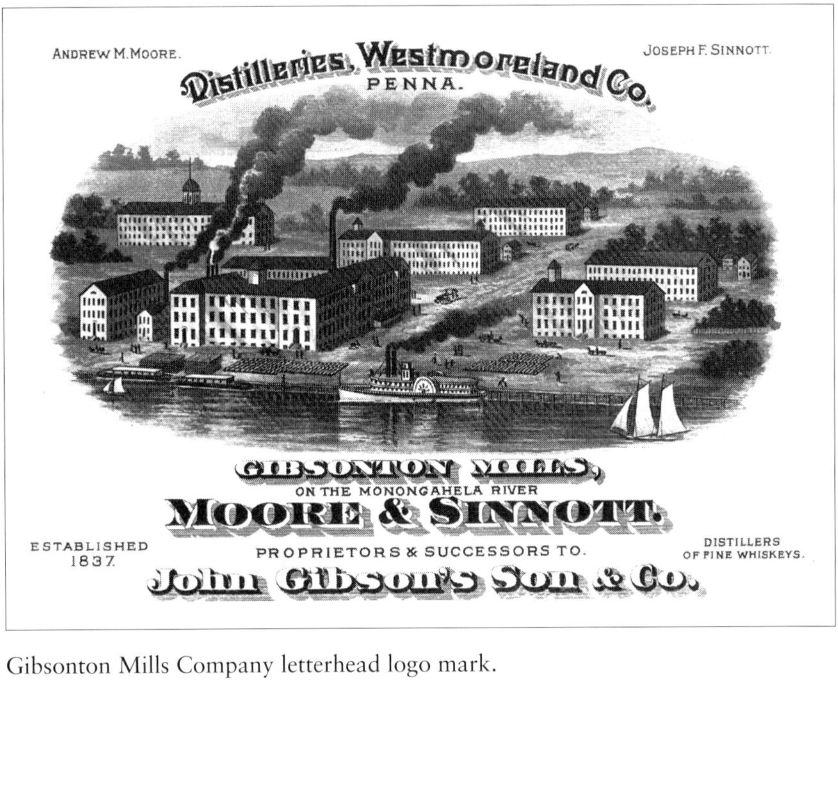

Gibsonton Mills Company letterhead logo mark.

2

Gray Coat—Blue Coat

While little is known about William Daly's life between 1858 and 1860, evidence indicates he accompanied his older brother, John M. Daly, John's wife, Amanda (Lohnabock), and their children, Willie and John, to Henrico County, Virginia (greater Richmond area). In July 1860, they were all recorded in the national census. John Daly described his occupation as farmer.[1]

In the census, William is listed as one of six occupants of the Western Subdivision of the Henrico County, Virginia, household of John, Amanda, and their two sons. Twelve-year-old William White is also listed as part of the household, but other than his occupancy, it is not known if he was a relative of John and Amanda like William Hudson Daly, or someone who came to live with the family for another reason.

There was excitement in the air around Richmond at the time of the 1860 census. Many years of public discourse and political battles over slavery were evident throughout the country. Virginia, with slightly more than a quarter of its families holding slaves, was caught up in the debate. While not the largest slaveholder state at the time, anxiety was high and the general political atmosphere highly charged. Only nine months before the census, John Brown's raid on the United States arsenal at Harper's Ferry, Virginia, in October 1859 was still fresh in the collective memory. In a prescient moment that would later have immense consequence, President James Buchanan engaged Lieutenant Colonel Robert E. Lee to command the Marines sent to quell the uprising. It was one of Lee's last acts as a member of the United States Army.

As in many slave-holding states at the time, ongoing national discussion of slavery consumed political and economic discourse in Virginia. For more than a quarter century the debate had raged, and by the 1860s words began to turn into action and open hostility between pro-slavery and anti-slavery forces. The outcome would soon lead to the Civil War and change the course of American

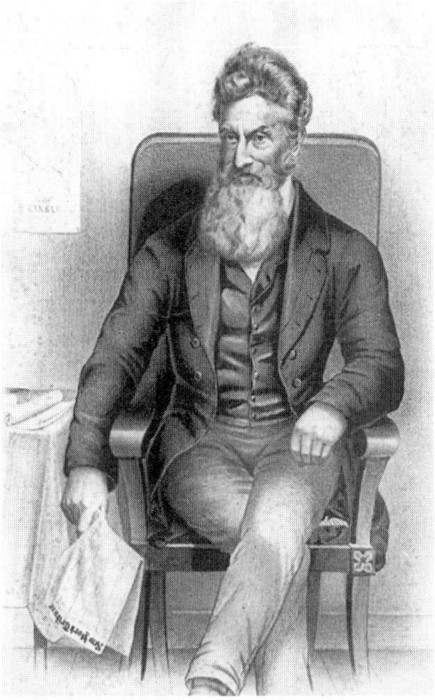

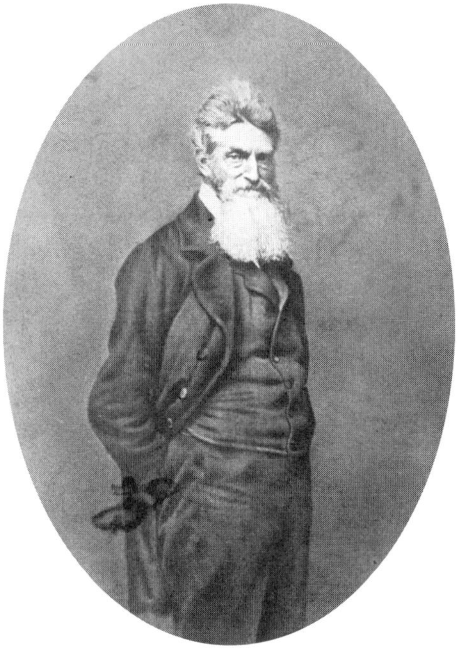

Above left: John Brown holding *New York Tribune* newspaper, 1859. (*Library of Congress*)

Above right: Portrait of John Brown, 1859. (*Library of Congress*)

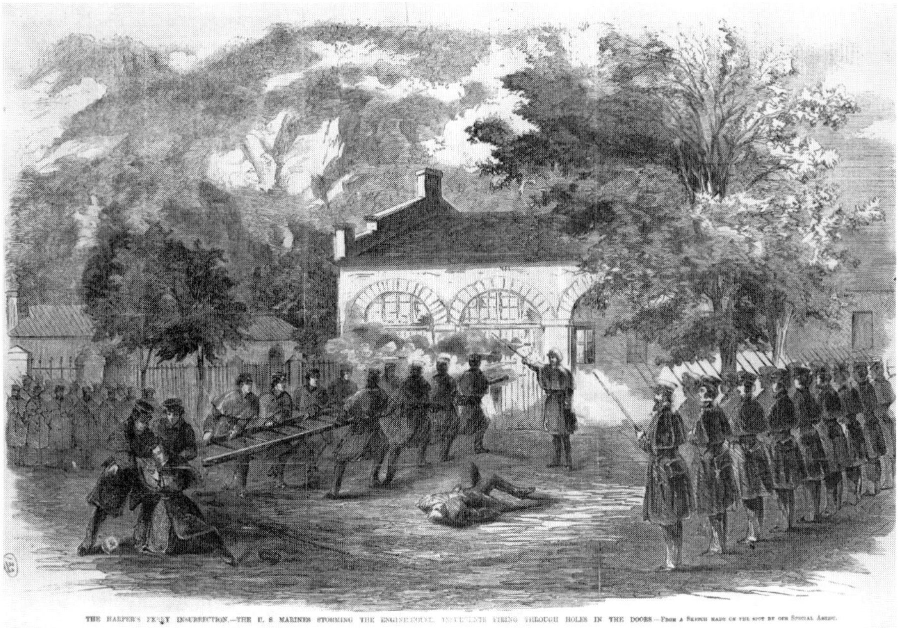

Harpers Ferry insurrection; U.S. Marines storming the engine house, 1859. (*Library of Congress*)

history. Through no fault of his own, William Hudson Daly (aged eighteen in 1860) was thrust into the debate in a most personal manner.

While there is no extant evidence indicating whether or not William Daly approved of slavery, it is hard to imagine his life and circumstances were not impacted by the discontent growing in the Richmond area at the time. On 06 November 1860, within months of the census, Abraham Lincoln was elected president even though his name did not appear on many southern state ballots. The shock of his election seemed to prompt a cascade of events that consumed the country in war.

Several weeks after Lincoln's election, on 20 December 1860, South Carolina seceded from the Union. On 26 December, federal troops from Charleston, South Carolina, were moved to Fort Sumter in anticipation of potential hostilities. On 09 January 1861, while on a mission to reinforce Fort Sumter, the *Star of the West* steamship carrying federal troops and supplies was fired upon in Charleston Harbor and turned away by southern forces. These were the first shots fired in the days preceding the bombardment of Fort Sumter and the official beginning of the Civil War on 12 April 1861.

In the time between South Carolina's secession on 20 December 1860 and the firing on Fort Sumter, the states of Mississippi, Florida, Alabama, Georgia, Louisiana, and Texas would follow suit and join the Confederacy. The remaining four states—Virginia, Arkansas, North Carolina, and Tennessee—that would comprise the eleven Confederate States would soon follow.

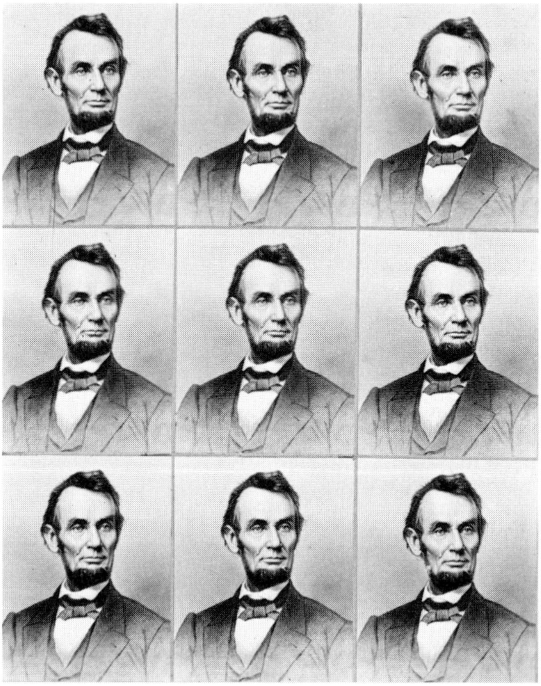

President Abraham Lincoln, 1860. (*Library of Congress*)

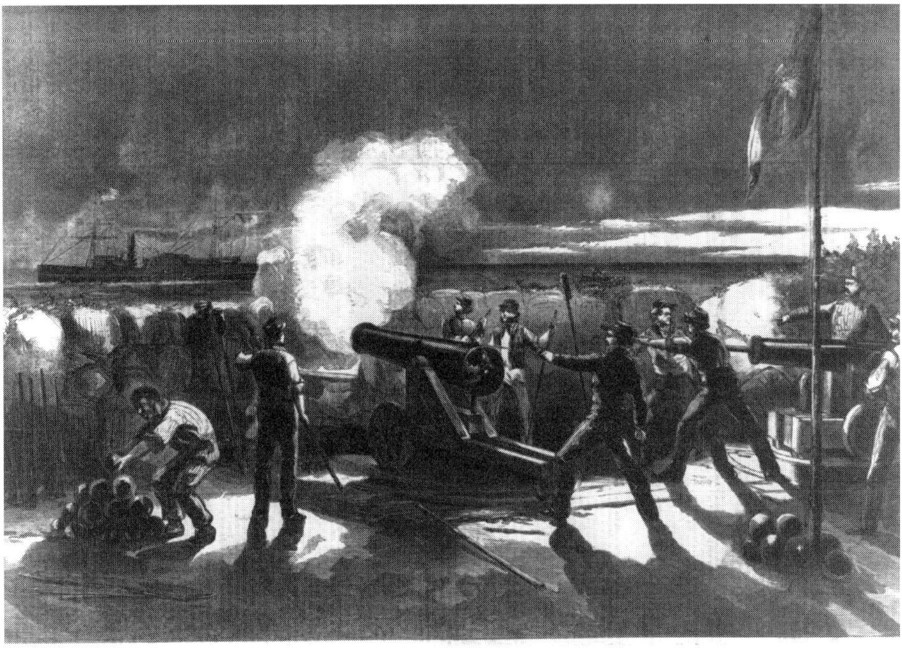

Firing on the *Star of the West* from the South Carolina battery on Morris Island, 10 January 1861. (*Library of Congress*)

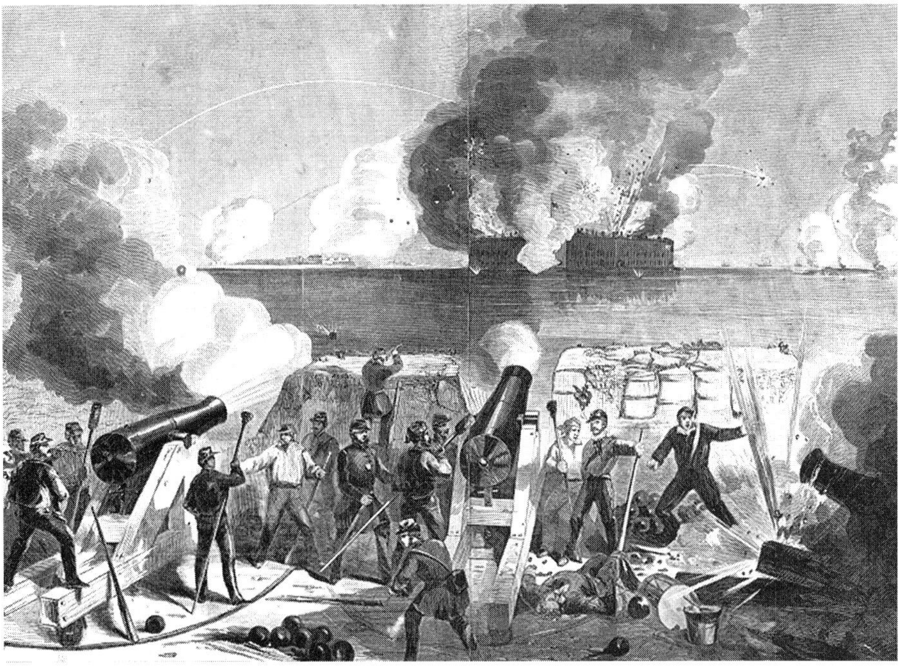

Bombardment of Fort Sumter by the batteries of the Confederate states, April 13, 1861. (*Library of Congress*)

New events would continue to unfold on an almost daily basis. The Provisional Constitution of the Confederacy was adopted on 08 February 1861. A day later, Jefferson Davis was elected president of the Confederacy and inaugurated on 18 February. Two weeks later, on 04 March, Abraham Lincoln held his presidential inauguration on the East Portico of the Capitol Building in Washington, D.C. Approximately forty-eight hours later, on 06 March 1861, the Congress of the Confederate States authorized the enlistment of an army of volunteers. The pace and significance of these events was staggering.

Within several weeks, the initial elements of the Confederate Army were mustered and ready for battle. Their first action would occur at Fort Sumter on 12 April. Three days later, Lincoln declared an insurrection had begun and put out a call to the northern states for 75,000 volunteers to supplement the small regular army that was woefully inadequate to answer the Union's immediate needs. Lincoln's proclamation read:

> BY THE PRESIDENT OF THE UNITED STATES OF AMERICA.
> A PROCLAMATION.
>
> Whereas, on the 15th day of April, 1861, the President of the United States, in view of an insurrection against the Laws, Constitution, and Government of the United States, which had broken out within the States of South Carolina, Georgia, Alabama, Florida, Mississippi, Louisiana, and Texas, and in pursuance of the provisions of the

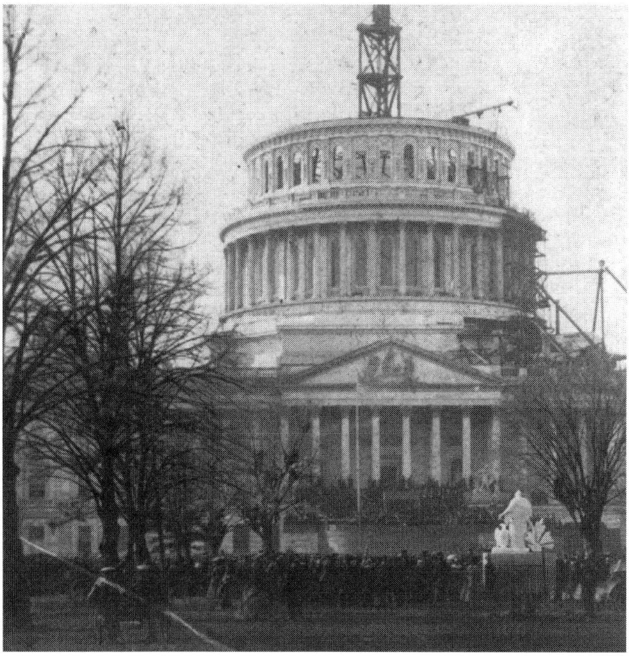

Inauguration of President Lincoln at U.S. Capitol, 04 March 1861. (*Library of Congress*)

act entitled "An act to provide for calling forth the militia to execute the laws of the Union, suppress insurrections, and repel invasions, and to repeal the act now in force for that purpose," approved February 28th, 1795, did call forth the militia to suppress said insurrection, and to cause the laws of the Union to be duly executed, and the insurgents have failed to disperse by the time directed by the President;

And whereas such insurrection has since broken out, and yet exists, within the States of Virginia, North Carolina, Tennessee, and Arkansas;

And whereas the insurgents in all the said States claim to act under the authority thereof, and such claim is not disclaimed or repudiated by the persons exercising the functions of government in such State or States, or in the part or parts thereof in which such combinations exist, nor has such insurrection been suppressed by said States:

Now, therefore, I, Abraham Lincoln, President of the United States, in pursuance of an act of Congress approved July 13, 1861, do hereby declare that the inhabitants of the said States of Georgia, South Carolina, Virginia, North Carolina, Tennessee, Alabama, Louisiana, Texas, Arkansas, Mississippi, and Florida, (except the inhabitants of that part of the State of Virginia lying west of the Allegheny Mountains, and of such other parts of that State and the other States hereinbefore named as may maintain a loyal adhesion to the Union and the Constitution, or may be, from time to time, occupied and controlled by forces of the United States engaged in the dispersion of said insurgents), are in a state of insurrection against the United States, and that all commercial intercourse between the same and the inhabitants thereof, with the exceptions aforesaid, and the citizens of other States and other parts of the United States is unlawful, and will remain unlawful until such insurrection shall cease or has been suppressed; that all goods and chattels, wares and merchandise, coming from any of said States, with the exceptions aforesaid, into other parts of the United States, without the special license and permission of the President, through the Secretary of the Treasury, or proceeding to any of said States with the exceptions aforesaid, by land or water, together with the vessel or vehicle conveying the same, or conveying persons to or from said States, with said exceptions, will be forfeited to the United States; and that, from and after fifteen days from the issuing of this proclamation; all ships and vessels belonging in whole or in part to any citizen or inhabitant of any of said States, with said exceptions, found at sea, or in any port of the United States, will be forfeited to the United States. And I hereby enjoin upon all district attorneys, marshals, and officers of the revenue and of the military and naval forces of the United States to be vigilant in the execution of said act, and in the enforcement of the penalties and forfeitures imposed or declared by it; leaving any party who may think himself aggrieved thereby to his application to the Secretary of the Treasury for the remission of any penalty or forfeiture, which the said Secretary is authorized by law to grant, if, in his judgment, the special circumstances of any case shall require such remission.

In witness whereof, I have hereunto set my hand, and caused the seal of the United States to be affixed.

> Done at the City of Washington, this sixteenth day of August, in the year of our Lord 1861, [L.S.] (place of seal) and of the Independence of the United States the eighty-sixth.[2]

With Lincoln's proclamation in place, there would now be a war the likes of which could never have been imagined, and the Commonwealth of Virginia would soon play an important role for both sides of the conflict. The Union and Confederate governments recognized the value of the state's significant industrial base, availability of plentiful natural resources, and prodigious farming capabilities. It also held the city of Richmond, the Confederacy's capital.

Upon taking office, President Lincoln and his primary military advisor Lieutenant General (and general-in-chief) Winfield Scott and other ranking members of his administration erroneously thought the insurrection could be quelled in short order. It was anticipated they could "overrun and subjugate Virginia in ninety days."[3] Their initial plans were to defend Washington, D.C., and safeguard Lincoln's inauguration, while offensively moving troops toward Richmond. Defense of the capital was relatively easy to achieve. However, the movement toward Richmond quickly failed as the Confederates anticipated the move and worked aggressively to thwart any northern offensive.

The idea of capturing Richmond was a critical element of Scott's broader "Anaconda Plan." His strategy called for the Union to blockade Southern

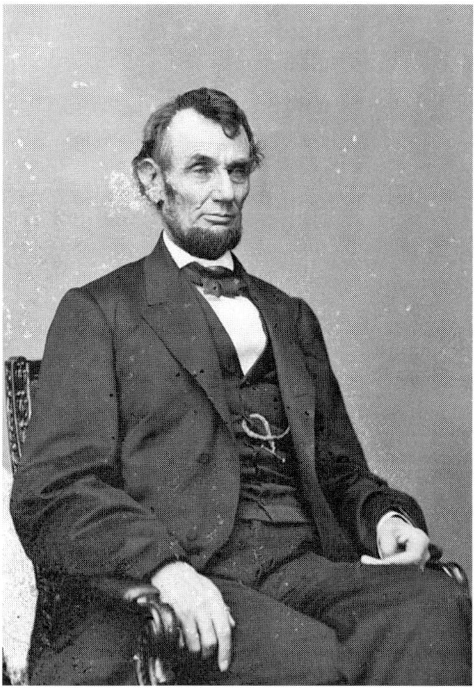

Abraham Lincoln, President of the United States, 1864. (*Library of Congress*)

ports while deploying large numbers of troops down the Mississippi River, effectively splitting the Confederate states in half. In the weeks between Lincoln's inauguration (04 March 1861) and the firing on Fort Sumter (12 April 1861), both armies made numerous offensive and defensive moves, with many focused on Maryland and the Chesapeake Bay, and the northern Virginia cities of Arlington and Alexandria. The movement and counter movement of troops played out much like a game of chess, with each side seeking geographic advantage. On 24 May, the Union Army crossed the Potomac River to take possession of Arlington Heights, Virginia, which included the property of Robert E. Lee. Within a matter of a few weeks, Lee would become commander of the Confederate Army of Northern Virginia.

Union and Confederate tactical movements would soon move further south into Virginia. The Union Army used the Chesapeake Bay and Atlantic coastline for offensive tactical purposes, while the Confederates amassed troops and built fortifications inland to deny access to Richmond and other key cities along the Virginia Peninsula. Meanwhile, on 03 June 1861, near the city of Philippi in Western Virginia, a skirmish between the northern and southern troops took place and marked the first land battle of the Civil War. The fight was short, with an immediate goal of the winner taking possession of an area that was critically located near vital railroad connections. The South lost on two counts that day: George B. McClellan's Union Army won the battle, and the citizens of Western Virginia showed their preferred allegiance to the Union cause. Two weeks after the battle, on 20 June, the northwestern counties of Virginia severed ties to the state and officially became West Virginia; the thirty-fifth state of the Union.

On Monday 13 May 1861, the *Richmond Daily Dispatch* newspaper ran an advertisement seeking to recruit volunteers for the Virginia Life Guard regiment. The ad read:

> The VIRGINIA LIFE GUARD will be mustered into the service of the State on TUESDAY MORNING next 14th inst. In consequence of the order of the Governor prohibiting Railroad employees and Telegraph Operators from volunteering, there are some vacancies. Persons desiring to join will please hand their names to the Captain, Lieutenants, Sergeant B. Bates, at the Methodist Book Concern, or any member of the corps immediately.[4]

As noted earlier, William Hudson Daly joined the Confederate Army in Richmond, Virginia, on 14 May 1861. His enlistment took place exactly nine days before Virginia seceded from the Union on 23 May 1861; ten months after the census was taken; and one month after the firing on Fort Sumter. William was still living with his brother, John, and his family in Henrico County, Virginia, at the time. The county was strategically located; it surrounded the city of Richmond on all except its southern border and served as a buffer zone protecting the city during

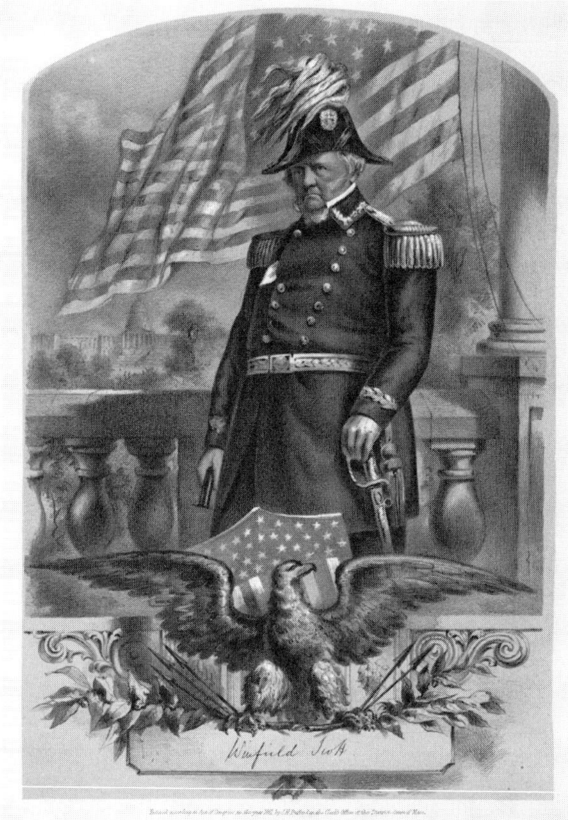

Left: Winfield Scott, 1861. (*Library of Congress*)

Below: General Winfield Scott and staff, 1861. (*Library of Congress*)

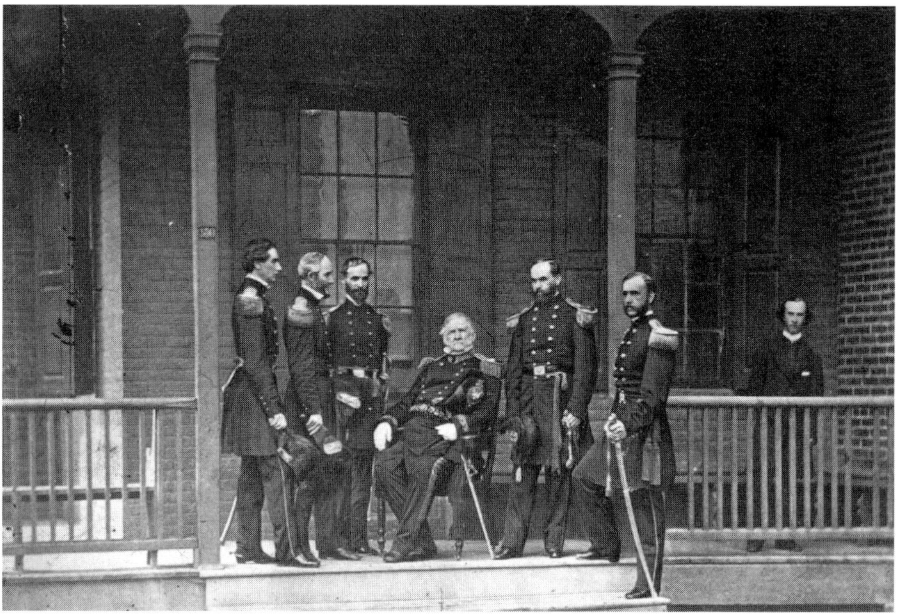

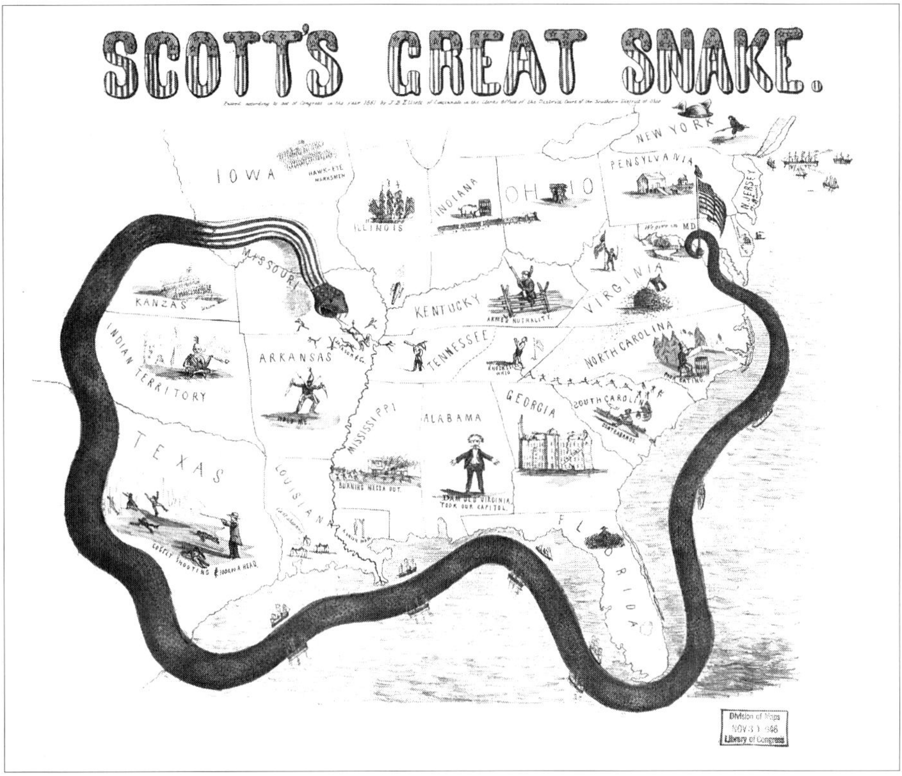

Above: Scott's great snake, Anaconda Plan 1861. (*Library of Congress*)

Right: General Robert E. Lee, 1861. (*Library of Congress*)

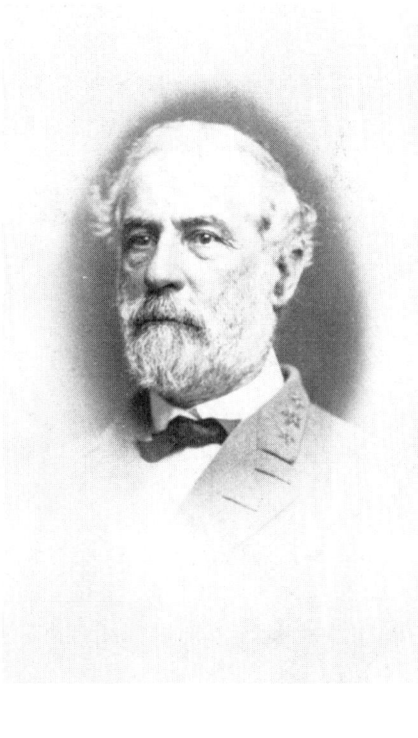

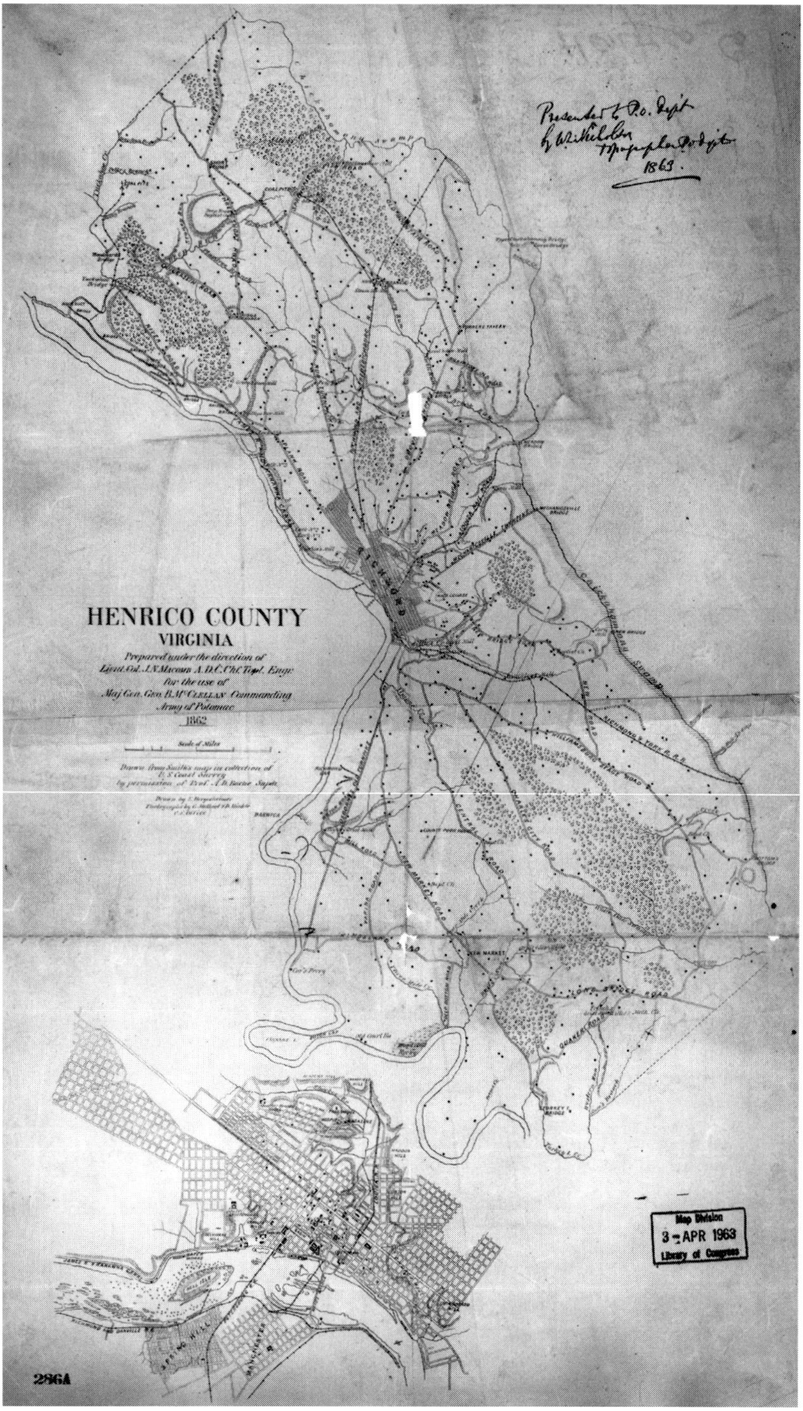

Henrico County, Virginia, map prepared under the direction of Lt. Col. J. N. Nacomb, A.D.C., for the use of Maj. Gen. George B. McClellan, commanding Army of Potomac, 1862. (*Library of Congress*)

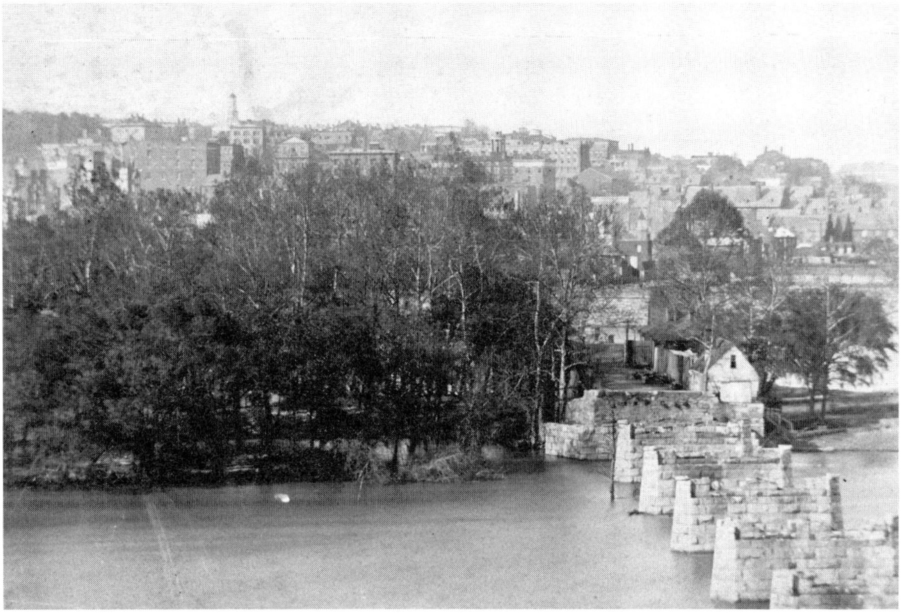

Richmond, Virginia, 1861. (*Library of Congress*)

the early part of the Civil War. It also provided a large number of early volunteers for the Confederate Army. In William's case, he joined the ranks of Company "B," 15th Virginia Volunteers. Not long before his enlistment, the regiment had been known as the 3rd Virginia, before reorganizing as the 15th Regiment. Company "B" was also known as the "Virginia Life Guard."

While William Hudson Daly left no written account of his early service in the Confederate Army, another member of the 15th Regiment kept a diary providing an extensive account of the regiment's activities between April 1861 and spring 1862. Like Daly, Claybrook Y. Lain was an early recruit. Lain was mustered into service as a private at Richmond on 21 April 1861, about one month before Daly's enlistment. Sometime in February 1862, Lain was promoted to 1st Sergeant of Company E. B. Albemarle Co., which was later integrated into the 15th Regiment. He subsequently held higher rank but died at the Battle of Drewry's Bluff on 16 May 1864. In his history of the 15th Regiment, Lain described its initial activities as follows:

> The 15th Virginia Regiment was formed about the middle of May 1861, and placed under the command of Colonel Harvie, and drilled by him for some weeks in the Hermitage Fair Ground near Richmond. It was then called the 3rd Va Regt, from its being the third Regt formed in that Camp. It was not a complete Regt while under his command as it contained only about six companies.
>
> The Camp at this time was under the command of Col Gilham of the Virginia Military Institute, who had as his aids the Cadets from the said place, for the purpose

> of drilling such as were sent to the camp for instruction. The Cadets as a general thing were very good drill masters, as they were well drilled themselves they were competent to drill others. They soon took the name of Heps from the fact of the word hep being used by them to call the men to attention when the step was lost by any in the ranks. It was quite strange to see a parcel of old and settled men trotting around at order of one of the smallest among the Heps. The companies which were in Camp at that time were drilled six times a day, which was enough to kill up any parcel of men, having only an hour to rest between drills.
>
> About the last of May [1861] the Camp was filled up with men from all parts of this state, so much so that looked almost impossible to travel about for the men. About this time the 3rd Regt was taken from Col Harvie and placed under the command of Col Thomas P. August of Richmond. The men were highly pleased to have him for their Col as he was a man known to a great many of the men and one who stood high as a military man and a gentleman. He was known to the greater portion of the men, as he was raised in the City of Richmond, and the Regt was formed of men from Richmond and the adjacent counties so that Col August was not a stranger to them, but in a measure a friend and associate.[5]

A day after William enlisted, the local newspaper reported that Company "B" (Virginia Life Guard) had arrived at the "Camp of Instruction." The article further noted: "The members are armed with the most efficient weapon, the Enfield rifle."[6] At the time, members of the Virginia Life Guard were considered very fortunate as the Enfield was deemed one of the best weapons in the world and few other units were equipped with such a fine rifle. Author Philip Schreier wrote about the gun in an article about the English Enfield rifles that were used by the Confederate Army. He noted:

> The Pattern 1853 Enfield rifle-musket (P'53) was then the standard arm of the British Army and was a percussion ignition, .577-cal. muzzle loading rifle with five-groove rifling cut with a progressive increase in depth toward the breech. It weighed 8 lbs., 15 ozs. without the triangular socket bayonet attached. The P'53 saw service with British troops in every corner of the globe and quickly became the standard by which all other firearms were measured.[7]

The *Daily Dispatch* newspaper reporter was not the only person who noticed the Enfield rifles. In his history of the 15th Regiment, Claybrook Lain did as well. Lain made a note of the rifles when describing the background and composition of the Virginia Life Guard (Company "B"):

> This company was formed in the City of Richmond and composed of young men who were members of the Young Men's Christian Association. It was formed and designed merely for home protection and malitia [*sic.*] service, it was quite a fine

> company as most of the men were young, but I may say for the most part delicate, and did not seem able to stand the many hardships of a soldiers life, but I am happy to say that a one who looked delicate made good soldiers and performed good service. It seemed as if they held themselves above the men in other companies of the Regt, from the fact of their having the Enfield instead of the common musket, with which a greater portion of the Regt was armed, and which proved on trial to be superior to the Enfield gun [*sic.*]. They were well drilled and a fine looking company and was for the most part of the time well uniformed. This Company is Commanded by Captain Walker who is a very good officer and one who takes pride in doing all he can for his men, by which means he has gained the love and esteem of all.[8]

It is worth noting that, around this time, the Confederate Army began receiving many shipments of weapons from abroad. The Confederate States were initially a step ahead of the Union government; its purchasing agents were able to buy up large quantities of arms and munitions from Great Britain, Belgium, and other European countries well in advance of their northern counterparts. It was not surprising to find that foreign nations generally treated the transactions as a business without picking sides. Weapons were eagerly sold to those willing to pay the best prices. Most importantly, those who arrived with funds in hand were always given preferential treatment. In some cases, however, there was some happiness expressed by those who sold guns and munitions and embraced the

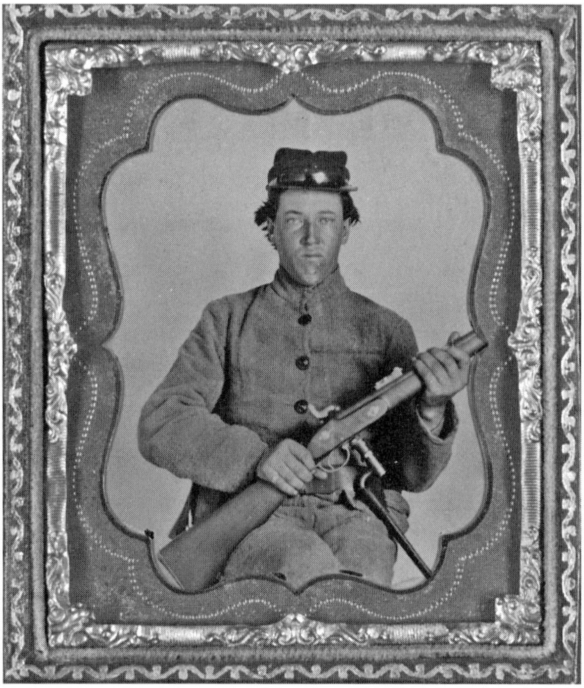

Unidentified soldier in Confederate uniform with Enfield rifle. (*Library of Congress*)

Confederate cause. In Great Britain, in particular, there were many who wished to see the United States deconstruct as retribution for previous military defeats.

Nine days after Daly enlisted on 14 May, and with only several days of basic military training, he and his fellow infantrymen prepared for deployment. The day was memorable because it was the exact day that Virginia chose to secede from the Union. Claybrook Lain described the regiment's preparations:

> Orders were issued for the 23rd of May [1861] to be the day for the Regiment to leave the Camp for some field [word(s) missing] which they could better show their courage [torn] enable them to fight in defence [*sic.*] of their [word(s) missing] and for their Country.
>
> At the appointed time the Regt formed on the ground, up to this time but few knew of what companies the Regt was formed. When the line was formed it was found that it consisted of five companies from Richmond, two from Henrico County (one of which was Daly's Virginia Life Guard regiment) and three from Hanover County, as they stood they were a fine set of men, as fine as any that had been seen anywhere around up to that time. Wagons were sent out to take the baggage of each Company and were loaded and in readiness to move off when the order was given. After some delay, all was in readiness to start, and the Regt (headed by Smith's Band, which was playing a lively march) moved out of the Camp by way of Broad St gate, and from thence down Broad to Third down Third, to Main, down Main to the wharf of the steamer Glen Cove, which was in readiness to transport them down James River for parts unknown. As the companies came in the formation of the Regt they were marched aboard and their baggage along with them, while on the march from the Fair Grounds to the Boat, the streets were thronged with those who were eager to see them and bid them God speed, while from many windows white handkerchiefs could be seen waving from the hand of the ladies. And a large crowd stood about the wharf, among whom were many who had come to bid their friends a last adieu. After a short time, all were aboard, and the bell was wrung to give all a warning that the Boat was ready to start, after giving all time to get ashore who did not belong aboard she loosed her moorings and pulled out into the stream.[9]

Later that day, the regiment disembarked at a wharf on the James River approximately 4 miles from Williamsburg, Virginia. Daly's unit, Company "B," was assigned duty at the dock guarding provisions, while the rest of the regiment marched toward Williamsburg. Lain noted the road to Williamsburg was a "dark and lonesome one," and the troops were anxious and fully expecting they would encounter Yankee soldiers on the way. Luckily, that was not the case, and the regiment made it safely into the town and established quarters at William and Mary College. They arrived during the evening hours, which frightened townspeople who thought the Union Army had arrived. The next morning, they were delighted and heartened to learn the previous evening's commotion was caused by the arriving elements of the Confederate Army.

That same morning, soldiers of the regiment learned their immediate mission was to construct fortifications near the city in anticipation of a Union assault. Under Confederate Colonel (later General) John B. Magruder's direction, William Daly and members of Company "B" were among the four companies deployed. With rifles never far away, picks, axes, and shovels soon became the tools of defense. Before they commenced work on fortifications, however, their orders were changed, and the regiment was told to begin preparations for pending action near Yorktown, at a distance of approximately 10 miles southeast of their position. They were then sent on a scouting mission to an area near Big Bethel, Virginia. Big Bethel (also known as Bethel Church and Great Bethel) was a church located less than 8 miles from Newport News and Hampton, Virginia. In both places, garrisons of Union soldiers under the command of Major General Benjamin Butler were staging for an anticipated assault on Richmond.

Confederate Colonel R. G. Lowe recalled in March 1900: "The defense of Richmond against the advance of McClellan by way of the peninsula in the spring of 1862 was one of the most remarkable achievements that occurred during the whole period. It is in keeping with Magruder's style in every way. 'Prince John' knew no such word as retreat."[10, 11]

In early June 1861, Samuel Phillips Day, a special correspondent of the British *Morning Herald* newspaper, spent time in the Big Bethel area. He noted: "The military ardour and aptitude of the Southerners struck me as remarkable. It is surprising how, in so short a time, tens of thousands of men could have been drilled, uniformed, and equipped, and prepared to meet the enemy in open field."[12] Describing the movements of the Confederate army in the area, he explained the preparations being made:

> The Confederate troops having advanced from Yorktown took up an entrenched position at Great Bethel Bridge, situated between the boundary line of York and Elizabeth City counties, under command of Colonel Magruder. Bethel is fifteen miles from Yorktown, nine from Hampton, bordering upon Fortress Monroe, and lies nearly in a direct line between the two points. Colonel Magruder's forces consisted of 500 strong, one artillery corps, numbering 100 men and 6 field pieces, and a cavalry corps of 100 men, in addition to 300 riflemen and infantry.
>
> General Butler, who commanded the military department of Virginia, having ascertained the position of the Confederate troops, and that they were gradually extending their outer line made instant preparations for driving them back. Orders were accordingly dispatched for several regiments to hold themselves in readiness for the march, and at the same time, the chief of the Ordnance Bureau received instructions to prepare a battery of howitzers, consisting of four 12-pounders, with a detachment of artillery. Ere long a force of about 3,000 strong, commanded by

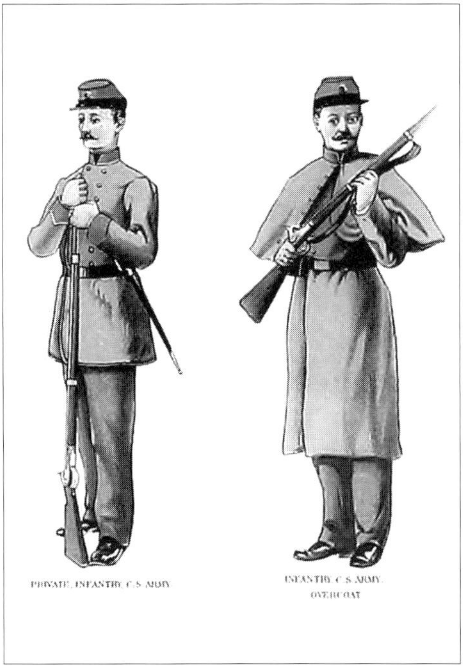

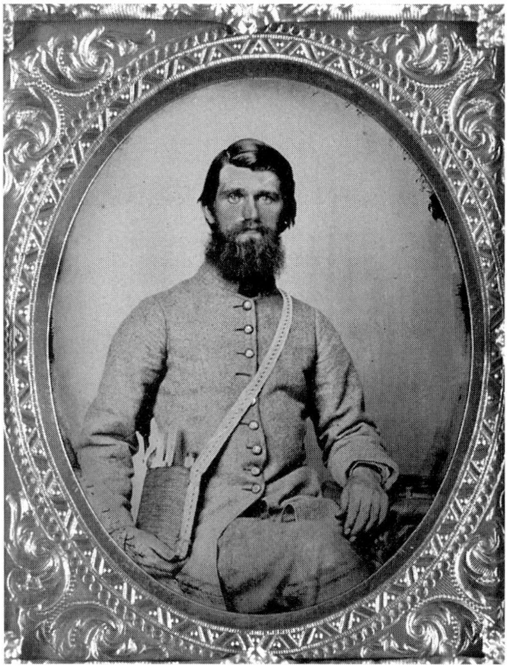

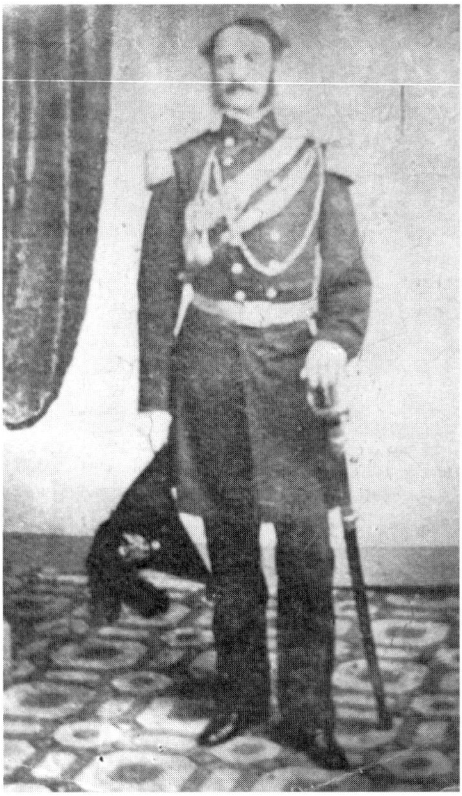

Above left: Confederate army infantry uniforms; Uniforms of officers and enlisted men, U.S. War Department Atlas to Accompany the Official Records of the Union and Confederate Armies, 1891–1895. (*Government Printing Office*)

Above right: Dr. Alexander Harris of 15th Virginia Infantry Regiment in uniform. (*Library of Congress*)

Left: General John Bankhead Magruder (Prince John) in dress uniform. (*Library of Congress*)

> Brigadier-General Pierce, were on their way, having struck their tents shortly after midnight on Sunday, June 9th. This force comprised the New York Zouaves (Colonel Duryea), the Albany Regiment (Colonel Townsend), the 7th Regiment (Colonel Benedix), with a few companies drawn from other regiments. The Zouaves started fully an hour before the other troops.[13]

On 10 June 1861, the day of the Battle of Big Bethel, correspondent Day reported on the action that day, including the involvement of Daly's Virginia Life Guard unit. He wrote:

> Although Colonel Magruder fully expected the approach of the foe, he was not, however, exactly prepared for his immediate presence. The troops were engaged in erecting a battery to intercept the advance of General Butler on Yorktown, when the arrival of a wounded picket, who had been shot from his horse, gave the alarm that the Unionists were in close proximity to the Southern lines. Six guns were immediately planted near the bank of the stream, or creek, which flowed in a south-easterly direction by the field of battle, while four additional guns were mounted in front, and two others a short distance in the rear, on the hill-side.
>
> The infantry and riflemen took up positions in the unfinished trenches on each side of the road behind the creek, and in front of it, on the right-hand side, looking towards the southwest—from which point the enemy advanced—while the cavalry fell back as a reserve. Right in front of the line stood a large orchard, some five or six yards distant, with a house or two adjacent. Under the shelter thus afforded the enemy opened fire from Lieutenant Greble's battery. The action commenced at a quarter past nine on the morning of Monday, June 10th, and raged fiercely until one in the afternoon. The Zouaves operated under cover against the one gun placed in front of the creek, on the right-hand side of the road, which was protected in flank by the North Carolina troops of Captain Walker's Virginian Guard [Day mistakenly connected the Virginia Life Guard (15th Virginia Regiment) with the 15th North Carolina Regiment which was also present]. This gun was captured by the enemy, but it was eventually recovered by the dashing bayonet charge made by two North Carolina companies. The Zouaves fled in confusion even before the bayonets got within dangerous proximity!
>
> After repeated and desperate attacks, which were effectually repulsed, the issue of the conflict was decided by a brilliant charging column of 1,000 men, whose destructive fire drove the enemy before them, until he was compelled to retire from the field. It was while crossing the creek and ravine, thereby endeavoring to turn the Confederate flank, that General Pierce's command met with such resistance as decided the fate of the engagement. Completely dispirited and demoralized, they were beaten from every position, and finally forced to retire, when they were hotly pursued to within a few miles of Hampton. The same evening the Confederate troops fell back upon Yorktown. The loss on the side of the enemy was computed

at 400, including killed, wounded and missing, although some accounts represented this number as far below the truth. The Confederates had only one man killed and six wounded; a circumstance which was regarded as a special interposition of Providence.[14]

Another correspondent, using the initials C. P. R., associated with the Richmond *Daily Dispatch* newspaper, was embedded with Daly's Virginia Lifeguard regiment and reported on the Battle at Bethel Church of 10 June. A day after the battle, he reported:

Battle at Bethel Church
Headquarters Virginia Lifeguard, Yorktown, June 11, 1861.

When I wrote last, we were in the country at a place called Bethel Church, and it was Sunday. We spent the day pleasantly until at night when there was an alarm given, caused by canon firing down towards Hampton. We afterwards learned that one of the county companies had encountered Federal troops, and had a fight—nothing more than a scrimmage. At 2 o'clock we were startled by the bugle sounding the "assembly call." In two minutes every soldier in the encampment was in arms and ready for duty, having previously been instructed to sleep with the accouterments on and arms by the side.

THE MARCH
In half an hour the North Carolina Regiment, under command of Col. Hill, a brave cool commander, and confident leader, were ordered with three guns of Major Randolph's Battery, to march toward Hampton, while the Virginia Lifeguard, Henrico Southern Guard, and Young Guard, under Lt. Col. Stewart, were ordered to move lower down the encampment and take the position vacated by the North Carolina regiment, which was promptly done. It was a noble sight, as we stood near the outer limits of our encampment, in the gray at the morning, to see the Howitzers and the North Carolina Regiment, those worthy sons of noble States, under the command of our gallant Col. Magruder, defile past us and advance to meet the mercenary legions of a besotted Government. They were soon lost to sight in the woods, and all was still, except the occasional challenge of a sentinel or an outpost; all the men were expecting some great event.

THE RETURN
Col. Magruder and his command had only gone three miles down the road when they learned that the enemy they were in pursuit of had retired to reinforce, and intended making an attack on us in a short time, as soon as they return. The entire camp was arranged for the assault.

POSITION OF OUR TROOPS

The encampment was a parallel formation, the corner of the fortifications lying nearly due East and West, North and South, and was protected by embankments thrown up on four sides, the strongest of which was on the southeast side, which commanded the road, the bridge and the field, through which troops must pass coming from Hampton, and was well fortified. To the defense of this position a howitzer battery of three guns, under the command of Major George W. Randolph, and four companies of the N.C. Regiment on the northwest side; the remainder of the N.C. Regiment were stationed from East to West. On the south side was a ravine 30 feet deep, and very marshy. This position was defended by a battery of one howitzer gun, under the command of Capt. J. Thompson Brown on the left, and an earthwork and trench made and occupied by the companies of Lieut. Col. Stewart's command, consisting of the Virginia Life Guard, Capt. Walker; Henrico Southern Guard, Capt. Childrey; and Young Guard, Capt. Charters—the remainder of the troops, of infantry and cavalry, were stationed inside the enclosure, and completed the defence of the entire parallel. All was now in readiness, and with calm, determined countenances, the men awaited their coming.

THE APPROACH

In a few minutes our scouts and the videttes commenced firing and coming in, announcing the advance. The cannoniers and infantry in the line of fortifications were notified and stood ready, ammunition in hand. Our men (Col. Stewart's) were ordered in the trenches, when they were compelled to kneel, in order to escape observation, it being our object to conceal our position until the enemy advanced to the middle of the field, and then open fire. That approach to the fortifications can only be made through a field 600 yards wide, and by the bridge, spanning the creek running along the line southeast of our position.

THE ATTACK

Our Colonel stood with glass in hand and soon discovered the glistening of bayonets coming from cover of the woods and up the road. As soon as they had arrived about one thousand yards from us, they planted two cannons in the road, one in the woods and several in the field, to our left, all of them being guns of heavy calibre. As soon as they were seen in position, Maj. Randolph gave the command, and their splendid Parrot gun belched forth a shot which took effect on the column in the road and did considerable damage; this was replied to by the enemy from their gun in the road, and replied to by Captain Brown's Battery in the field. The action then became general, and the deafening roar of the guns was all that could be heard for an hour—our shot taking good effect, that of the other side not having hit a single man or gun, all being aimed too high, doing great damage among the boughs of the trees. Col. Stuart's command were placed fifty yards on the right of Capt. Brown's Battery, to serve as a protection to them, and we soon saw the approach of a company of Zouaves of a

New York Regiment, advancing under cover of some houses and a large orchard to the right of the field. The Virginia Life Guard were ordered to rise and shoot them, as our position had not been discovered; the men of the first platoon rose, and taking deliberate aim, fired; the shots had good effect, 7 of the Zouaves falling, two killed and remainder wounded, as we ascertained afterwards by finding the bodies of the dead. We immediately drew upon us the fire of the Zouaves and one piece of cannon; but our men were undaunted, and between every fire of the dastardly crew they rose by file and fired. Nearly every time a man was felled. Our guns being the Enfield rifle gun, were very effective. The entire force of both sides then came into action, and to men unaccustomed to such sights the scene was sublime. After the first fire all of the hesitancy and trepidation incident to the first battle was over, and every man felt eager to give them a salute. There was a cessation of firing for five minutes, when our guns commenced again, and constant and rapid firing was kept up for one hour or more, our guns working beautifully and doing great damage. The shot of the enemy wounded three of our Howitzer and one of the N.C. Regiment men.

During this engagement the Howitzer gun in the field was accidentally disabled by the breaking of the vent wire in the touch hole, and had to be hauled in the woods and abandoned; and Col. Stewart's command was ordered to close in upon the fortifications, and defend the interior of our camp as we moved off. A Regiment of infantry was seen to file up the road to the south of our position, in order to get to our rear, and several cannon were ordered to the road through which they must pass. The cannon were supported by the commands of Col. Stewart and Capt. Montague; but they did not make their appearance, and we remained interested spectators of the third attack, holding our position in the trenches, and prepared to defend the ravine and the road to the south and west of our fortifications.

This attack was made a few minutes after 12 o'clock and was the most severe of all the day's work. Our guns commenced again, and after exchanging shots for fifteen or twenty minutes, the enemy formed in column, one thousand strong, and under command of a brave looking General, well mounted, advanced over the road, over the bridge, and up to the embankment on the southeast. Every man looked on with breathless interest, as the charge was a brilliant one. As soon as they were in good range, our battery opened, and the first fire struck the head of the advancing column and crashed through from rank to rank. They attempted to mount the embankment, but our infantry rose, and they were repulsed with great loss, and so discomfited that they returned with a double-quick movement down the road. The Colonel commanding in this charge was seen to reel in his saddle. The battery again exchanged shots, and the action closed with six men wounded on our side.

It was now one o'clock, and the enemy showing no disposition to commence again, the dragoons were ordered out, and found the enemy retreating with all speed toward Hampton. As they pursued them, they scattered like sheep, and the wounded and dying fell on every side of the road. It was a pitiable sight, and as our men came back they were picked up and carried on litters to our camp and cared for.

The battle was now over, having commenced at 9½ A.M., and continued till 1 P.M. One of the wounded of the enemy said he would tell the truth before he died, and say four thousand five hundred were engaged on the part of the Federal troops, and five hundred held in reserve, and the dead and wounded were over two hundred; while on our part there were only twelve hundred men, and at no time were there more than 800 engaged.

During the entire engagement Col. Magruder was in every part of the field, and displayed consummate generalship and courage, directing every movement in person and exposing himself with a recklessness of danger, which was seen and admired by all in camp.

INCIDENTS OF THE BATTLE

The enemy, when they first approached, tried to keep up their courage by repeated cheering, yelling like so many savages, which the writer of this heard distinctly, while our men said not a word; but, with uplifted hearts to the God of Battles, stood silent and courageously, awaiting them.

One of the Captains of the advancing column of the enemy approached near the N.C. Regiment's lines, and, standing on a log, cheered his men. He was seen, and a private in one of the companies took deliberate aim, and he fell dead. The man ran out and secured his sword as a trophy of his valor.

The Howitzer Battery, under superintendence of Major Randolph, elicited the cheers of the entire soldiery, every man performing his part with the celerity of practiced gunners, and often exposing themselves upon the parapet to see, as they said, the enemy's eyes, so as to take aim. In a word, no man on the ground could express how much of the result of our victory is due the Howitzers.

Late in the evening the encampment was broken up and we returned to Yorktown. Long live Magruder, Hill, Stewart, and Allan, illustrious leaders in this, our first great battle and glorious victory! while to God thanks be given for His providential care and support.[15]

A Union account of the battle included the following details:

Big Bethel, Va., June 10, 1861. 1st, 2nd, 3rd, 5th and 7th New York, 1st Vermont, and 4th Massachusetts Infantry, and 2nd United States Artillery. About 8 miles from Newport News were two churches known as Big and Little Bethel. At the former there was a considerable force of Confederates, under Col. J. B. Magruder, and works of more or less strength were in process of construction, while at the latter there was a Confederate outpost, from which a squad of cavalry was nightly sent out to annoy the Federal pickets, impress Union men into the Confederate army, carry away slaves who had been left in charge of farms, and take them to Yorktown and Williamsburg to work on the fortifications. Gen. B. F. Butler, therefore, determined to destroy the outpost and drive the enemy from his position at Big Bethel.

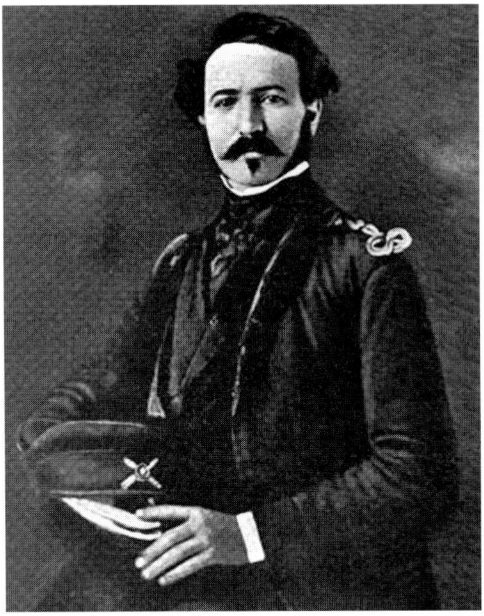

John Bankhead Magruder, *c.* 1848. (*Wikimedia Commons*)

An expedition, under the command of Brig.-Gen. E. W. Pierce, was planned on the evening of the 9th and at 1 o'clock on the morning of the 10th the 7th N. Y. (Duryea's Zouaves) was ferried across the creek and ordered to march to New Market bridge in the enemy's rear. At 2 o'clock the 3rd N. Y. under Col. Townsend, and the 7th N. Y., with the Massachusetts and Vermont troops under Col. Bendix, marched by different roads, intending to effect a junction at the forks of the road about a mile and a half from Little Bethel, the purpose being to attack that place at daybreak. Bendix reached the rendezvous first and his men, mistaking Townsend's force, as it approached in the dim light of the early dawn, for Confederates, fired upon them, killing 2 and wounding 21. The sound of the firing made it impossible to surprise the enemy and some of the officers favored a return to Camp Hamilton, but Pierce, knowing that reinforcements were coming to his assistance, pushed on to find Little Bethel deserted.

The church was burned, the artillery, under Lieut. Greble, was brought to the front and the whole column advanced on Big Bethel. By a peculiar coincidence Col. Magruder had planned an attack on Camp Hamilton for that morning, had aroused his men at 3 a.m., and when the first firing was heard was three and a half miles from his works. He returned to his position at Big Bethel and disposed his forces to resist any assault likely to be made. When Pierce came up about 9 o'clock he found the ford on the Hampton road guarded by two companies of North Carolina sharpshooters, while on the opposite side of the road, protected by earthworks, were Stuart's cavalry and the 3rd Va. infantry with a howitzer commanding the road. Beyond the creek were two more howitzers, well supported, trained on the ford.

> After some skirmishing Pierce, seeing the strength of the Confederate position, withdrew his forces with a loss of 18 killed, 53 wounded and 5 missing.[16]

Colonel Daniel Harvey Hill, who was in command of the 1st Regiment of the North Carolina Volunteers that also fought at Bethel Church, delivered an official report to the Governor of North Carolina after the battle. His report included mention of the soldiers of the Virginia Regiments. On 11 June, he wrote from Yorktown:

> Sir, I have the honour to report that 800 men of my regiment and 360 Virginians were engaged for five hours and a quarter with four and a half regiments of the enemy at Bethel Church, nine miles from Hampton, this afternoon. The enemy made three distinct and well sustained charges, but were repulsed with heavy loss. Our cavalry pursued them for six miles, when their retreat became a total rout. Fearing that heavy reinforcements would be sent up from Fortress Monroe, we fell back at nightfall upon our works at Yorktown. I regret to report the loss of one man killed, Private Henry L. Wyatt, Edgecombe Guards, and seven wounded. The loss of the enemy, by their own confession, was 150, but it may be safely estimated at 250. Our regiment behaved most gallantly. Not a man shrunk from his post or showed symptoms of fear.[17]

Shortly after the Battle of Big Bethel, Hill was promoted in quick order to the rank of Lieutenant General; by spring 1862, his rank was elevated to Major General.

The battle was a clear victory for the Army of the Peninsula and did much to promote a favorable public impression of the entire Confederacy. Although later proven misguided, it suggested the Confederate States could put a quick and successful end to the war. The battle, however, did forestall further Union incursions into the Virginia Peninsula until McClellan's Peninsula campaign the following year. The battle was also significant in that Lieutenant John T. Greble was the first Union Army officer killed in the war.

Brigadier General H. T. Douglas, C.S.A., recalled in an article published in December 1903: "The Army of the Peninsula was composed of the flower of the South: troops from Virginia, North Carolina, South Carolina, Georgia, Alabama, Florida, Mississippi, and Louisiana filled its ranks. It received its baptism of fire on the field of Big Bethel."[18]

Based on Private Lain's diary, while Daly participated in the battle, it appears he was never under direct fire. Lain's account stated:

> Four Companies were detailed from the Regt for the purpose of being sent to other posts, for defense and working duty. They were Companies A, B, G, and H, which were marched into Yorktown and quartered until further orders. We find that instead of having been sent as first ordered they had been sent with other forces below on

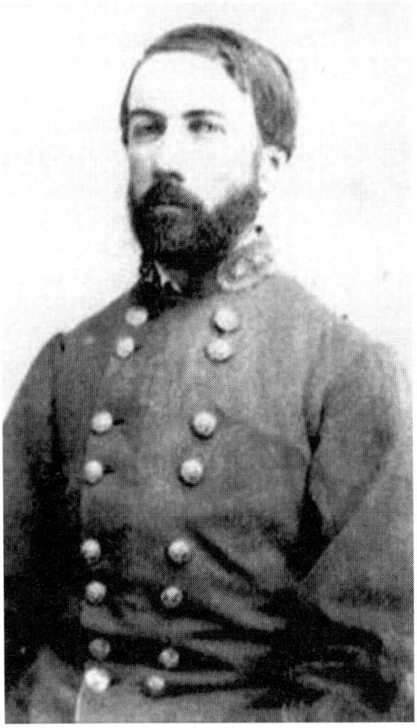

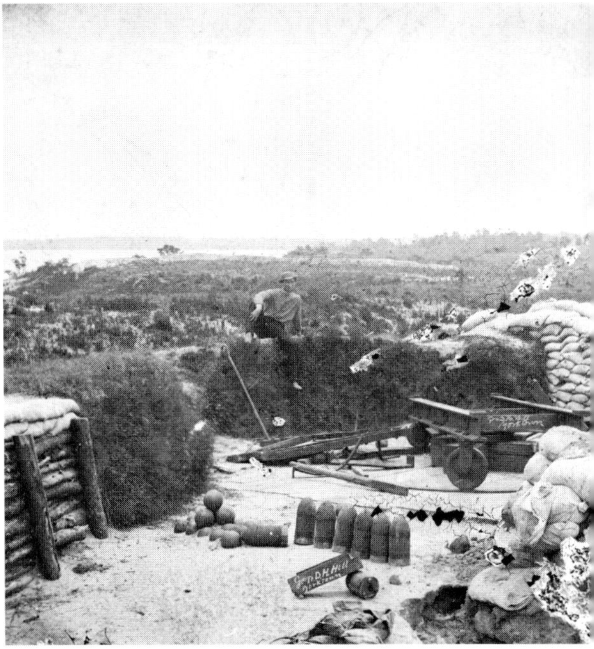

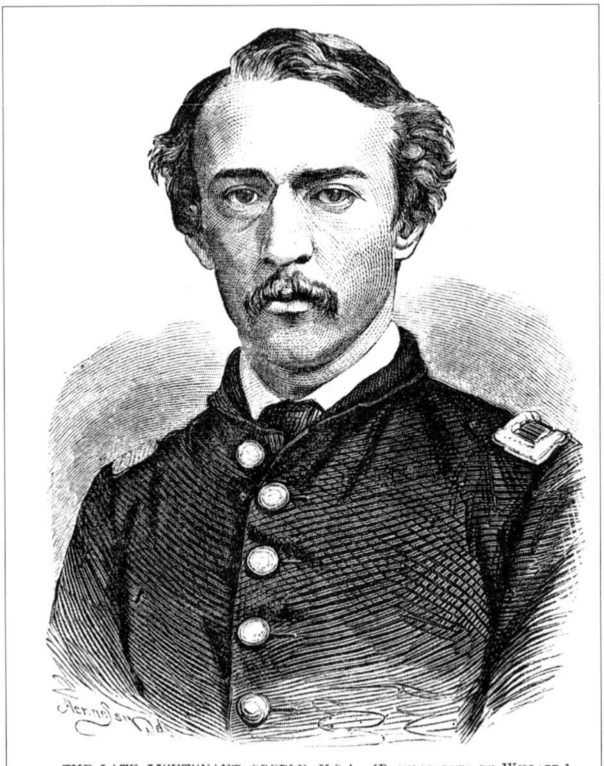

THE LATE LIEUTENANT GREBLE, U.S.A.—[PHOTOGRAPHED BY WILLARD.]

Above left: General Daniel Harvey Hill. (*Wikimedia Commons*)

Above rigt: Confederate fortifications near Yorktown, Virginia. (*Library of Congress*)

Left: The late Lt. Greble, U.S.A., *Harper's Weekly*, 29 June 1861. (*Library of Congress*) a scout, and it so happened that they were present at the Bethel fight, though they did not have a chance to take any part in it, as they were on a post which was not attacked.[19]

Also included in Lain's diary is a copy of a song written by Sergeant Wade of Young's Guard. Along with Daly's 15th Regiment, Young's Guard was one of the other regiments of Brigadier General Lafayette McLaws' Brigade that fought at Bethel Church that day:

Bethel Song
(Air Happy land of Canaan)

The Yankees came to Bethel Church, T'was on the 10th of June
The Southern Boys they thought they would give training
But we gave them such a beating, they never stopped retreating
Till we drove'em from the Happy land of Canaan

When they got to great Bethel, they thought they'd try our mettle
With prisoners they would go home full laden
But Gen'l Magruders Boys, they kicked up such a noise
That it scared 'em from the Happy land of Canaan

They had a lot of men, they called the Zouaves,
Penitentiary are the place, they got their training
They come to steal our chickens, but we gave 'em other fixings
And we sent 'em from the Happy land of Canaan

There was one among the whole, who showed a manly soul
He tried to get the Hessians, to sustain him
But the North Carolina boy, he popped him off the fence,
And he sent him from the Happy land of Canaan.[20]

Lain added:

Such is the song made on the Bethel fight and it gives within itself as good a description of the fight as could be given in a large volume should it be written. On Sunday the 16th of June orders were received for the Regt to leave Williamsburg again, and this time it was to be divided into three parts and each part to hold a post. Four companies were ordered to Grove Wharf, four to Kings Wharf and two to Sprudlies farm, which is somewhere near Jamestown. So all left Williamsburg for their different posts and arrived there in due time.[21]

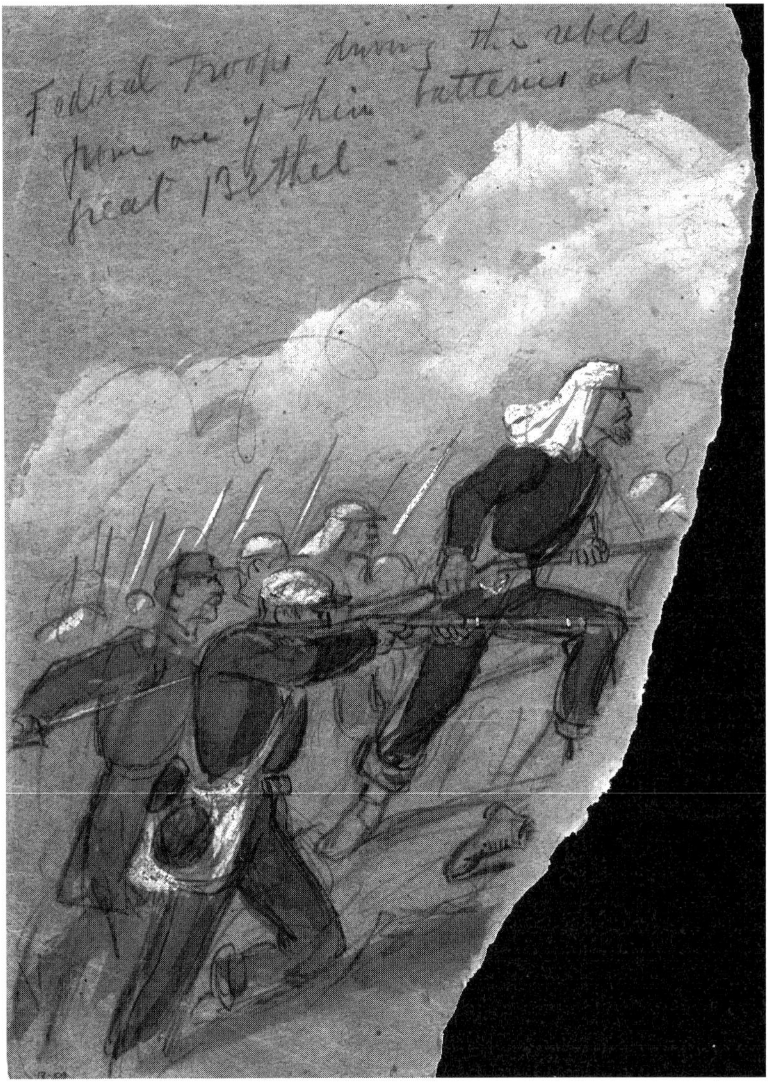

Left: Federal troops moving rebels from their batteries at Great Bethel. (*Library of Congress*)

Below: Battle of Big Bethel sketch by Thomas Nast, showing Duryee's Zouaves, Fifth New York Regiment, during their final charge into battle. (*Library of Congress*)

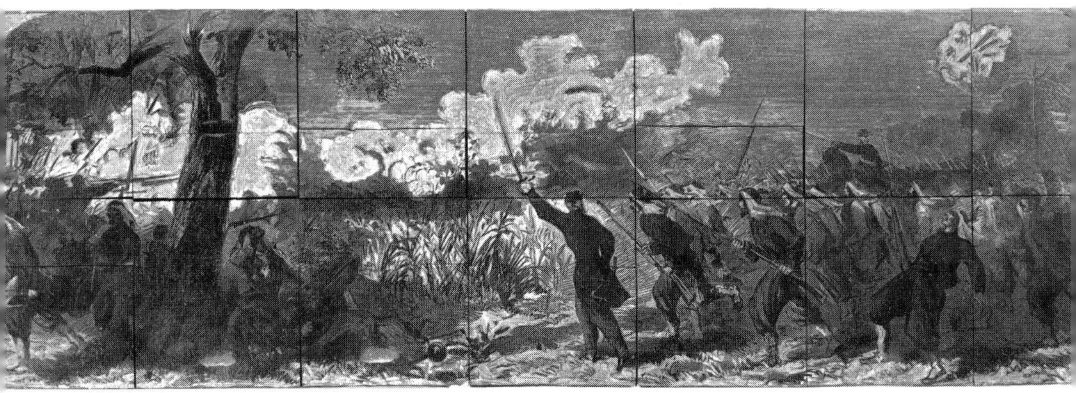

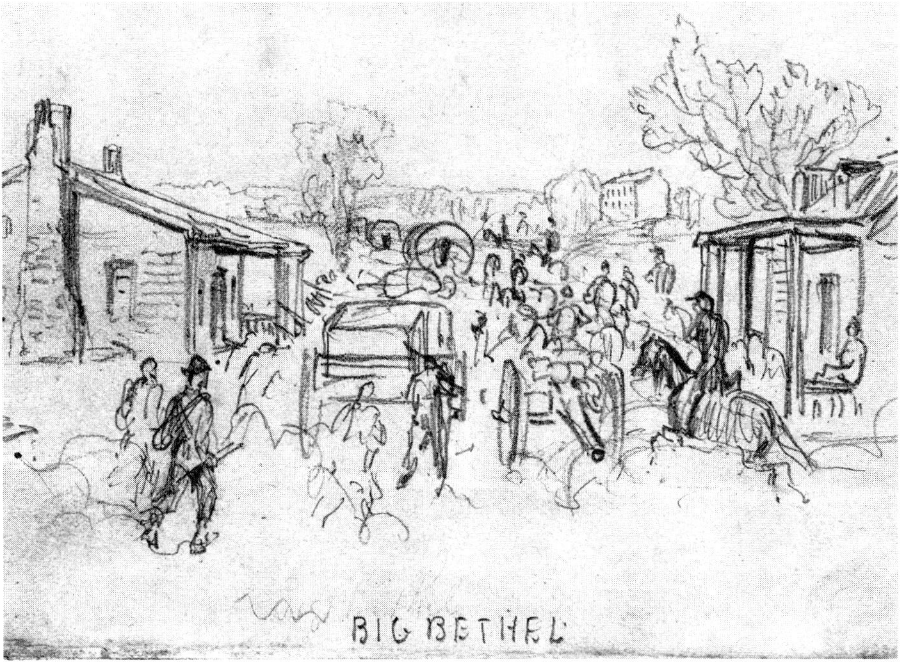

Battle of Big Bethel—Soldiers, caissons, and covered wagons moving through town, 1861. (*Library of Congress*)

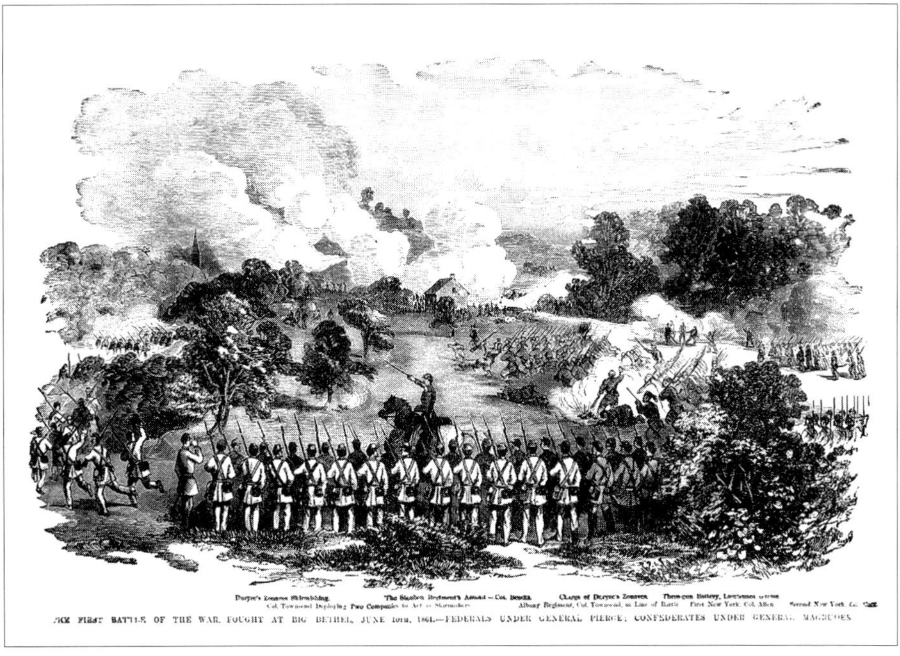

Big Bethel, the first battle of the War. (*The Soldier in our Civil War: a pictorial history of the conflict, 1861–1865*)

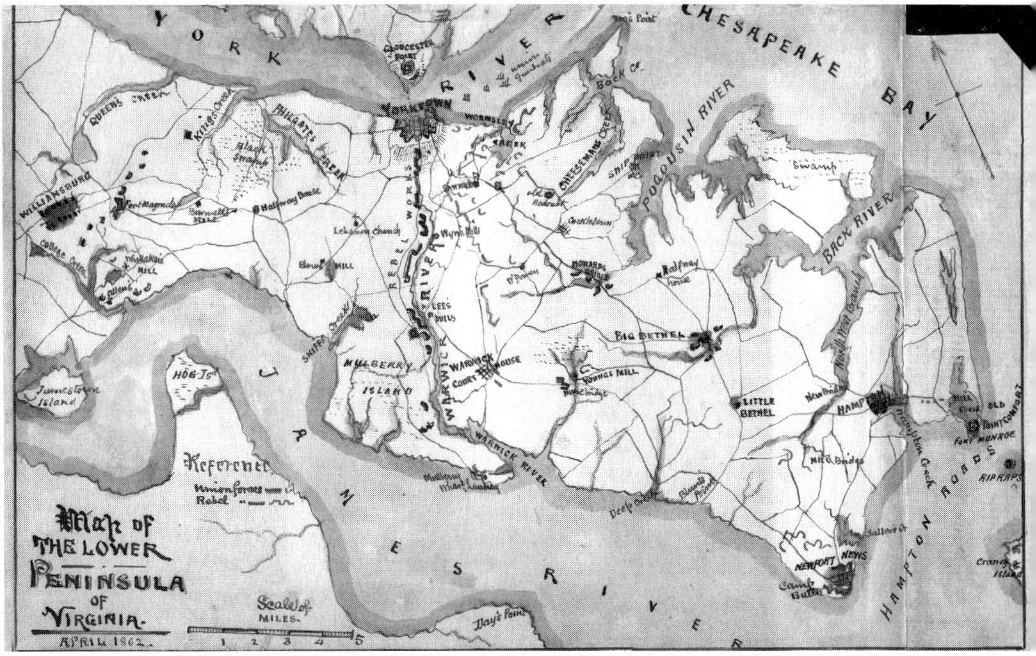

Map of the Lower Peninsula of Virginia, April 1862. (*Library of Congress*)

He further noted:

> Those at Kings Wharf (Companies A, B, E, and D) were camped on the hill beyond the wharf, it was a very fine place for a Camp, but it was very much exposed to the sun as there was not any shade near by, so the men were forced to resort to artificial means and for the purpose set out trees around their tents so as to shade them during the heat of the day. There was a fine spring of most excellent water near their Camp.[22]

Little is known about the 15th Regiment's specific activities during late summer 1861 other than they continued to drill and fortify defensive positions around Yorktown and Williamsburg in preparation for further incursions. In his 1903 "Reminiscences of the Peninsula" article in the *Confederate Veteran* journal, Brigadier General Douglas offered some general insight into the activity that Daly's regiment engaged in during the fall and winter of 1861. Douglas wrote:

> After the repulse of the Federal army at Bethel, the Army of the Peninsula was kept actively employed for the next year in constructing defences of the Peninsula at Gloucester Point, and Yorktown and along the Warwick River, and in constantly

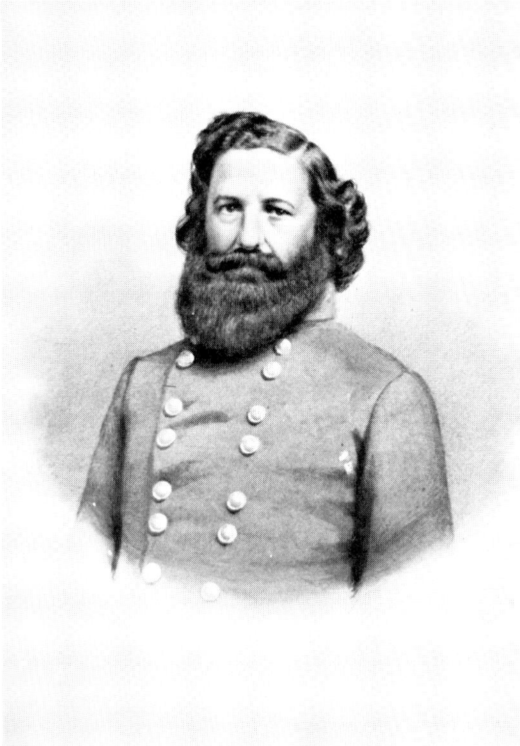

Lafayette McLaws, 1860.
(*Library of Congress*)

> moving from point to point, watching and skirmishing with the enemy and keeping him well within his intrenchments at Newport News and Fort Monroe.[23]

He added: "The Peninsula became the drill ground and training school for a part of that army to become so famous as the Army of Northern Virginia, and to the lessons taught it by its able commander may be attributed to a large degree the distinguished career of the soldiers of this gallant little army."[24]

Private Lain likewise made general notes of the period in his diary. As the 15th Regiment moved between drills and entrenchment details, he described the situation during August: "On Sunday the 4th of August, they left Camp Adams for a march into the lower country, starting at five in the evening and reaching Lee's Mill about midnight."[25] Taking stock of what the regiment found there, he wrote: "… Lee's Mill was nothing more than a common country mill situated in the fork of a road."[26] "The men by this time were the hardest looking set it has ever been my luck to see, for they had been out for nearly two weeks without a change of clothes, and sleeping on the ground during that time, and they had worn the worst they had when they left camp, so they presented anything but a fine appearance as they were ragged and dirty and some near naked."[27]

On 04 September, there is a record of Daly being admitted to Williamsburg Seminary Hospital.[28] He was suffering from a case of nephritis and was hospitalized for a few days. His recovery lasted for several weeks, and on 23 October 1861, he rejoined his company after six weeks' sick leave.[29]

Thanks to the efforts of Letitia Tyler Semple, daughter of President John Tyler, and other prominent women of Williamsburg, Seminary Hospital is considered the first hospital in Virginia to serve sick and wounded soldiers.[30] It was housed in a female seminary and reportedly contained seventy-five beds. Daly was, therefore, one of the hospital's earliest patients.

The 15th Regiment and others under Magruder's command made the best of the time. Lain noted that work on the batteries and trenches went so well that Magruder assessed what had been accomplished in a matter of a few months and reportedly stated: "… they were about the best he had seen and that the men deserved praise for the way in which they had constructed them and for the shortness of time they had been at work on them."[31] After reporting Magruder's comments, Lain went on to note: "There is not anything worthy of mention during the winter months so we will leave them until spring opens and then see what may be their fate."[32] His assessment would prove correct, as the Union's second campaign on the peninsula would soon commence.

In March 1862, Union Army General George B. McClellan began another attempt to dislodge the Confederates from the Virginia Peninsula with the intention of capturing Richmond. In preparation for the Peninsular Campaign of 1862, large contingents of Union forces were landed at the southern end of the peninsula at Fort Monroe. Their first order of business was a planned siege of Yorktown. Over the next several weeks, the Northern Army's movement northwest into the interior resulted in numerous battles with each side claiming small victories. Initially, however, Confederate General John B. Magruder serving under General Joseph E. Johnston had sufficient time to make plans to disappoint McClellan's troops. Magruder was given command of the "right of the position commencing at Dam No. 1 and extending to the river."[33]

Reporting from Lee's Mill for the period 05–07 April 1862, the 2nd Division of the Union's 4th Army Corps reported:

> During the operations at the beginning of the siege of Yorktown, Gen. McClellan gave orders on the 4th for Gen. Keyes, commanding the 4th corps, to "move forward Smith's division at 6 a.m. via Warwick Court House and the road leading near the Half-way House on the Yorktown and Williamsburg road." Pursuant to this order Smith moved promptly at the designated time from his camp at Young's mill. After advancing about 4 miles the enemy's pickets were encountered and driven back, and some 2 miles beyond Warwick Court House the advance came within sight of the Confederate works at Lee's mill. The 7th Me. was thrown forward as skirmishers and the rest of Davidson's brigade was ordered to deploy out of sight along the edge

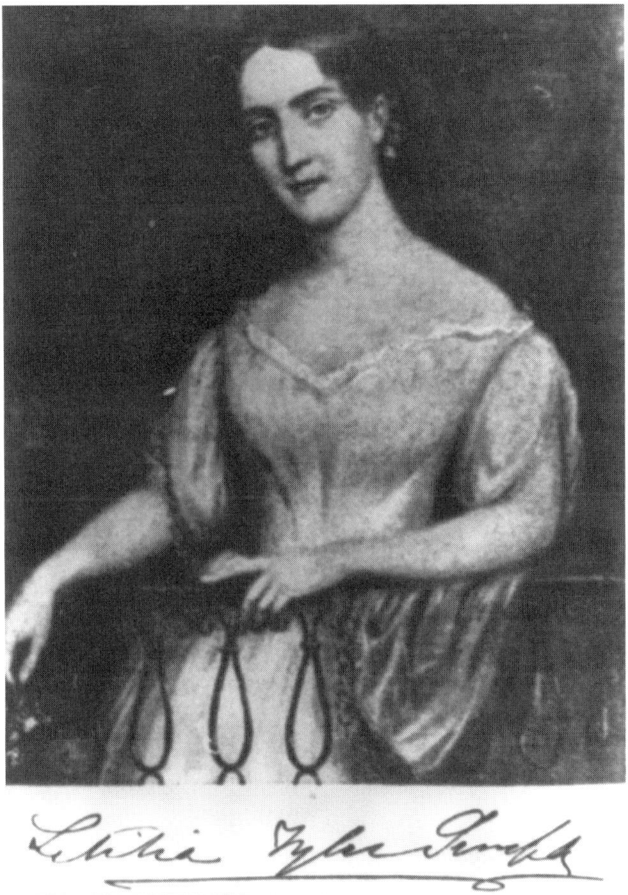

Right: Letitia Tyler Semple, daughter of President John Tyler, 1850. (*Library of Congress*)

Below: A view in Williamsburg, Virginia, 1862. (*Library of Congress*)

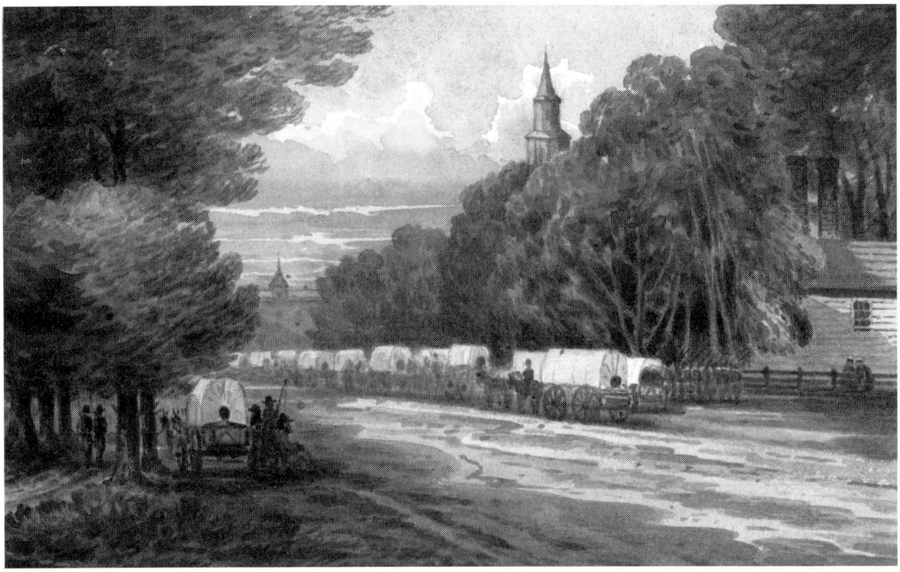

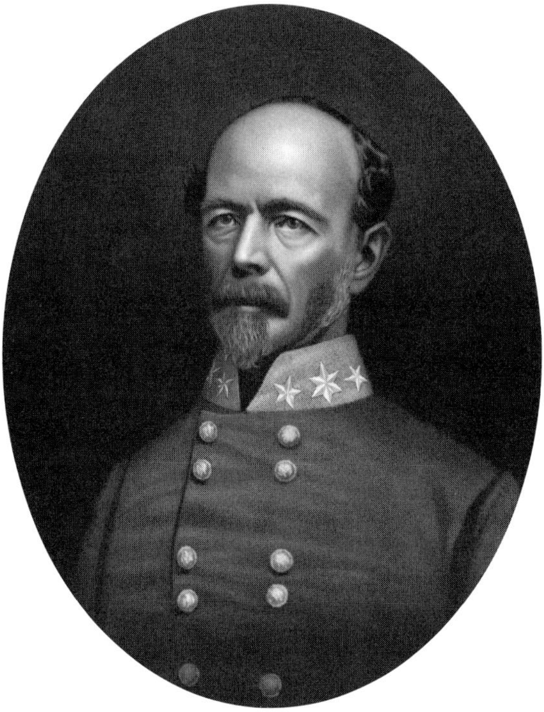

General Joseph E. Johnston.
(*Library of Congress*)

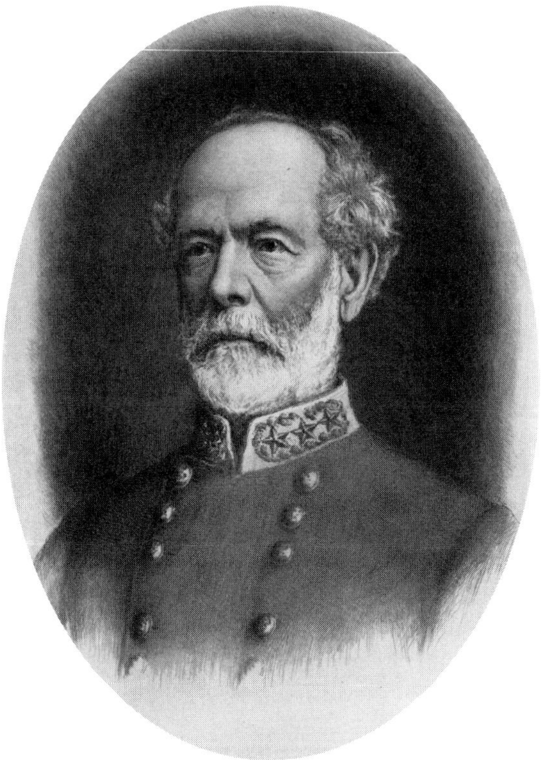

Joseph E. Johnston, 1860.
(*Library of Congress*)

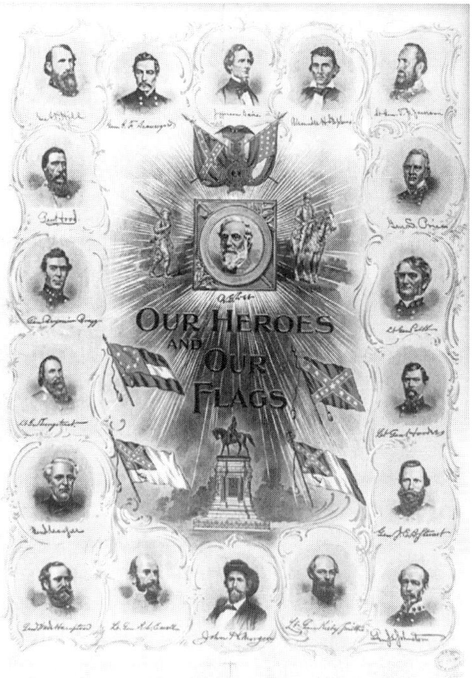

"Our Heroes and our Flags," memorial print for the Confederacy, 1895. (*Library of Congress*)

> of the woods, Hancock's brigade supporting his right and Brook's brigade in reserve. Wheeler's battery was then brought up and opened fire on the enemy. An attempt as made to turn Davidson's left, but it was frustrated by the 49th N. Y., which was thrown back at an obtuse angle to the rest of the line. The division then remained in this position, under fire a good part of the time, until the 7th, when it was withdrawn about a mile to the rear. Davidson's brigade lost 3 men killed and 12 wounded.[34]

The following week, on 11 April 1861, Major-General Magruder issued a proclamation from his Headquarters of the Army of the Peninsula at Lee's Farm, near Lee's Mill, to the "Citizens of the Peninsula and south side of James River." It read:

> McClellan, at the head of 100,000 men, is threatening our whole lines. To meet this force successfully our main reliance is to be placed upon breastworks. Soldiers cannot be expected to work night and day and fight besides.
>
> Our negro force now at work on fortifications is too small to accomplish this object before the enemy may attempt to carry us by assault when it will be beyond the power of all the force in the country to remedy that which earlier could have been effected with a slight additional assistance.
>
> Under these circumstances I am sure that no patriotic citizen, with the issue truly at heart, would hesitate to respond most cheerfully to the call which I now make, *viz*., one

negro man, with his ax or spade, to be furnished at once by each proprietor. Without the most liberal assistance in axes, spades, and hands to work, we cannot hope to succeed, and the Northern army will be in possession of your farms in a few days.

Mr. Junius Lamb is my authorized agent to receive the negroes. Send them at once, under overseers, to Colonel Ewell, at Williamsburg.[35]

Magruder's call for civilian assistance paid off. His advanced planning strategically placed fortifications around Lee's Mill and Yorktown and his resourceful troop placements outwitted and foiled McClellan's early advances. Another report of the 2nd Division of the Union's 4th Army Corps described the situation from the northern perspective:

> Lee's Mill. Va., April 16, 1862. 2nd Division, 4th Army Corps. Brig.-Gen. William F. Smith with his division proceeded to Lee's mill (or Burnt Chimneys) at Dam No. 1 on a reconnaissance. The troops were deployed and the infantry to the right opened fire on the Confederates working on their intrenchments [*sic.*]. The enemy's artillery at once replied, the Union pieces were brought into action, and after an hour the Confederate battery was silenced. About 3 p. m. the enemy's musketry fire slackened, when four companies of the 3rd Vt. were pushed across the stream and up to the works. On arriving at the crest of the parapet they were met by the enemy in force, and as their ammunition had been dampened in the passage of the stream, they were obliged to fall back. Later in the day another reconnaissance was made further up the stream, but with little success. The Federal loss in this engagement was 35 killed, 121 wounded and 9 missing. The Confederate casualties were not reported. This affair was an incident of the siege of Yorktown.[36]

Reporting as Major-General, Commanding, Right Wing, from his headquarters at Lee's Farm on 19 April 1862, Magruder offered the following account of the situation and recognized the valiant efforts of his outnumbered troops by writing:

> In making known to the right wing of the Army of the Peninsula the foregoing orders of the general commanding, Major-General Magruder deems it a duty he owes to the soldiers of the Army of the Peninsula to express publicly the approval with which their uniform good conduct has inspired him.
>
> Duty has exacted many sacrifices of them and they have been cheerfully made.
>
> The spade and the ax have been no less familiar to their hardy hands than the musket and the sword.
>
> Placed by the determination of our Government upon a narrow tongue of land, washed on three sides by navigable waters and ever menaced in front by the frowning fortress of Monroe, the soldiers of the old Army of the Peninsula have ever kept faithful ward and vigil over that avenue to the heart of the Confederacy intrusted [*sic.*] to their watchful care.

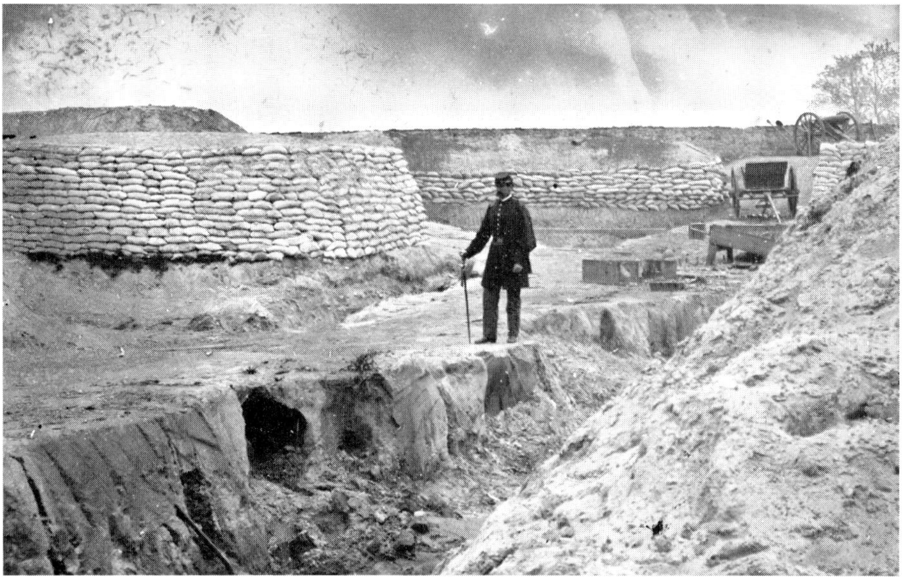

Above: Yorktown, Virginia, vicinity fortifications. Defensive ditch originally constructed by Gen. Cornwallis in 1781 was deepened by Gen. Magruder in 1862. (*Library of Congress*)

Below: Magruder's defense of the Virginia peninsula. (*Library of Congress*)

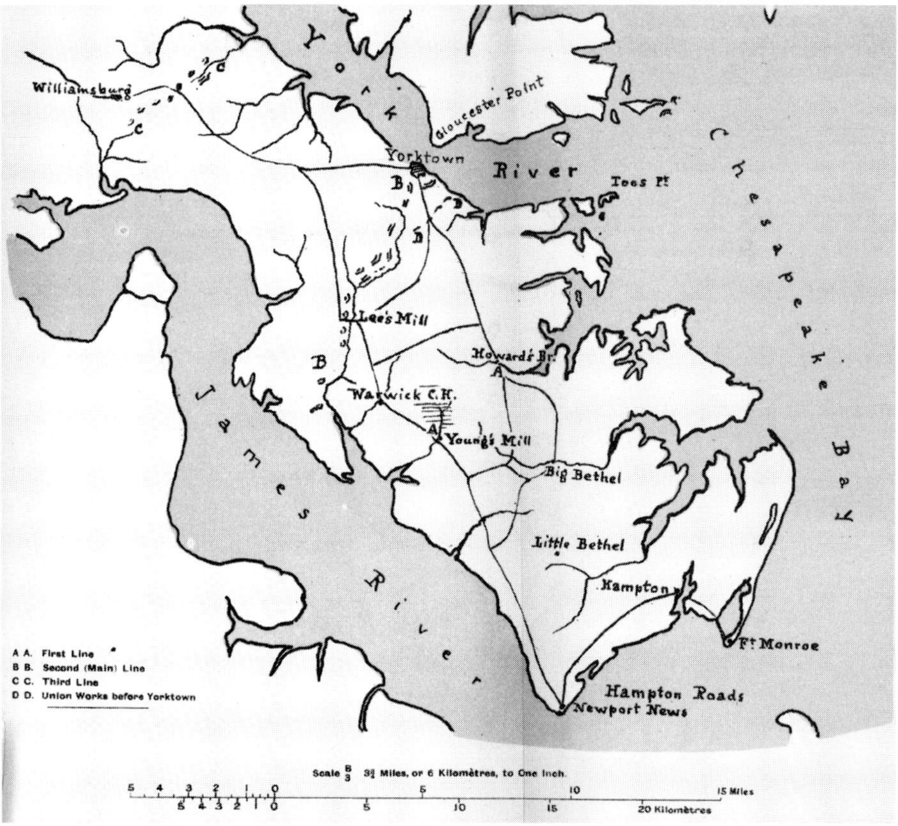

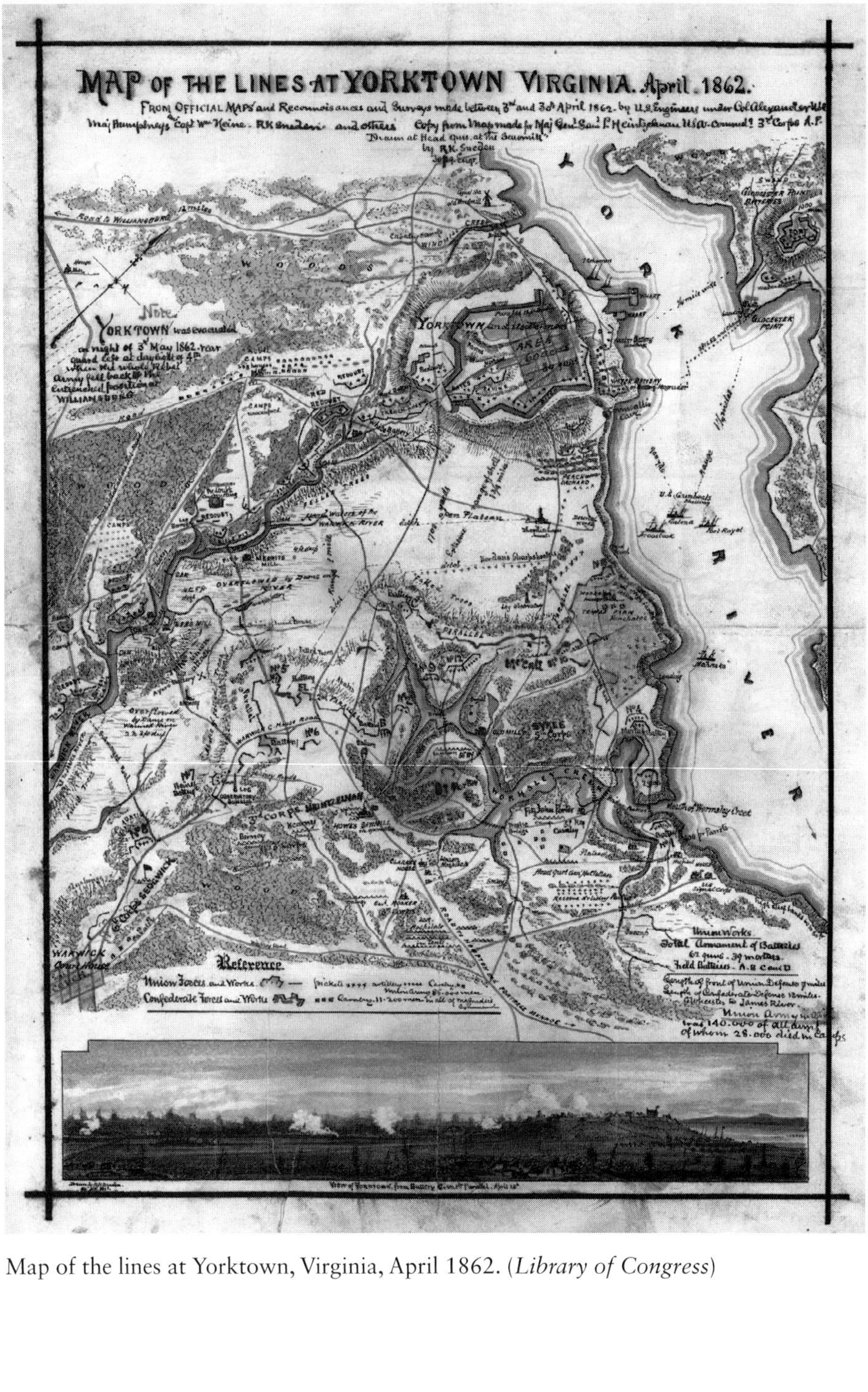

Map of the lines at Yorktown, Virginia, April 1862. (*Library of Congress*)

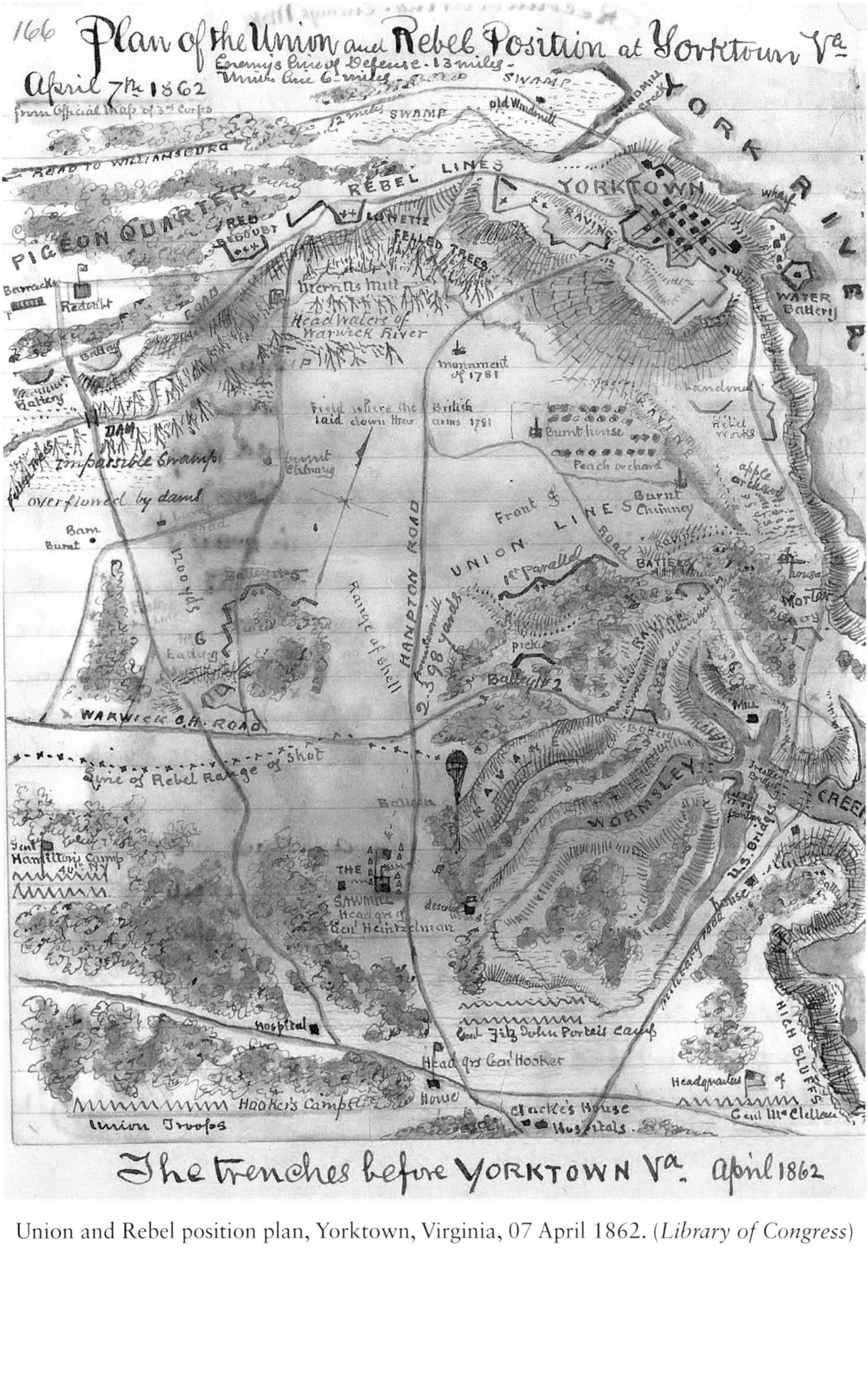

Union and Rebel position plan, Yorktown, Virginia, 07 April 1862. (*Library of Congress*)

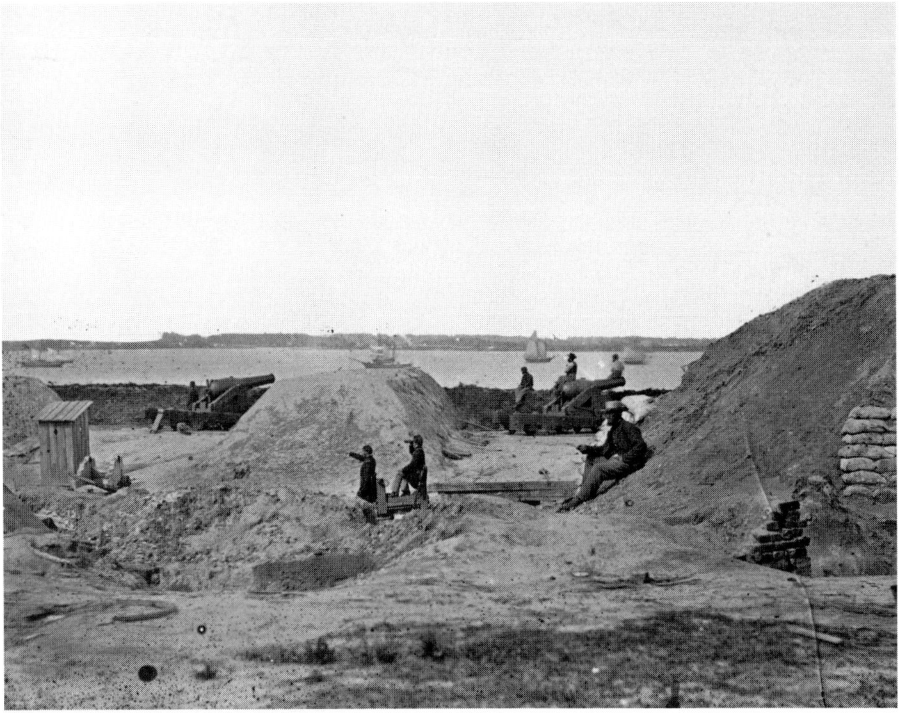

Confederate fortifications Yorktown, Virginia, 1861. (*Library of Congress*)

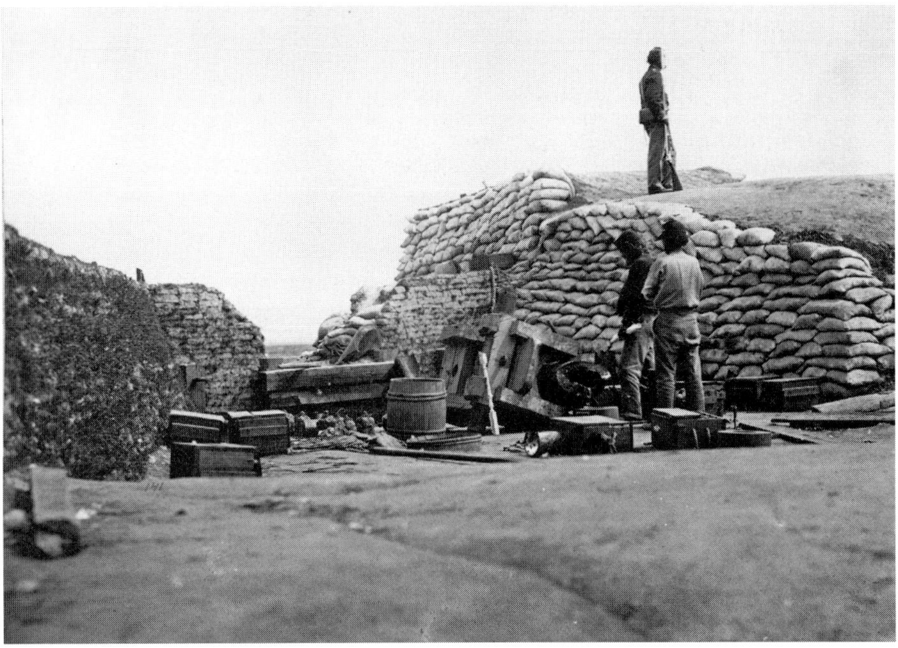

Confederate fortifications Yorktown, Virginia, 1861. (*Library of Congress*)

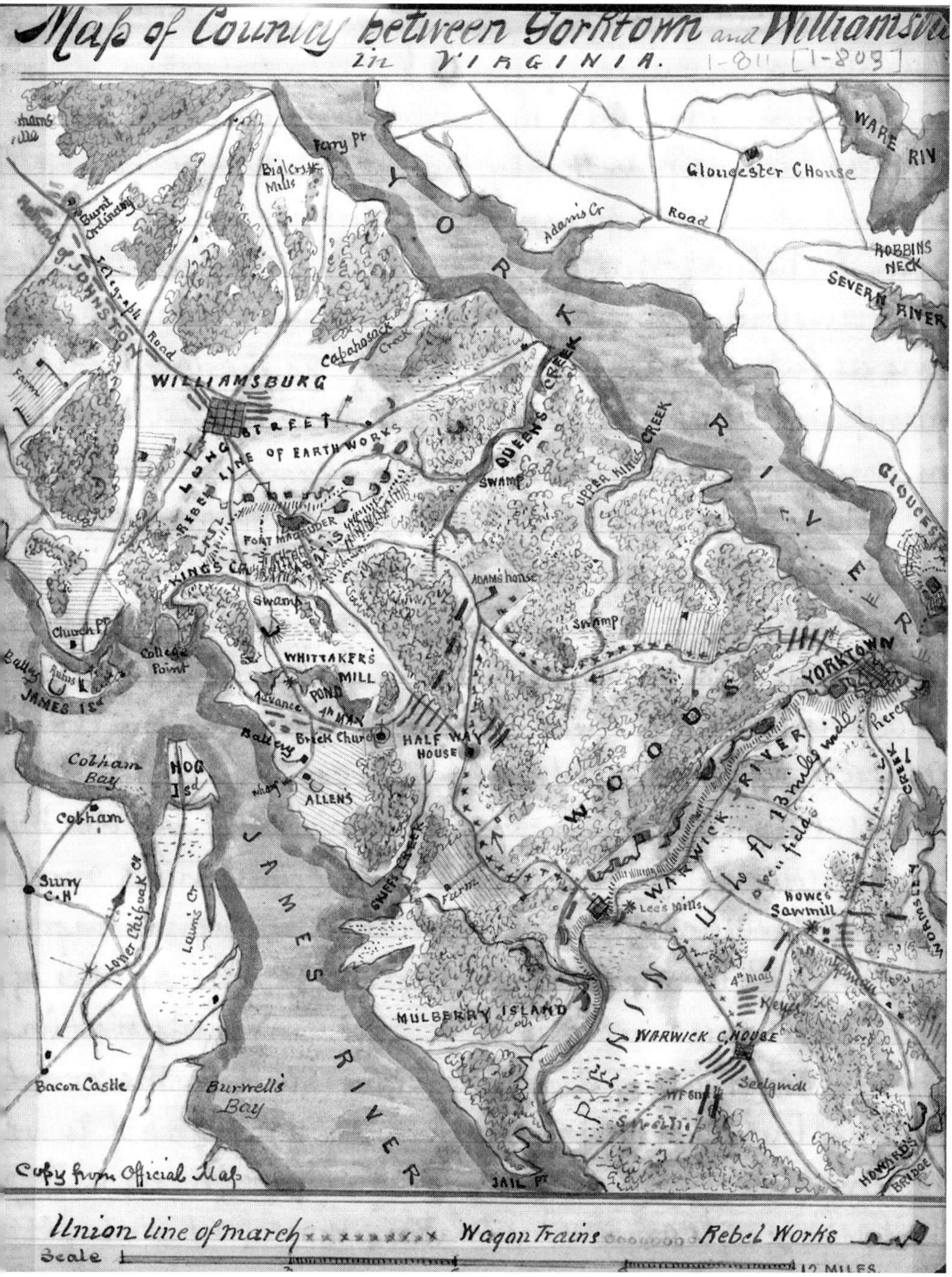

Map of country between Yorktown and Williamsburg, Virginia, 1862. (*Library of Congress*)

By their labors, skill, and courage the broad waters of York and James Rivers have been locked to the progress of the invaders by iron gates, which his energy and fertility of resources have yet been unable to unlock; and when pressed back by overwhelming numbers from that advanced line of defense, which, with a fourth of the army now present under our flag, would have been impregnable even to the vast hordes of our enemy, the little Army of the Peninsula fell back with its front to the marching enemy until it reached the Warwick River, along which its skill and energy had constructed a line of defense sufficient to temporarily stay the swelling advance of invasion.

The major-general late commanding this little army cannot refrain from declaring his gratification at the conduct of the troops, when, on Saturday, the 12th of this month, the immense legions of the enemy made their first demonstration along our line, embracing a front of 10 miles, and defended by a force, exclusive of the fixed garrison of Yorktown and Mulberry Island, of scarce half as many thousand men as there were miles to defend. Whenever along this line the enemy ventured to approach he was met by the roar of your artillery and the unwavering ranks of your soldiery.

To accomplish this almost incredible result, when an army of twenty times your numbers was checked and held at bay along a front of 10 miles, you hesitated at no marches or vigils, by night or by day, and you shrank from no encounter, however unequal, which your general asked at your hands. And now, when you have fulfilled our whole mission, when you have checked the advance of an exultant enemy, until a breathing spell of countless value to our country could be obtained, during which adequate preparations have been made to meet our foe upon any field he may choose, you can with pride turn over to your gallant and patriotic comrades the position which you have firmly held and protected against such terrible odds, and gladly share with them the duty of guarding this road to the capital of the Confederacy, the arduous labors of which had become too great for the unaided efforts of our little band.

Everything looks bright. We have a gallant army, led by a general whose courage and skill approve him worthy of the universal confidence in which he is held, and the major-general late commanding feels every assurance that in the great drama about to be enacted on this Peninsula the soldiers of that little army which he so long had the honor to command will prove themselves worthy comrades of those gallant warriors who have made the names of Manassas and Leesburg illustrious in Southern history.

By the new arrangements which the exigencies of the service require the late major-general commanding finds himself separated from a portion of the old Army of the Peninsula. How painful this separation is to him he will not venture to express, but he begs to assure them that his heart will follow them in the perils of the coming conflict though it be not his fortune to lead them, and he feels confident that their courage and gallantry will win the esteem and affection of their new general, as it has already done that of their old commander.

> To those of his ancient comrades who still remain under his command, he can only express the hope that the future, like the past, will only strengthen those kindly ties which unite soldiers in arms for the service of their country.
>
> Comrades, the hour of the decision of our liberties is approaching, and during its eventful minutes let no man rest satisfied with the performance of his duty, for our country demands of each of us that he do more.[37]

In his 1903 *Confederate Veteran* journal article, Brigadier General Douglas recalled the situation:

> In the spring of 1862 Gen. McClellan, with his grand army splendidly equipped and organized, began his march from Fortress Monroe and Newport News on Richmond. The troops of our advance guard fell back slowly as McClellan moved up until our lines at Yorktown and on the west bank of the Warwick River, stretching from Yorktown to Mulberry Island, on the James River, were reached and occupied. The Army of the Peninsula comprised at the time about 12,000 men of all arms, and its thin gray line interposed to its giant foe the only barrier to the Confederate capital.[38]

On 16 April 1862, the same day the Union's 2nd Division, 4th Army Corps' report on the Battle of Lee's Mill was filed, William H. Daly was captured.

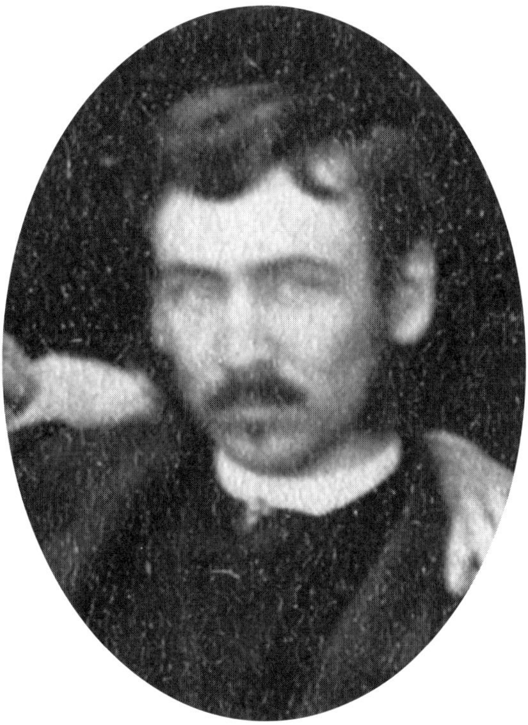

William Hudson Daly immediately after the Civil War; University of Michigan Medical School graduating class 1865–1866. (*University of Michigan Bentley Historical Library*)

3

A Galvanized Yankee

When the 15th Regiment's muster roll was filed on 26 April 1862, Daly was listed as a "prisoner of war."[1] On the regiment's final report of 1862, dated 31 December, he was described as "having been taken prisoner at Lee's Mill." The report further noted that Daly "Never returned, he taking Oath of Allegiance to the U.S."[2] An example of an oath used at the time read:

> I do solemnly swear (or affirm) that I will support, protect and defend the Constitution and Government of the United States against all enemies, whether domestic or foreign, and that I will bear true faith, allegiance and loyalty to the same, any ordinance, resolution or law of any State, convention or legislature to the contrary notwithstanding; and further, that I do this with a full determination, pledge and purpose, without any mental reservation or evasion whatsoever: So help me God.[3]

Little is known about the location where Daly was held prisoner. However, evidence suggests he may have been detained at Fort Monroe since the stronghold served as the Union's closest prison camp.

The 15th Regiment's 31 December 1862 report suggests Daly was in the right place at the right time. Within three months of his capture, new regulations were enacted on prisoner exchange and parole. While likely very distressing for him, his internment occurred during a period that was perhaps the best time in the war for such a thing to occur. It was not long after Daly's capture that northern and southern public and government debate forced both sides to make decisions about how they were going to handle the growing numbers of prisoners of war each side was holding. In the north, President Lincoln and Secretary of War Stanton agreed to formalize prisoner exchanges. In the south, Confederate leaders concurred.

During the early months of the war, military commanders on both sides had accomplished prisoner exchanges, albeit on a small scale and in an *ad hoc* manner. As the war progressed and the burden of holding, feeding, clothing, and providing medical care for a burgeoning numbers of prisoners soon became a problem for both sides, something had to be done on a larger and more permanent basis. On 12 July 1862, Lincoln assigned Major General John Adams Dix to meet with Confederate General Robert E. Lee's representative, Major General Daniel Harvey Hill, to develop a prisoner exchange agreement. Dix was the commanding officer at Fort Monroe at the time. Hill, Stonewall Jackson's brother-in-law, was division commander of the Army of Northern Virginia.

The generals met a number of times at Haxall's Landing on the James River in Virginia before they concluded an agreement on 22 July 1862.[4] The generals used an old agreement between American and British forces during the War of 1812 as the basis for what became known as the Dix-Hill Cartel. The "Cartel established a sliding scale to calculate the relative values of officers and enlisted personnel. Excess prisoners would be paroled and not permitted to take up arms until properly exchanged. The agreement called upon each side to appoint an agent of exchange to oversee the process."[5] Within days of the Cartel signing, large numbers of prisoners on both sides were released. When formally "exchanged," soldiers returned to duty with their regiments. Under terms of the Cartel, others who were not exchanged could be released by parole. Conditions of parole required that soldiers could no longer take up arms until such time as they might be formally exchanged. Article 6 of the Cartel specified that not only could soldiers not take up arms, it also prohibited "the performance of field, garrison, police, or guard, or constabulary duty."[6] In other words, they were of little use to either army. At that point, the United States also formally started to recruit black soldiers, which caused much consternation in the Confederacy. Supplementary articles of the Cartel included Article 7, stating:

> All prisoners of war now held on either side and all prisoners hereafter taken shall be sent with all reasonable dispatch to A. M. Aiken's, below Dutch Gap, on the James River, Va., or to Vicksburg, on the Mississippi River, in the State of Mississippi, and there exchanged or paroled until such exchange can be effected, notice being previously given by each party of the number of prisoners it will send and the time when they will be delivered at those points respectively; and in case the vicissitudes of war shall change the military relations of the places designated in this article to the contending parties so as to render the same inconvenient for the delivery and exchange of prisoners, other places bearing as nearly as may be the present local relations of said places to the lines of said parties shall be by mutual agreement substituted. But nothing in this article contained shall prevent the commanders of two opposing armies from exchanging prisoners or releasing them on parole from other points mutually agreed on by said commanders.[7]

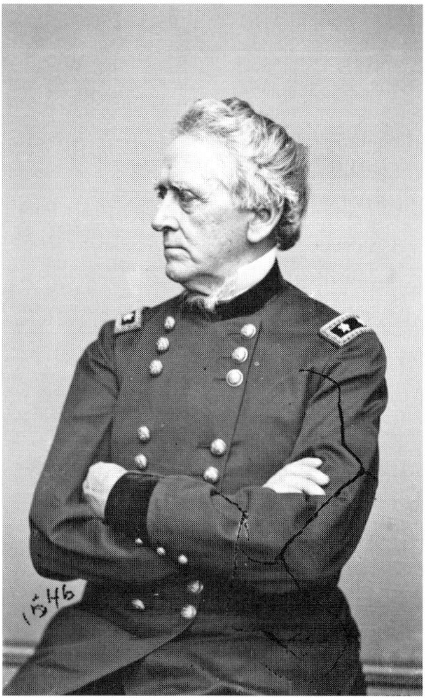

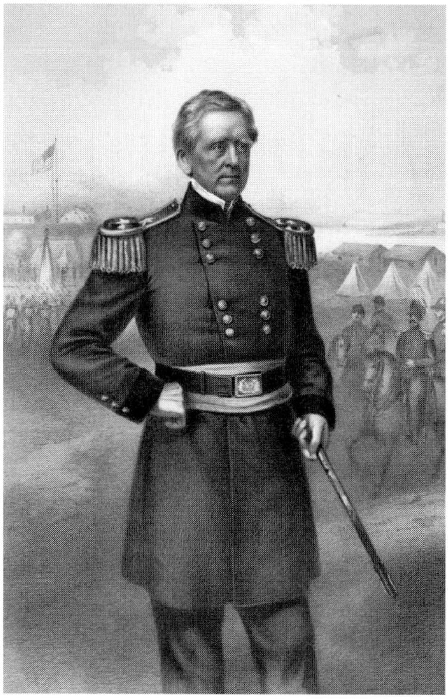

Above left: Gen. John A. Dix, 1855. (*Library of Congress*)

Above right: Maj. Gen. John A. Dix, 1862. (*Library of Congress*)

Below: Union guards at Sally port, Fort Monroe, Virginia, 1864. (*Library of Congress*)

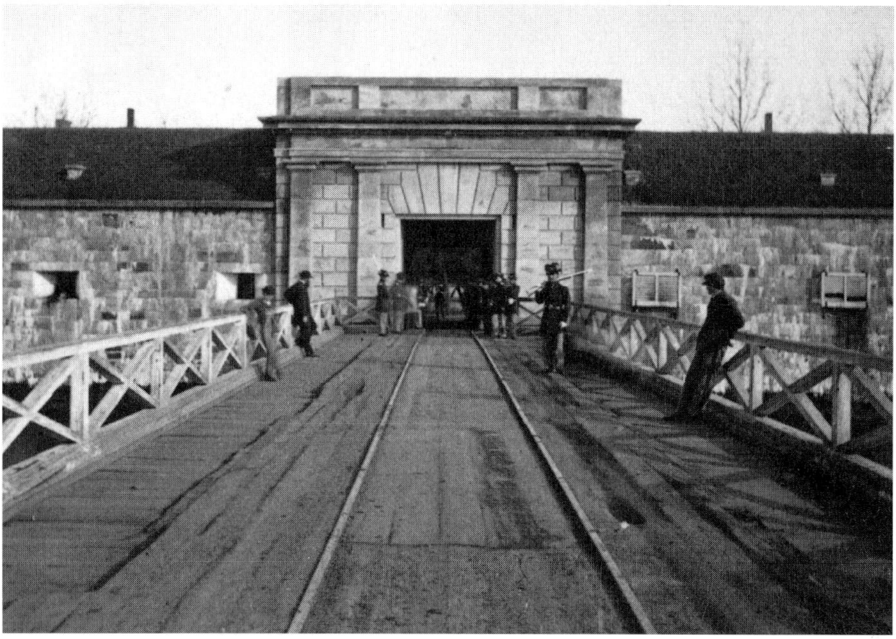

With Daly's capture at Lee's Mill, he was in the immediate area where the negotiations took place, and prisoners in that region were some of the first to benefit from the exchanges and paroles sanctioned by the Cartel.

Several weeks after the Cartel was signed, in September 1862, President Lincoln issued the Emancipation Proclamation. It became effective 01 January 1863. In April 1863, the Federal government issued General Order 100, known as the "Lieber Codes."[8] It stipulated the United States government expected all prisoners to be treated equally, regardless of color. One month later, in May 1863, the Confederate Congress passed a joint resolution formalizing Jefferson Davis' proclamation that black soldiers taken prisoner would not be exchanged.[9] President Lincoln reacted by issuing Order 252 on 30 July, officially suspending the Dix-Hill Cartel until such time as the Confederates agreed to treat black prisoners the same as whites. Large-scale prisoner exchanges were not formally resumed until August 1864.[10] Thus, Daly's parole occurred during a brief window of favorable opportunity.

The exact date of Daly's parole and his geographic whereabouts immediately following his liberation remain unknown. Several months after his capture and release, however, he began attending a course of medical lectures at Jefferson Medical College in Philadelphia, Pennsylvania. It is also known that sometime in 1863 he began serving as a U.S. Army medical cadet at Philadelphia's Germantown (Cuyler) Hospital. Once again, his timing appears to have been impeccable.

Formation of the U.S. Army medical cadet corps was originally approved by an Act of Congress on 03 August 1861, but the number of positions was limited to fifty and competition for openings was intense. Section 5 of the Act was entitled "An Act for the Better Organization of the Military Establishment," and it formally established a corps of medical cadets to be attached to the medical staff of the army. It read:

> And be it further enacted, That there be added to the medical staff of the army a corps of medical cadets, whose duty it shall be to act as dressers in the general hospitals and as ambulance attendants in the field, under the direction and control of the medical officers alone. They shall have the same rank and pay as the military cadets at West Point. Their number shall be designated by the exigencies of service, at no time to exceed fifty. It shall be composed of young men of liberal education, students of medicine, between the ages of eighteen and twenty-three years, who have been reading medicine for two years, and have attended at least one course of lectures in a medical college. They shall enlist for one year, and be subject to the rules and articles of war.[11]

Daly was indeed fortunate his capture and release coincided with Congress further expanding the number of medical cadets on 16 April 1862. Daly's reason for pursuing a medical career at this point remains unknown, but it was a decision that would influence the rest of his life. Now that he was a "galvanized Yankee," his move from the gray uniform of the Confederacy to the blue uniform of the Union was opportune.[12] As a medical cadet, he was now among a very select

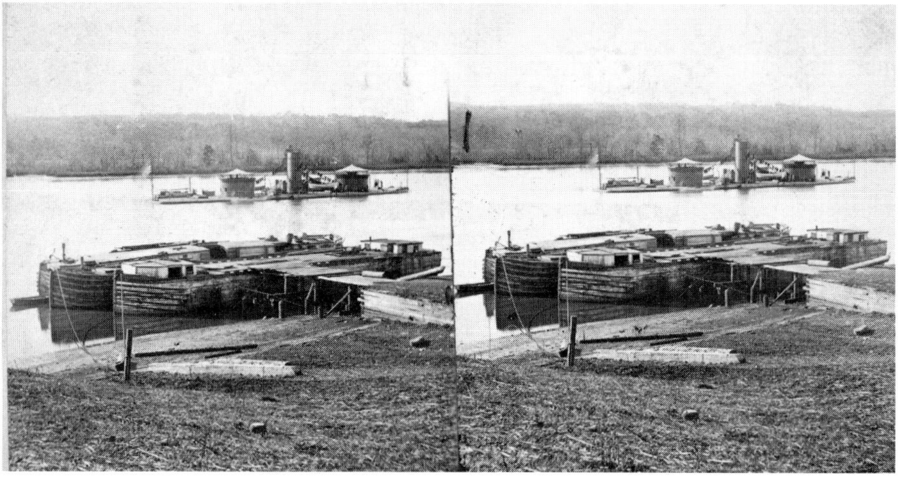

Aiken's Landing, Virginia, showing canal boats docked at the wharf where Union prisoners were exchanged for Confederate prisoners. The Union double-turreted monitor U.S.S. *Onondaga* is in the distance, 1864. (*Library of Congress*)

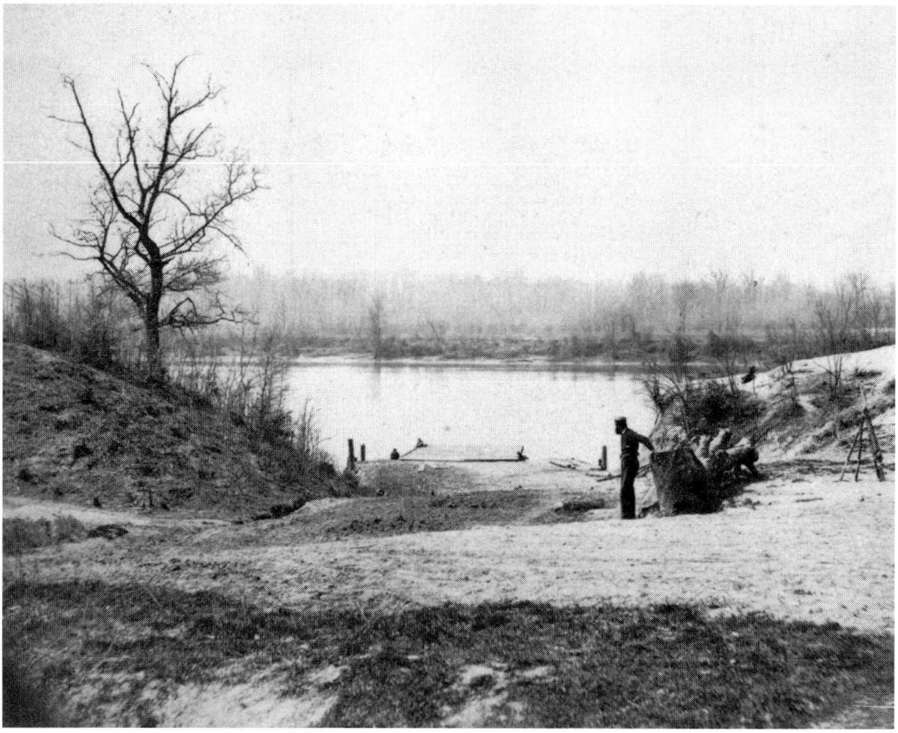

Soldier standing at landing where prisoners were exchanged, James River, April 1865. (*Library of Congress*)

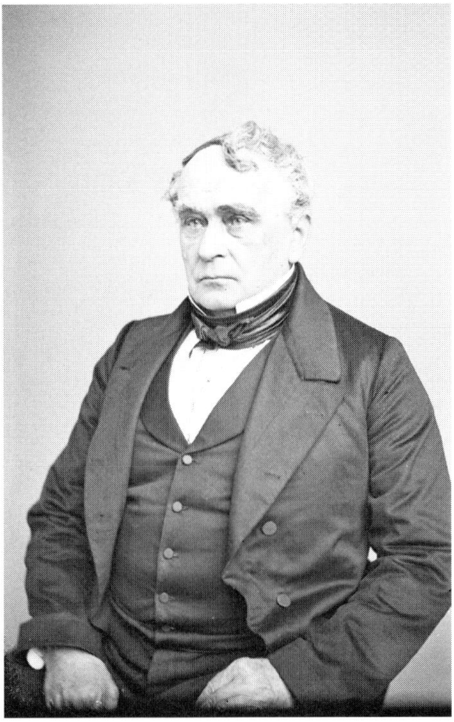

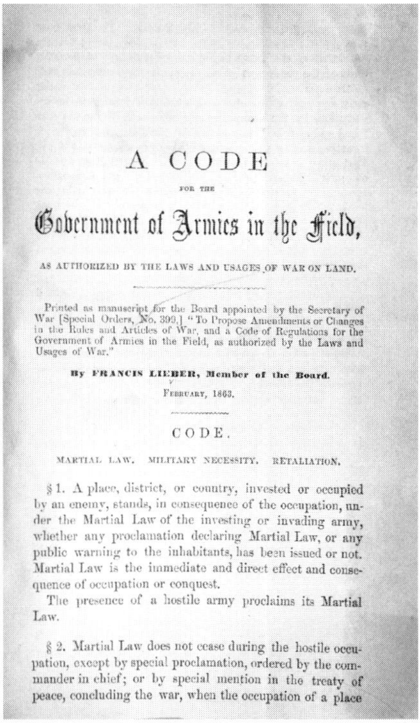

A CODE

FOR THE

Government of Armies in the Field,

AS AUTHORIZED BY THE LAWS AND USAGES OF WAR ON LAND.

Printed as manuscript for the Board appointed by the Secretary of War [Special Orders, No. 399,] "To Propose Amendments or Changes in the Rules and Articles of War, and a Code of Regulations for the Government of Armies in the Field, as authorized by the Laws and Usages of War."

By FRANCIS LIEBER, Member of the Board.

FEBRUARY, 1863.

CODE.

MARTIAL LAW. MILITARY NECESSITY. RETALIATION.

§ 1. A place, district, or country, invested or occupied by an enemy, stands, in consequence of the occupation, under the Martial Law of the investing or invading army, whether any proclamation declaring Martial Law, or any public warning to the inhabitants, has been issued or not. Martial Law is the immediate and direct effect and consequence of occupation or conquest.

The presence of a hostile army proclaims its Martial Law.

§ 2. Martial Law does not cease during the hostile occupation, except by special proclamation, ordered by the commander in chief; or by special mention in the treaty of peace, concluding the war, when the occupation of a place

Above left: Professor Frances Lieber, principal author of U.S. General Order No. 100—Instructions for the Government of the Armies of the United States in the Field, commonly recognized as the "Lieber Code." (*Library of Congress*)

Above right: Front page of the "Lieber Code," a code of regulations for the government of armies in the field. (*National Library of Medicine*)

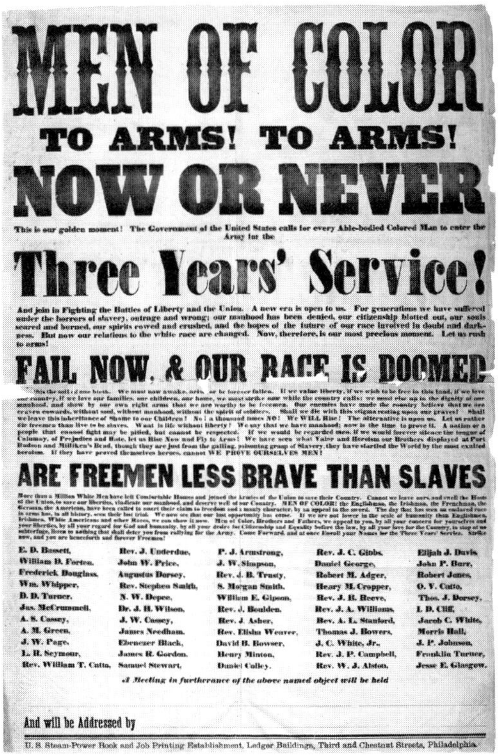

MEN OF COLOR

TO ARMS! TO ARMS!

NOW OR NEVER

This is our golden moment! The Government of the United States calls for every Able-bodied Colored Man to enter the Army for the

Three Years' Service!

And join in Fighting the Battles of Liberty and the Union. A new era is open to us. For generations we have suffered under the horrors of slavery, outrage and wrong; our manhood has been denied, our citizenship blotted out, our souls seared and burned, our spirits cowed and crushed, and the hopes of the future of our race involved in doubt and darkness. But now our relations to the white race are changed. Now, therefore, is our most precious moment. Let us rush to arms!

FAIL NOW, & OUR RACE IS DOOMED

...this the soil of our birth. We must now awake, arise, or be forever fallen. If we value liberty, if we wish to be free in this land, if we love our country, if we love our families, our children, our home, we must strike now while the country calls; we must rise up in the dignity of our manhood, and show by our own right arms that we are worthy to be freemen. Our enemies have made the country believe that we are craven cowards, without soul, without manhood, without the spirit of soldiers. Shall we die with this stigma resting upon our graves? Shall we leave this inheritance of Shame to our Children? No! a thousand times NO! We WILL Rise! The alternative is upon us. Let us rather die freemen than live to be slaves. What is life without liberty? We say that we have manhood; now is the time to prove it. A nation or a people that cannot fight may be pitied, but cannot be respected. If we would be regarded men, if we would forever silence the tongue of Calumny, of Prejudice and Hate, let us Rise Now and Fly to Arms! We have seen what Valor and Heroism our Brothers displayed at Port Hudson and Milliken's Bend, though they are just from the galling, poisoning grasp of Slavery, they have startled the World by the most exalted heroism. If they have proved themselves heroes, cannot WE PROVE OURSELVES MEN!

ARE FREEMEN LESS BRAVE THAN SLAVES

More than a Million White Men have left Comfortable Homes and joined the Armies of the Union to save their Country. Cannot we leave ours, and swell the Hosts of the Union, to save our liberties, vindicate our manhood, and deserve well of our Country. MEN OF COLOR! the Englishman, the Irishman, the Frenchman, the German, the American, have been called to assert their claim to freedom and a manly character, by an appeal to the sword. The day that has seen an enslaved race in arms has, in all history, seen their last trial. We now see that our last opportunity has come. If we are not lower in the scale of humanity than Englishmen, Irishmen, White Americans and other Races, we can show it now. Men of Color, Brothers and Fathers, we appeal to you, by all your concern for yourselves and your liberties, by all your regard for God and humanity, by all your desire for Citizenship and Equality before the law, by all your love for the Country, to stop at no subterfuge, listen to nothing that shall deter you from rallying for the Army. Come Forward, and at once Enroll your Names for the Three Years' Service. Strike now, and you are henceforth and forever Freemen!

E. D. Bassett,	Rev. J. Underdue,	P. J. Armstrong,	Rev. J. C. Gibbs,	Elijah J. Davis,
William D. Forten,	John W. Price,	J. W. Simpson,	Daniel George,	John P. Burr,
Frederick Douglass,	Augustus Dorsey,	Rev. J. B. Trusty,	Robert M. Adger,	Robert Jones,
Wm. Whipper,	Rev. Stephen Smith,	S. Morgan Smith,	Henry M. Cropper,	O. V. Catto,
D. D. Turner,	N. W. Depee,	William E. Gipson,	Rev. J. B. Reeve,	Thos. J. Dorsey,
Jas. McCrummell,	Dr. J. H. Wilson,	Rev. J. Boulden,	Rev. J. A. Williams,	I. D. Cliff,
A. S. Cassey,	J. W. Cassey,	Rev. J. Asher,	Rev. A. L. Stanford,	Jacob C. White,
A. M. Green,	James Needham,	Rev. Elisha Weaver,	Thomas J. Bowers,	Morris Hall,
J. W. Page,	Ebenezer Black,	David B. Bowser,	J. C. White, Jr.,	J. P. Johnson,
L. R. Seymour,	James R. Gordon,	Henry Minton,	Rev. J. P. Campbell,	Franklin Turner,
Rev. William T. Catto,	Samuel Stewart,	Daniel Colley,	Rev. W. J. Alston,	Jesse E. Glasgow.

A Meeting in furtherance of the above named object will be held

And will be Addressed by

U. S. Steam-Power Book and Job Printing Establishment, Ledger Buildings, Third and Chestnut Streets, Philadelphia.

Right: Men of Color Civil War Recruitment Broadside, written by Frederick Douglas, 1863. (*Wikimedia Commons*)

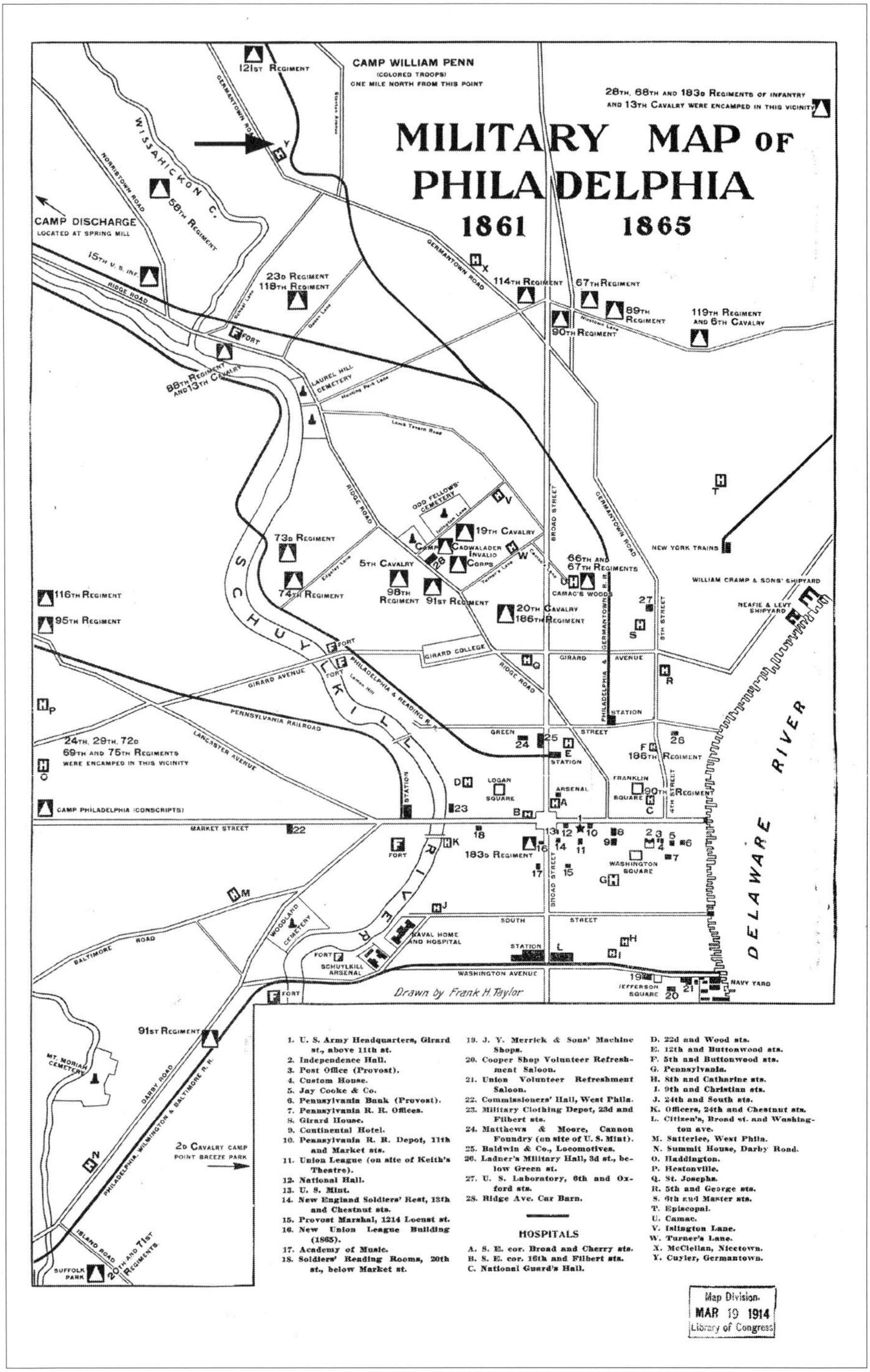

Military map of Philadelphia 1861–1865 created in1914. (*Library of Congress*)

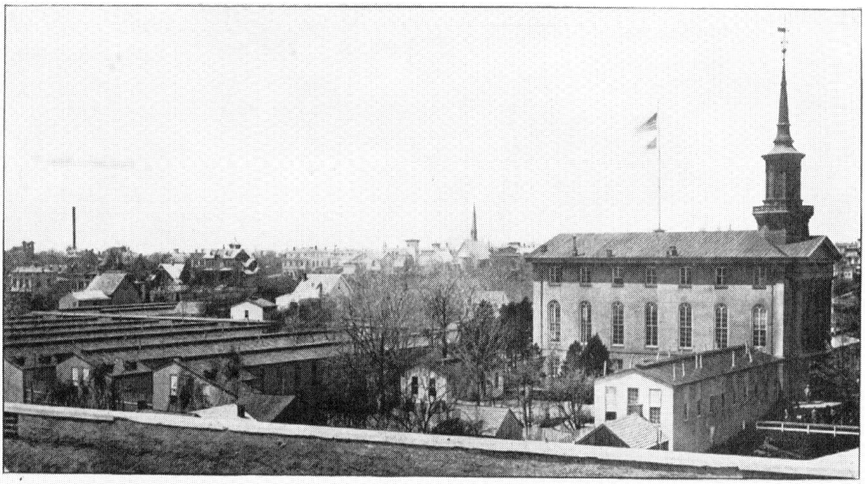

Cuyler Hospital. (*Taylor, Frank H. Taylor, Philadelphia in the Civil War 1861–1865: City of Philadelphia, 1913*)

group of young men without formal medical degrees or apprenticeships to be given a unique opportunity to engage in the practice of medicine.

As Guy R. Hasegawa noted in his study on Civil War medical cadets, "Applicants for a position as medical cadet provided their date and place of birth, place of residence, period of medical studies, certification of attendance at one full course in a medical college, and testimonials of character and physical fitness."[13] If accepted, they would "act under the direction and control of medical officers alone as dressers in general hospitals and as ambulance attendants."[14] Hasegawa further noted a majority of cadets served in Army hospitals, and "Philadelphia's medical schools proved to be a particularly rich source of medical cadets; at least 23 medical students from the University of Pennsylvania and 18 from Jefferson Medical College, for example, enlisted in the corps."[15] He also made note: "Becoming a military surgeon was undoubtedly on the mind of many medical cadets. Of the 247 men who served up to one term as medical cadet, 94 (38%) became a commissioned or contract surgeon, and of the 26 men who served more than one term, 17 (65%) made that progression."[16]

It is interesting to find one of the other medical cadets who served during this period was Frank LeMoyne. In contrast to Daly, LeMoyne served in the field rather than in a Philadelphia military hospital. Within a decade, they would end up as physicians in Pittsburgh working together at Western Pennsylvania Hospital. Daly and LeMoyne would each go on to have extraordinary medical careers.

Records indicate Daly progressed quickly in his role as a medical cadet and he was among those that became contract surgeons with the U.S. Army. On 05 July 1864, Daly signed a contract as acting assistant surgeon and was assigned duty at U.S. General Hospital White Hall, near Bristol, Pennsylvania, just a few miles northeast of Philadelphia.[17] His contract read:

CONTRACT WITH A PRIVATE PHYSICIAN

This Contract, entered into this 5th day of July, 1864, at Philadelphia, in the State of Pennsylvania, between Surgeon, John Campbell of the United States Army, and Dr. Wm. H. Daly, of Belle Vernon, in the State of Pennsylvania, Witnesseth: That for the consideration hereafter mentioned, the said Dr. Wm. H. Daly promises and agrees to perform the duties of a Medical Officer, agreeably to Army Regulations, at White Hall, Pa. or elsewhere, and to furnish and keep in good order, and accessible at all times, complete sets of amputating, trephining, and pocket instruments; and the said Surgeon John Campbell promises and agrees, on behalf of the United States, to pay, or cause to be paid, to the said Dr. Wm. H. Daly, the sum of one hundred dollars for each and every month he shall continue to perform the services above stated, and one hundred and thirteen 83/100 dollars per month, and transportation in kind, when performing service in the field, which shall be his full compensation, and *in lieu* of all allowances and emoluments whatever;

And it is further agreed, that in case the said Dr. Wm. H. Daly be unable to provide the aforesaid instruments, they shall be furnished to him by the Medical Department of the U.S. Army, and the cost price thereof deducted from his monthly pay. This contract to continue at least three months, if not sooner determined by the Commanding Officer for the time being, the Medical Director, or Surgeon General.[18]

The contract was appropriately witnessed and countersigned by John Campbell, surgeon and medical director, and Acting Assistant Surgeon William H. Daly. Several months later, Daly's contract was extended and he was transferred to General Hospital No. 2 in Savannah, Georgia, for the period 12 February to 03 May 1865. On 04 May, Daly was sent as an acting assistant surgeon to Jacksonville, Florida, where he served for a short time until 26 May. While his stay was short, his work there was challenging. During his tenure, he assisted in providing medical care for the last 5,000 Union prisoners released from the notorious Andersonville Prison in Georgia.[19]

His next tour of duty, which began on 03 July 1865, was at Provost Hospital at Hilton Head (Port Royal), South Carolina, where he served as medical officer in charge. This assignment was again short-lived as he resigned on 21 August. The next day, on 22 August, the medical director of the Department of South Carolina sent a letter to Surgeon General Joseph K. Barnes reporting that, due to Daly's resignation, he had annulled his contract.[20] With his resignation accepted, Daly was now a physician without a formal medical degree, and a veteran of both the Confederate and Union Armies. His Civil War experiences with the military and medicine would serve as a prelude for the remarkable achievements he was about to accomplish.

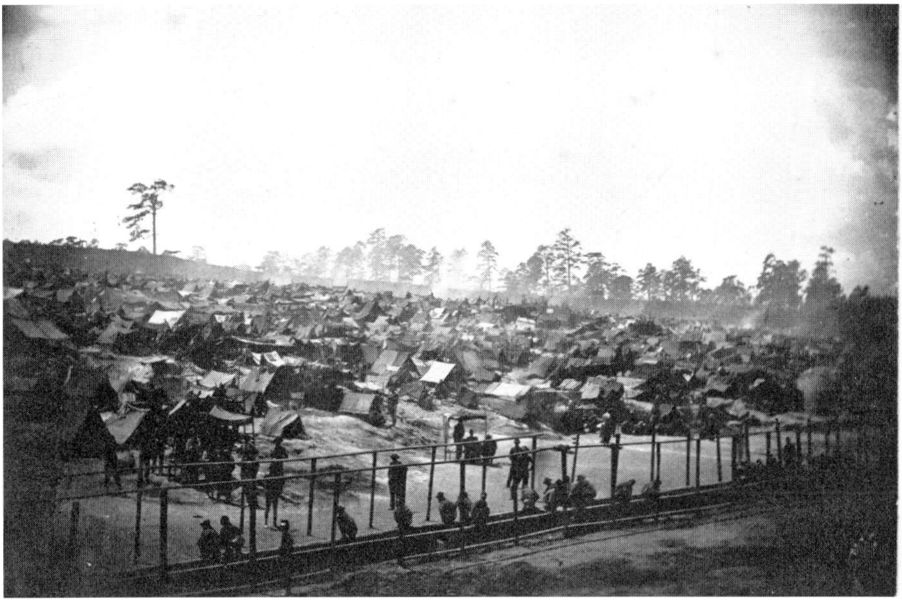

Andersonville Prison, Georgia. Southeast view taken from the stockade. (*Library of Congress*)

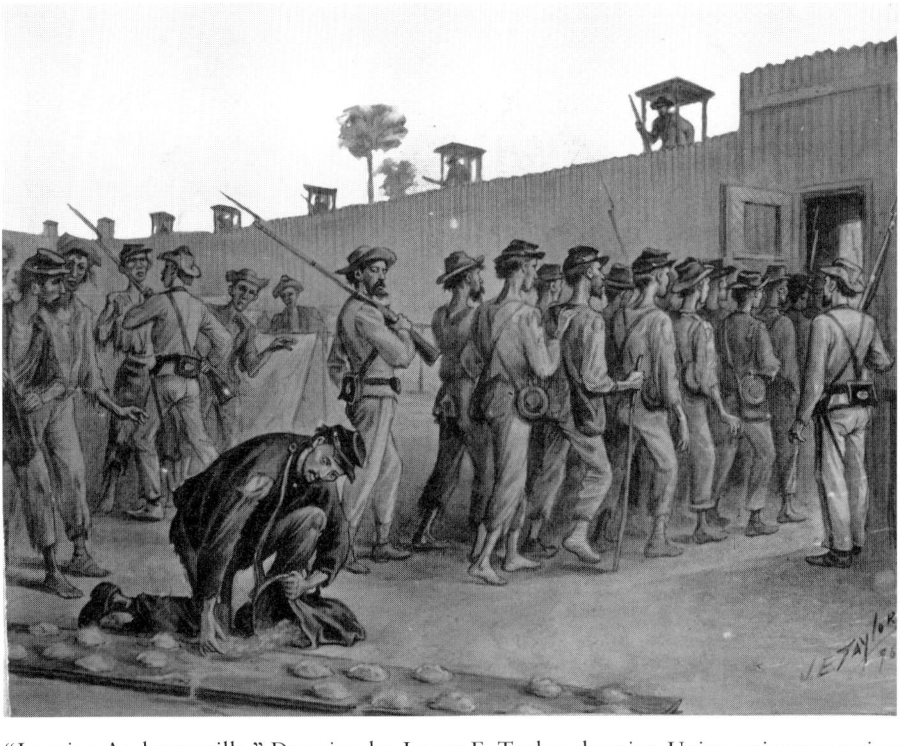

"Leaving Andersonville." Drawing by James E. Taylor showing Union prisoners going through stockade wall door as one prisoner collects a cake of bread. (*Library of Congress*)

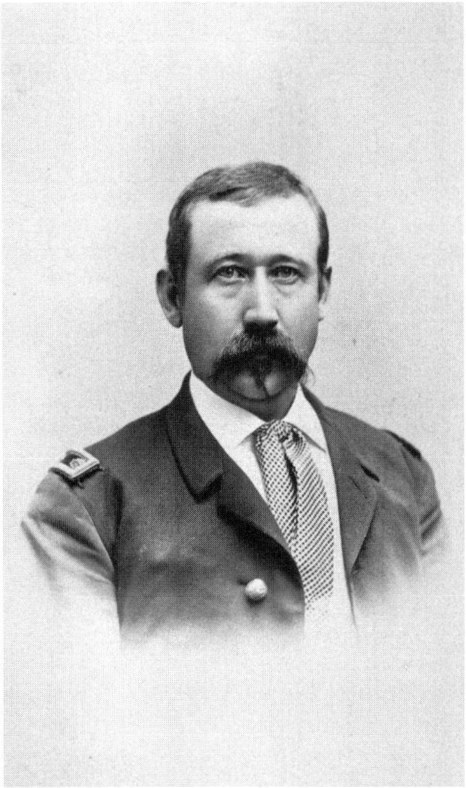

W. H. Forward commanded White Hall General Hospital near Bristol, Pennsylvania, when William H. Daly served as acting assistant surgeon. (*National Library of Medicine*)

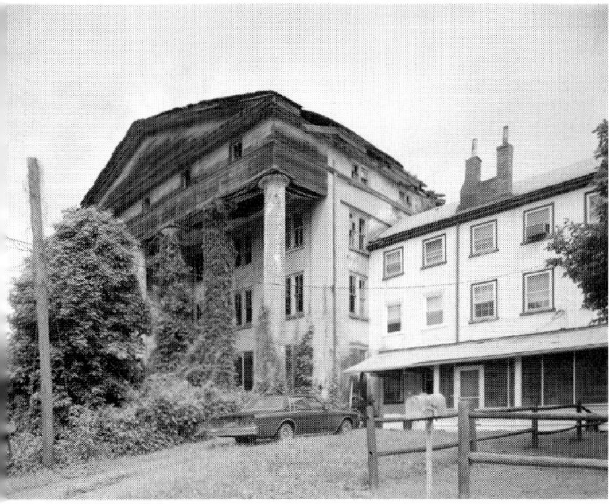

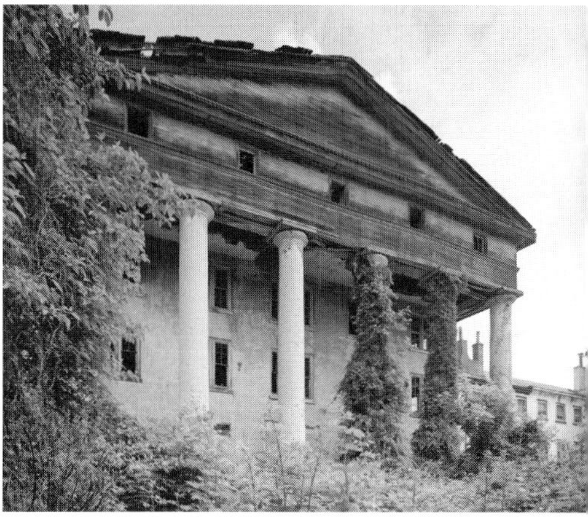

Above left: White Hall at Bristol College, Bucks County, Pennsylvania, served as a hospital during the Civil War. View is of south front elevation taken from the southeast. (*Library of Congress*)

Above right: White Hall at Bristol College, Bucks County, Pennsylvania, served as a hospital during the Civil War. View is of south front elevation taken from the southwest. (*Library of Congress*)

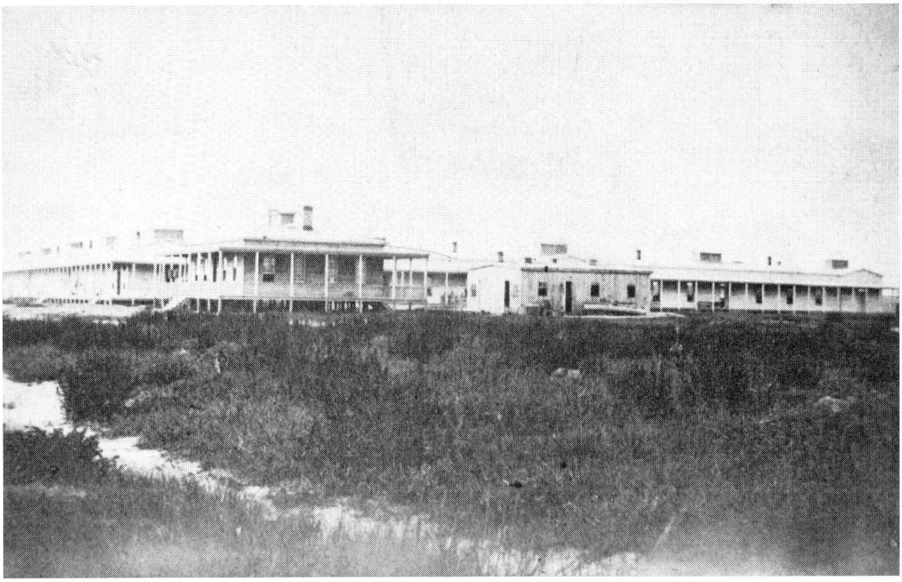

U.S. Army General Hospital at Hilton Head, South Carolina. Built facing the ocean on Broad River, Port Royal Bay. The residence of the medical director is located in the left foreground. (*Library of Congress*)

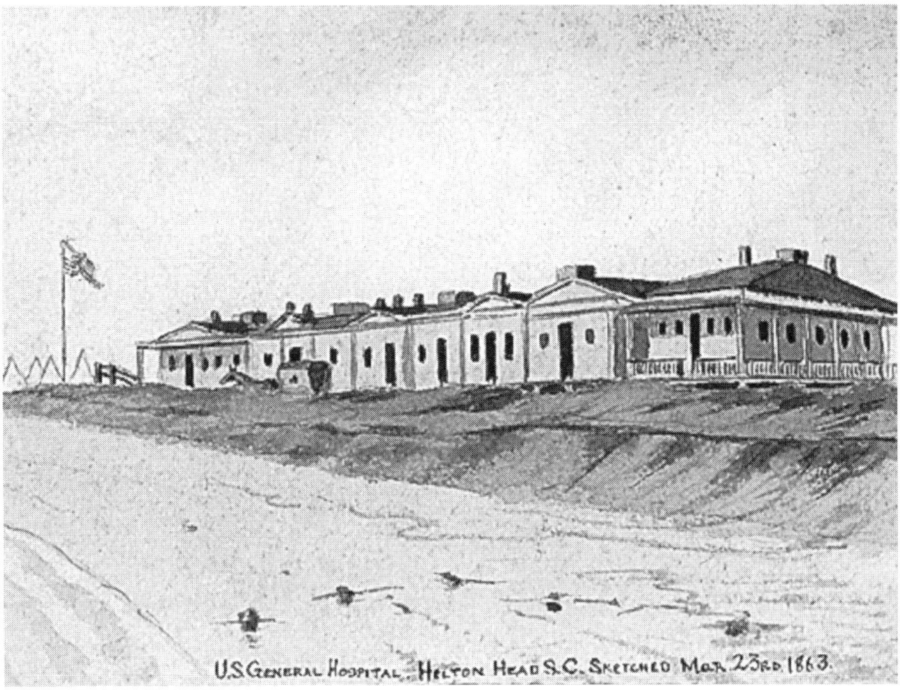

Drawing of U.S. Army General Hospital at Hilton Head, South Carolina, March 1863. (*Library of Congress*)

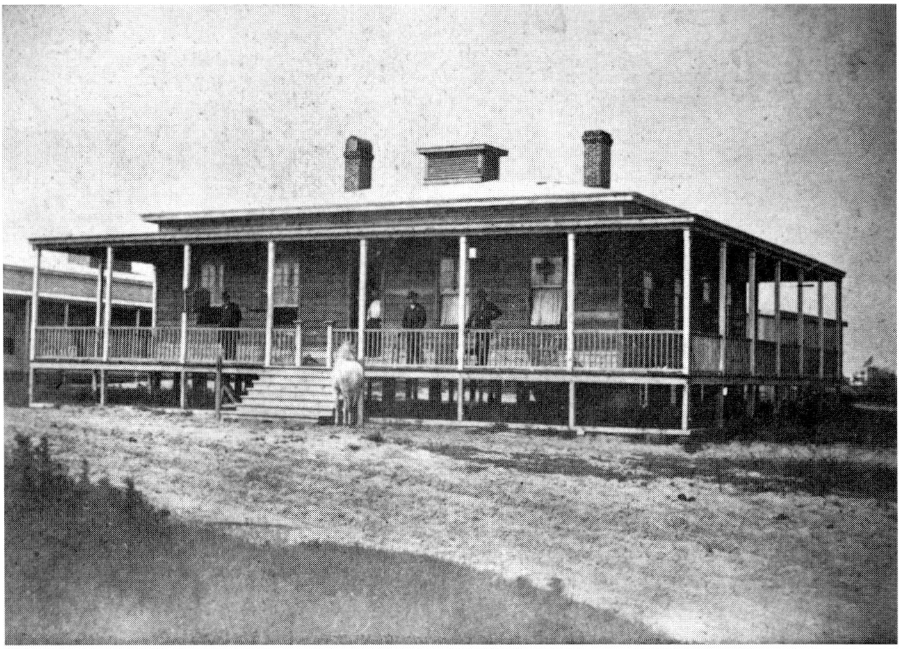

Residence of the medical director of the U.S. Army General Hospital at Hilton Head. (*Library of Congress*)

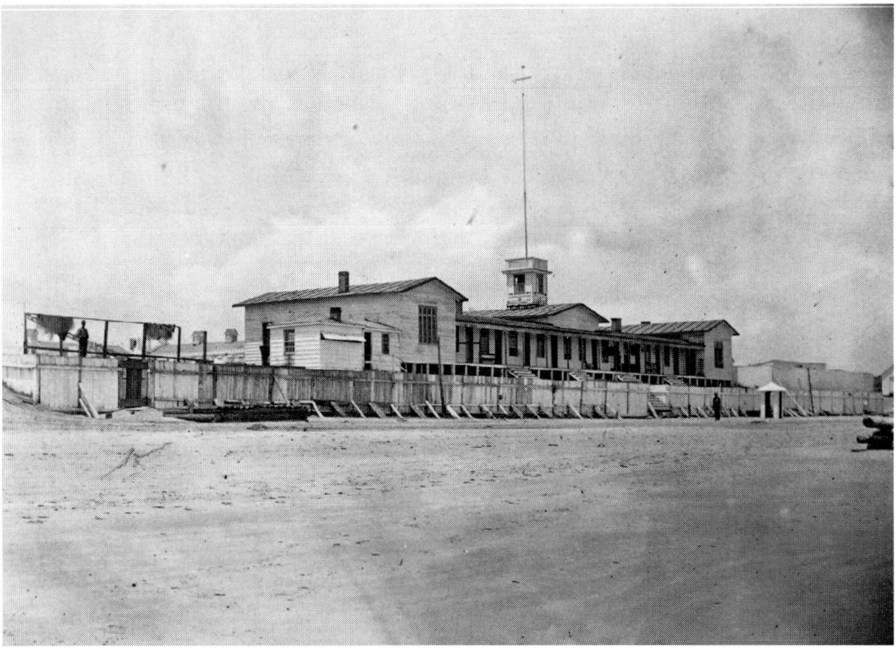

Provost Guard Buildings, Hilton Head, South Carolina. (*The J. Paul Getty Museum, Los Angeles*)

4

Doing Things Worth the Writing

The medical experiences Daly gained during his military service, particularly those at hospitals in Philadelphia, were incredibly valuable. Like many individuals who served in a medical capacity and survived the war—whether under a Union or Confederate flag—their battlefield or hospital service served as a kind of new coin of the realm for entry into post-war medical practice.

Before the war, physician education in the United States typically consisted of training that had not changed for more than a century. For a majority of practicing physicians, pre-war medical instruction was essentially comprised of a three- to seven-year apprenticeship to an established physician who had likely been similarly trained. Few physicians had taken the next step of enrolling in one of the few medical colleges or universities that were established in this country before the 1860s. Even when they did, medical school training was principally achieved through didactic lectures lasting for one or two semesters over a period of two years. For the most part, the instruction was repetitive over the two sessions. Even fewer aspiring physicians had the opportunity to travel abroad—to England or continental Europe—to study at leading medical schools. Generally, the vast majority of physicians trained in the United States never had an opportunity to set foot into a hospital or learn anatomy through dissection of a human body. The situation changed dramatically with the start of the Civil War:

> At the beginning of the war, many physicians had not seen or used a stethoscope, thermometer, syringe, ophthalmoscope, laryngoscope, or any other advanced instruments widely utilized in Europe. Although many were unacquainted with these modern diagnostic tools, things changed quickly. Ultimately, they were capable of bringing about significant changes in medical care for soldiers during the war, and for the civilian population afterward. These "*nouveau* surgeons" needed to learn quickly. General battlefield conditions offered a quick education. The seemingly

endless hands-on surgical experience they gained became the great equalizer between those educated in medical schools and those who were trained through apprenticeship.[1]

Daly's tenure as a U.S. Army medical cadet along with his participation in classes at Jefferson Medical School essentially equated to an apprenticeship. Although he did not possess a medical degree, the firsthand practical knowledge and skills he acquired through his service at a half-dozen military hospitals between 1863 and 1865 provided the credentials and impetus he needed to pursue a formal medical degree after the Civil War.

As noted earlier, in April 1865, Daly resigned his position as a medical officer in charge of Provost Guard Hospital at Hilton Head, South Carolina. His appointment to the position indicates that even without the benefit of a medical degree, his skills were thought of highly.

Little is known about where he was and what he did during the summer of 1865 after he resigned his post at Provost Guard Hospital, but evidence suggests he used the time to explore medical school enrollment. By the fall of 1865, he was registered at University of Michigan Medical School.[2] He attended two semesters at Michigan, which complemented his earlier "partial course of study" at Jefferson Medical School at Philadelphia, Pennsylvania, in 1863–1864.[3] His preceptor at Michigan was Dr. H. B. Rupp.[4] Based upon the medical school's requirements, Rupp had to be a practicing physician with whom Daly could study and work when school was not in session.

The 1865–1866 medical school class was the largest since the school's founding in 1848. At 467 students, the size of the class was largely attributed to the ending of the Civil War and the high number of people who, like Daly, wished to translate their war experience into a medical career.[5]

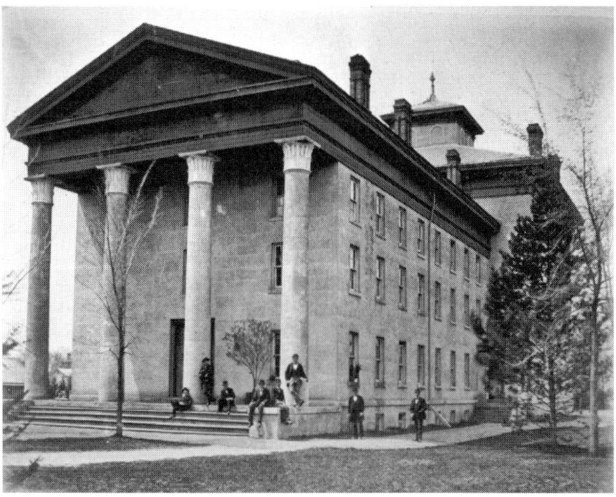

University of Michigan Medical School built in 1850. (*University of Michigan Bentley Historical Library*)

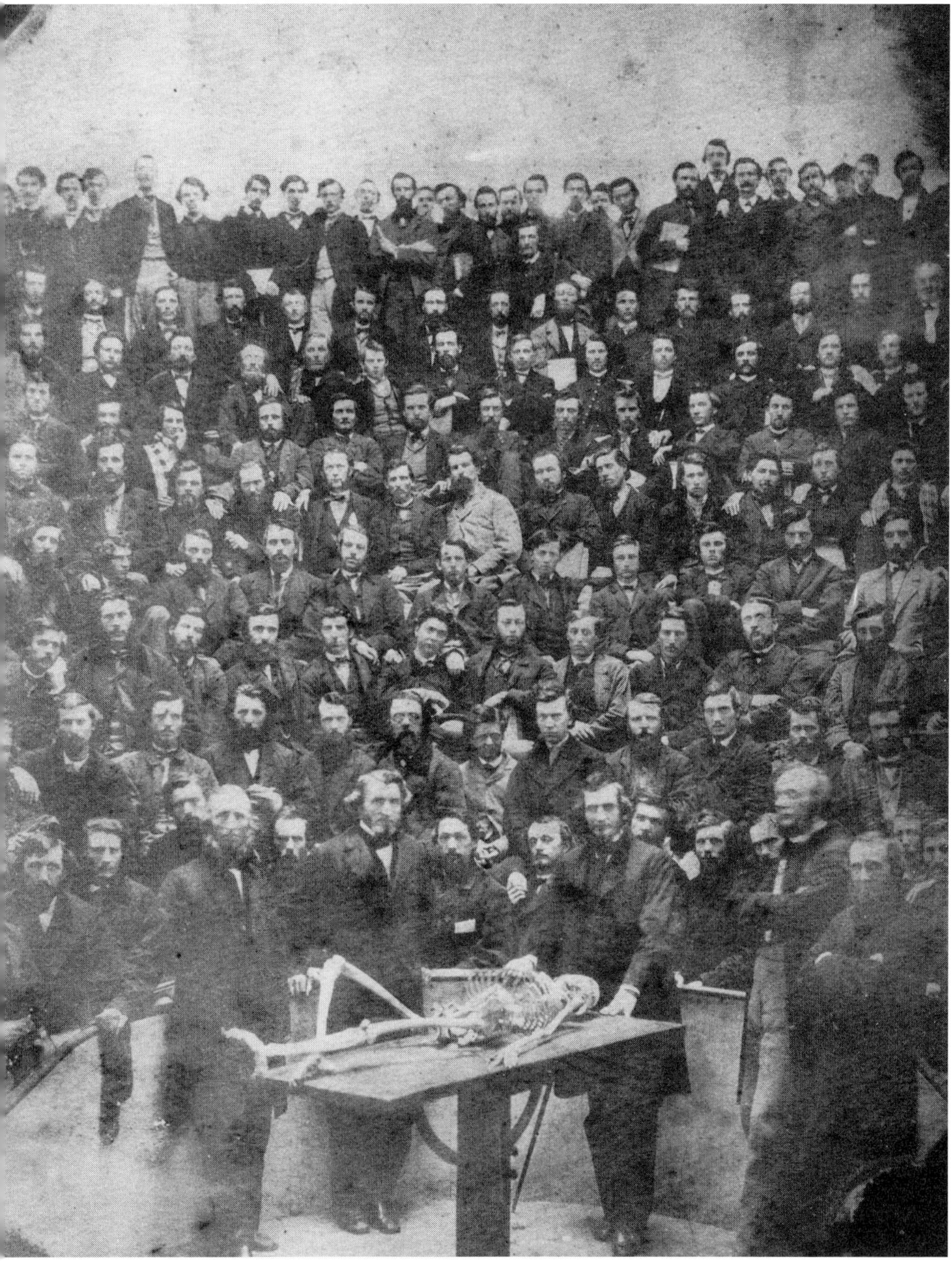

University of Michigan Medical School. Students in amphitheater with skeleton on table. (*University of Michigan Bentley Historical Library*)

Daly undoubtedly enjoyed being a well-practiced and well-informed student. His experience as a medical cadet in Philadelphia presented him with opportunities that medical students and a majority of practicing physicians could not have easily obtained before the war. Most notably, he had access to large volumes of patients and participated in countless surgeries. The number of amputations alone that occurred during one month as a cadet, or his subsequent service as an acting assistant surgeon, would have been more than most regular physicians would see during their entire careers. He would also have gained a much better understanding of anatomy and disease.

Anatomy was an area that was always an issue for students without military medical experience. At the University of Michigan, School of Medicine, it was noted: "... in the first years of medical instruction (1850) fifteen or twenty cadavers annually had met all needs, the much larger classes after the Civil War required at least 125 to 140 bodies a year."[6]

After completing his course of medical study and submitting his thesis, "Sympathetic Pruritus with More Special Reference to that Form Affecting the Scrotum of the Male," Daly graduated and received his Doctor of Medicine degree on 28 March 1866.[7,8] The *Students in Medicine, Catalogue of the Students for 1865–1866* offers a clue to Daly's whereabouts during the summer of 1865. In the catalogue, he lists his residence as Belle Vernon, Pennsylvania, which suggests he either had returned to his childhood home during the summer or planned to return upon graduation.[9]

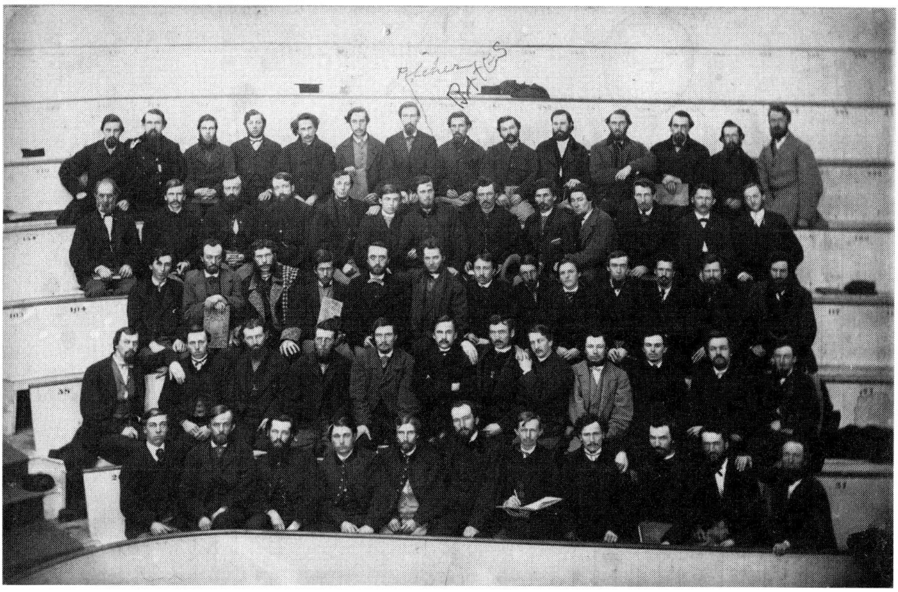

Medical School graduating class University of Michigan 1865–1866. William H. Daly seated second row, sixth person from right. (*University of Michigan Bentley Historical Library*)

With his newly minted medical degree in hand, Daly left Michigan and moved back to Pennsylvania. It is easy to assume his return was influenced by a desire to re-engage with his family in the Belle Vernon area, but there was another reason motivating him. Instead of opting for the familiar, he instead chose the city of Pittsburgh as the place he wished to establish a medical practice. While he had never been to Pittsburgh before, there were many other compelling reasons for selecting the city.

Post-Civil War Pittsburgh was a thriving city. Before the war, it was already well known as a place of business and industry. Its three rivers—the Allegheny, Monongahela, and Ohio—had long served as a key gateway to the west. Many thousands of people had come and gone from the city over the previous hundred years. Over those years, others had stayed and made the city their home. Those who stayed and created businesses actively participated in supplying materials needed for the war. All commercial activities expanded dramatically to meet the requirements of war; food and manufactured goods were being transmitted by river and rail throughout the country, as were arms and munitions, like never before.

During this period, thousands of soldiers, including many drawn from the city and its environs, moved through the area on the way to battle. Those that survived war likewise traversed the streets, railways, and rivers upon discharge from military duty. Among those that returned during and after the war were thousands of ill and wounded warriors who sought relief and care.

Pittsburgh responded to their needs by sending physicians to the battlefields, creating relief organizations, establishing a soldiers' home, and expanding hospital services. In less than four years, the exigencies of war had transformed medical care in the city. The old ways of dealing with disease and resolving surgical issues had given way to new treatments and procedures. The lessons learned from the human carnage of war paved the way for a new, more modern, system of medical care in the city. Physicians and related medical personnel, like nurses, were now better-trained and qualified to offer hope and recovery where little existed before. Pre-war methods of diagnoses and treatment now looked primitive by comparison. Hospitals previously relegated to intermittently housing those afflicted by epidemic diseases, the poor, and the insane were now places of optimism and healing. While sick and wounded soldiers were the primary beneficiaries of this evolution in care, the general public benefitted as well.

Once again, Daly was in the right place at the right time. His arrival in Pittsburgh in 1866 was fortuitous as opportunities for starting a new medical practice in the city may have never been better. He likely felt right at home in a city where discharged soldiers were evident at every turn. Some had returned to resume pre-war careers; others who had traveled in or out of the city elected to stay and call Pittsburgh their home. Those who had been ill or injured and received care in the city did likewise. Countless others needed longer-term care.

Admirably, the city's three established hospitals worked hard to meet their needs, and they would continue to do so for many years after the war. Of the three, the Western Pennsylvania Hospital assumed a more vital role and Daly would soon become inexorably linked to the institution.

Western Pennsylvania Hospital first opened its doors to receive patients in 1853. Originally designed to serve the general medical needs of the local population it soon found the provision of care for the insane a more pressing demand. Based upon the understanding of the needs of the mentally ill at the time, the hospital's geographic location near the center of the city was not well suited for their care. In response, in 1858, with the assistance of Dorothea Dix, hospital leaders decided to build a new hospital for the insane on a more advantageously located site outside the city. Construction began in May 1860. In November 1861, seven months after the shelling of Fort Sumter and the start of the Civil War, Dixmont Hospital for the Insane opened and mentally ill patients from the Western Pennsylvania Hospital were transferred to the new facility.[10] With the transfer of patients, Western Pennsylvania Hospital was practically emptied.

Not long after the start of the Civil War, Secretary of War Edwin M. Stanton wrote to the managers of Western Pennsylvania Hospital, inquiring about what accommodations might be made for sick and wounded soldiers. Hospital managers responded and offered the old hospital to the War Department once the new hospital at Dixmont had been completed. In anticipation of the transfer, the War Department began assigning Army surgeons to the hospital in August 1861. Some alterations to the facility were initiated in preparation for care of a yet unknown volume of sick and wounded soldiers. In December 1862, Western Pennsylvania Hospital was formally transferred to the federal government and placed under the control of the U.S. Army Department of the Monongahela.[11] For military purposes, it was renamed the U.S.A. General Hospital, Pittsburgh, upon transfer. The general public, however, simply referred to it as the "Ninth Ward Hospital" during the period of military occupation. Once the hospital was returned to civilian control on 03 October 1865, the Western Pennsylvania Hospital name was restored.

Over the three years of military service, the U.S.A. General Hospital, Pittsburgh, frequently cared for 1,500 or more soldiers at the same time. That number represented more than three times the amount of beds in the hospital. To accommodate that many soldiers, the Army resorted to using tents placed on the hillside around the hospital. As one reporter noted, "there are some forty-nine tents arranged in six rows."[12]

While many soldiers suffering from major illness or required surgical treatment were cared for at the hospital, others without life-threatening wounds or illness received treatment at the Pittsburgh Sanitary Soldiers' Home. The home was specifically designed to deal with medical issues of traveling soldiers and those recently mustered out of service with an honorable discharge. It was created as an extension of work of the Pittsburgh Subsistence Committee, which provided

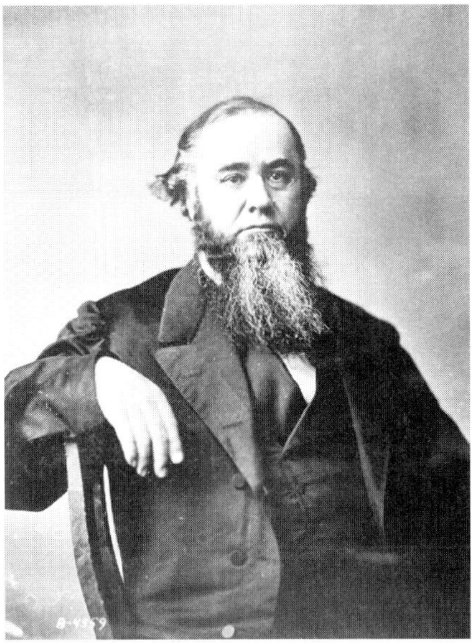

Edwin M. Stanton, U.S. Secretary of War. (*National Archives and Records Administration*)

nourishment, a place to rest between travel engagements, and provision of reading and writing materials through the entirety of the war. By the end of the war and after four and a half years of service, the home had provided care for more than 80,000 soldiers, roughly the equivalent of an entire Army Corps.

In early 1866, the Subsistence Committee disbanded, and the Pittsburgh Sanitary Soldiers' Home concluded its operations under its umbrella. In March 1866, the Pennsylvania State Assembly rechartered the home as an independent organization, and the medical services it previously offered were transitioned to the Western Pennsylvania Hospital, along with sufficient financial resources to continue the work:

> Under terms of the transfer, residual funds from the Pittsburgh Sanitary Fair were used to pay for care rendered at Western Pennsylvania Hospital. The agreement lasted until September 1877 when the remaining funds, in the amount of $198,383.71, were used to establish an endowment sufficient to guarantee veterans "of the Volunteer Armies of Western Pennsylvania," would continue to receive free medical care. A joint committee of the region's Grand Army of the Republic and hospital managers would administer the fund.[13]

With the stroke of a pen, Western Pennsylvania Hospital thereby became Pittsburgh's first veterans' hospital. Many newspapers reported on the transition and Daly could not have missed the news. The city's population was growing, business was booming, and assurances of a large group of sick and maimed veterans needing medical attention surely served as a clarion call to the twenty-four-year-old doctor.

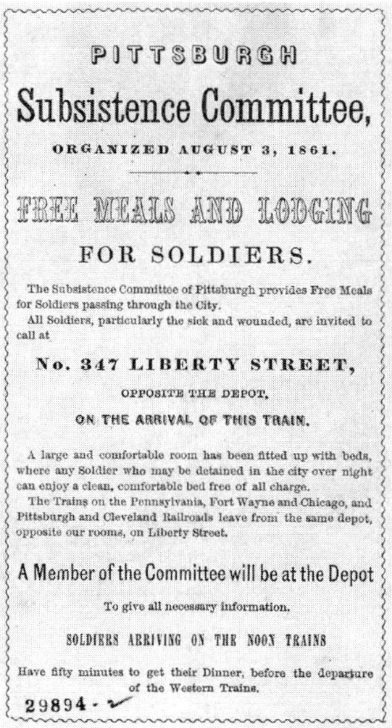

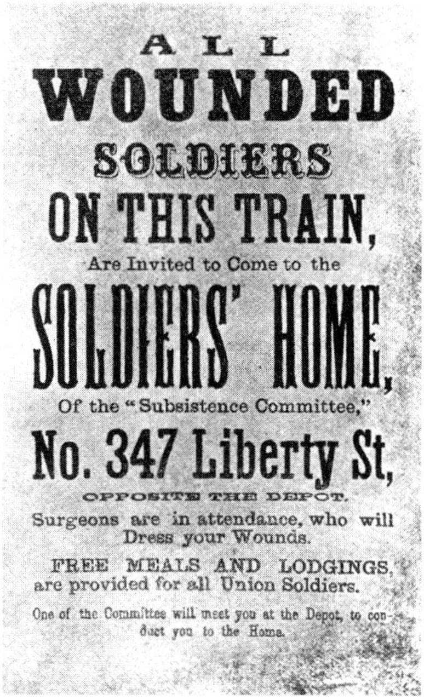

Above left: Pittsburgh Subsistence Committee advertisement 1864. Lincoln papers, Series 1, General Correspondence 1833–1916; W. P. Weyman to Abraham Lincoln, Wednesday, 27 January 1864, Pittsburgh Subsistence Committee. (*Library of Congress*)

Above right: Soldiers' Home Handbill. (*The 28th National Encampment of the Grand Army of the Republic, Official Program 1894*)

Below: Subsistence Committee members awaiting guests at City Hall, 1861. (*Heinz History Center, Pittsburgh*)

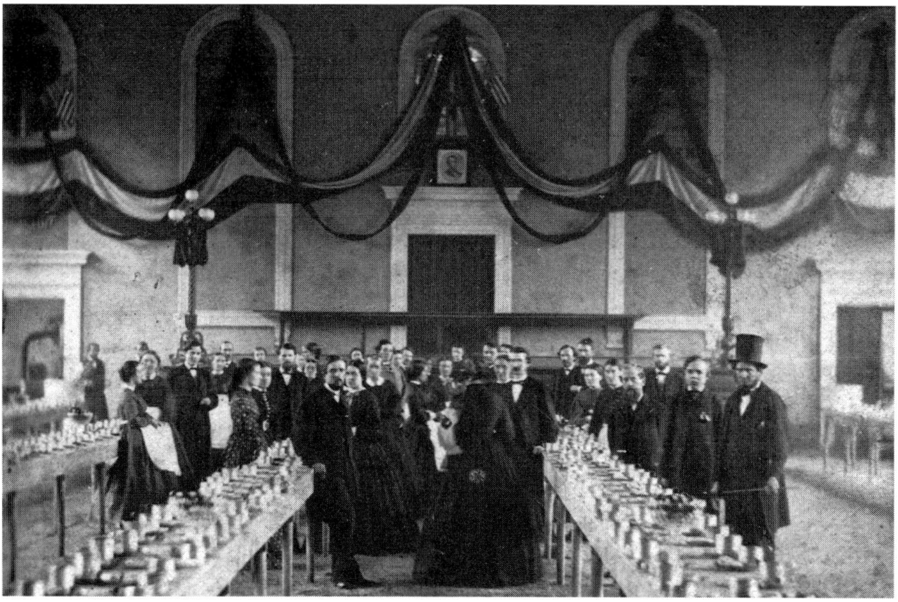

5

Writing Things Worth the Reading

Upon arriving in Pittsburgh after receiving his medical degree, Daly's initial whereabouts remain unknown. It is understood, however, his affiliation with Western Pennsylvania Hospital began immediately. Thus far, no records have been discovered that shed light on his place of residence during his first eighteen months in the city. While a number of people with the same last name resided in the city, surviving records do not indicate whether any were related to him.

In 1867, several months after he came to Pittsburgh, it is known he joined the Allegheny County Medical Society.[1] The Society was not the first professional medical organization to form in the city, but it was the first to survive for longer than a few years. Its organization took place on 20 April 1865, just eleven days after Robert E. Lee's surrender at Appomattox and the end of the Civil War. Many of its founders had served in the war as surgeons or lay volunteers providing medical-related services for soldiers. Daly fit right in with the group and undoubtedly felt at ease with its members as many had similar backgrounds and war experiences.

Interestingly, at Daly's first meeting, the subject of equality for women doctors was a main topic of discussion. It was decided members could confer with women doctors as long as the women "observe the code of ethics."[2] While women were required to follow the code of ethics, they were not permitted to be members. It would be many years before women were allowed to join the society as equals.

Daly's membership in the society would last for more than three decades. On 18 January 1870, after serving as a general member for less than three years, he was elected recording secretary. He held the position for ten years. Over the decade of service as secretary, Daly participated in the society's quarterly meetings, chronicling not only mundane business matters but also scientific presentations made at each meeting. His attention to recording meeting agendas and documenting scientific presentations served as a form of ongoing continuing medical education. The presentations covered clinical aspects of interesting cases reported by many of the city's leading physicians. They also included details of the latest medical and surgical treatments. In some cases, Daly was both recorder and presenter. During membership meetings, other subjects like the aforementioned discussion on inclusion of women frequently occurred. Water purity, epidemic diseases, patent medicine sales, regulation of "irregular" practitioners, the need for new hospitals, and other general medical related subjects were covered over the years.[3] The challenge of regulating irregular practitioners and controlling the sale of patent medicines would rage on for decades.

In addition to his election to the post of recording secretary in January 1870, Daly was one of several members designated to represent the group as a delegate to the Pennsylvania Medical Society. From this humble beginning, Daly would later be selected to serve as representative at countless other state, national and international medical associations. In 1881, he stepped down as recording secretary when he was elected president of the society.[4]

The written products of his work as recording secretary served him well. As his proficiency in recording Medical Society minutes and scientific sessions developed, so too did his medical practice. After his patient caseload had expanded, he began documenting myriad case files, which later served as the basis for independent research that led to his subsequent specialization in the fields of laryngology and rhinology. After a few years growing his skills in these domains, he became recognized as the pioneering practitioner of those specialties in Pittsburgh. Likewise, as his writing skills and medical acumen grew, so too did his interest in publishing and presentation.

Interestingly, his earliest known published articles were not medically related. Instead, they focused on nature, animals, and sports hunting, which became a passion of his in the early 1870s. Beginning in 1876 and for a period of a few years, he became a regular contributor to the nature magazine *Forest and Stream*. A list of his known contributions to the magazine include the following titles: "An Encounter with a Wounded Fox;" "Areca Nuts vs. Santonine;" "Quail Shooting Extraordinary;" "Was it Worms, Medicine, or Distemper?;" "The Question of Spaying or Ovariotomy in Dogs;" and "Forellen Fishing in Cheruskian Waters, Being a Sketch of Trout Fishing in Germany."[5]

There is also a record that Daly published two additional nature articles. However, the publication they appeared in remains unknown. The articles were "The Miseries of Summer Woodcock Shooting" and "Duck Shooting on the Kankakee."[6] Daly's love of nature and sports hunting would become more sophisticated over the years, and he would regularly travel throughout Pennsylvania, Maryland, Virginia, and the Midwest to engage in such activity.

Beginning in the late 1880s, he would also begin making hunting trips to mountain areas in western states in search of big game animals. It was during one of these western hunting expeditions that he once again found himself in

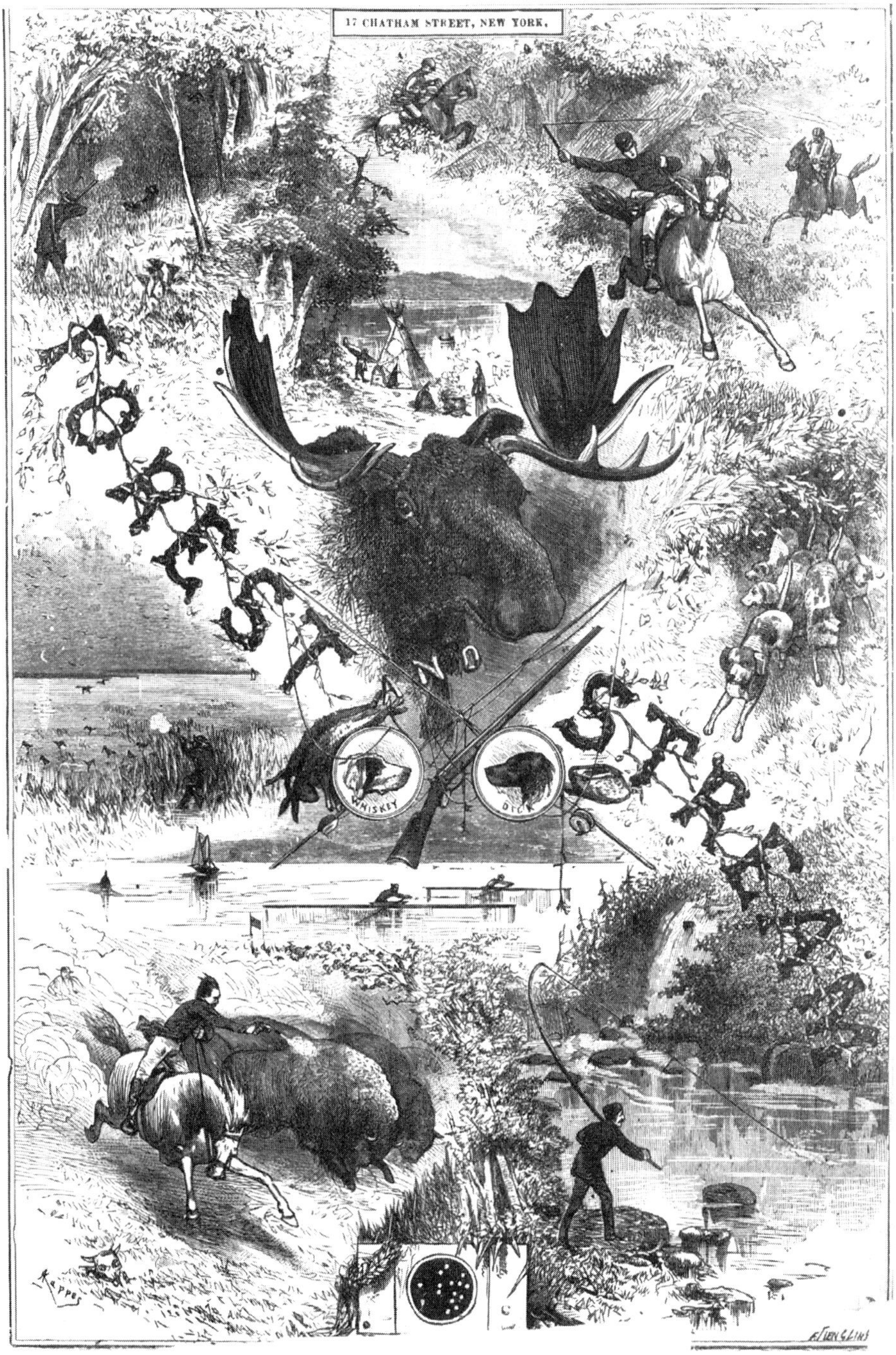

Forest and Stream magazine frontispiece, Volume 7, Number 1, 1876.

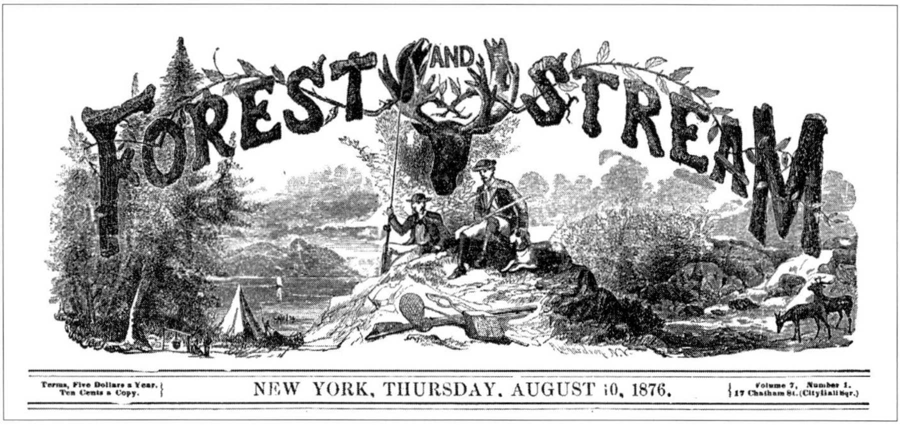

Forest and Stream magazine masthead, Volume 7, Number 1, 1876

the right place at the right time. On this trip, he encountered General Nelson A. Miles and Buffalo Bill Cody. Daly's introduction to Miles would soon bring him national notoriety and cause major changes in his life. Details of Daly's western expeditions and his encounter with Miles and Cody will be covered in greater detail in a later chapter.

City directories for 1868–1869 report Daly's affiliation with the House of Refuge, which was located on Woods Run Avenue in Allegheny City. The directories indicate he had both an office and home at that location.[7] The House of Refuge was originally incorporated in 1850; however, it did not open until 1854. The institution served the city's juvenile population as a reform school, orphanage, and a mental hospital for the "feeble-minded." After twenty years of operation, the facility on Woods Run Avenue was abandoned, and in 1876, the organization moved to the Morganza farm in Washington County, Pennsylvania. A primary reason for deserting the property was a typhoid epidemic that hit the city. The loss of life at the Reform School was devastating. It was reported 270 of the school's 300 juvenile residents were stricken with the disease. Daly advised school officials a main cause for the outbreak was the school's location in a low-lying area near the confluence of the Monongahela and Allegheny rivers, where sewage drained.[8] This would not be the last time Daly became involved in the study of waterborne diseases. His work at the end of the nineteenth century would prove to be years ahead of others in hypothesizing water instead of air was the medium by which malaria entered the human body.[9]

The property in Allegheny City was subsequently converted for use in establishing the Western Penitentiary. At the time of the House of Refuge's removal from the city, its name was changed to "Pennsylvania Reform School."[10] It subsequently became known simply as "Morganza" in the local community. Daly served as the institution's physician for eight years, ending his relationship when the school moved to Washington County. The last indication of Daly's connection to the House of Refuge was in 1875.

In 1869, Daly married Athalia Cooper, a young Pittsburgh socialite. The change in marital status prompted him to make changes in both his office location and residential living situation. City directory listings for 1870 show Daly having an office at 152 Fifth Avenue in the heart of downtown Pittsburgh. From 1870 until 1896, directories show he maintained offices on either Fifth Avenue or Sixth Avenue (No. 71) throughout the period.[11] During earlier years, his listings indicate the Sixth Avenue location served as both home and office. In 1887, his home address was listed as Howe Street, located in the Shadyside area of the city. Between 1887 and 1893, his home address was 6213 Howe. In 1894, he purchased the home next door and moved to 6211 Howe, a home address he would maintain until his death in 1901. During the last three years of the nineteenth century, he moved his office to Market Street, which was a short distance from his old office spaces on Fifth Avenue and Sixth Avenue.[12] In addition to seeing patients in his office, he also offered limited hours at his home.

The city directory for 1873 is the first year a formal association with the Western Pennsylvania Hospital is documented.[13] It noted Daly was a full-fledged member of the hospital's medical staff. It was also the first year since the end of the Civil War and the return of the hospital to civilian control that the hospital formally listed any of its medical staff. Between the end of the war and 1873, the only official medical staff member was a curator. During that period, all physicians in the city had admitting privileges. Daly was among them.

In April 1878, at the age of thirty-six, Daly applied for and received a passport to travel abroad. He intended to spend a year studying at leading medical institutions in London, Berlin, and Vienna.[14] The trip to Europe afforded him an opportunity to temporarily forego the routine of recording meeting minutes and documenting technical presentations for the Allegheny County Medical Society and focus on his personal scientific writing. Records indicate it was at this time he also elected to stop submitting articles to nature magazines.

Daly's first accounts of his travels in Europe began in July 1878 with a communication recorded in the *Medical and Surgical Reporter*. In the foreign correspondence section of the 27 July edition, Daly reported:

> While at one of Sir Henry Thompson's private lithotrity operations to-day, I observed that Mr. Clover, a surgeon of some note, was employed to administer the anaesthetic, which consisted of nitrous oxide followed by chloroform, by means of Mr. Clover's apparatus. This latter gentleman makes a specialty of the administration of anaesthetics, and is employed and paid by the operating surgeons of London requiring his services, and I am informed has all he can attend to in this branch. Sir Henry Thompson is a quick operator with the lithotrite, grasping one fragment of a calculus after another within the bladder, with a facility that can certainly only

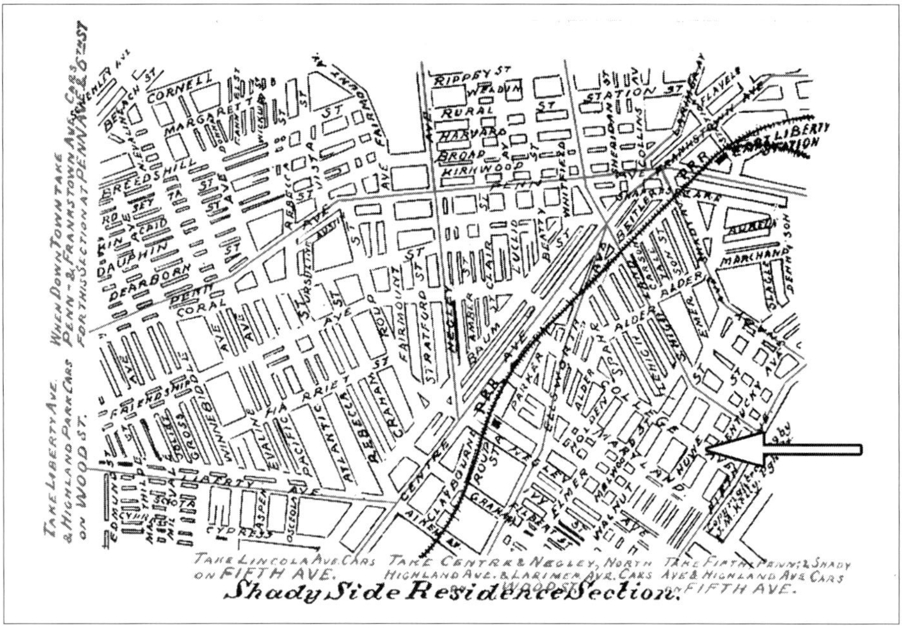
Take Liberty Ave. & Highland Park Cars on Wood St.
When Down Town take Penn- & Frankstown Ave. Cars for this Section at Penn Ave & 6th St
Take Lincoln Ave. Cars on Fifth Ave.
Take Centre & Negley, North Highland Ave. & Larimer Ave. Cars on Wood St.
Take Fifth & Penn; & Shady Ave & Highland Ave Cars on Fifth Ave.
Shady Side Residence Section.

"The Pittsburgh and Allegheny Blue Book." Howe Street where William H. Daly resided is marked with arrow. (*Historic Pittsburgh*)

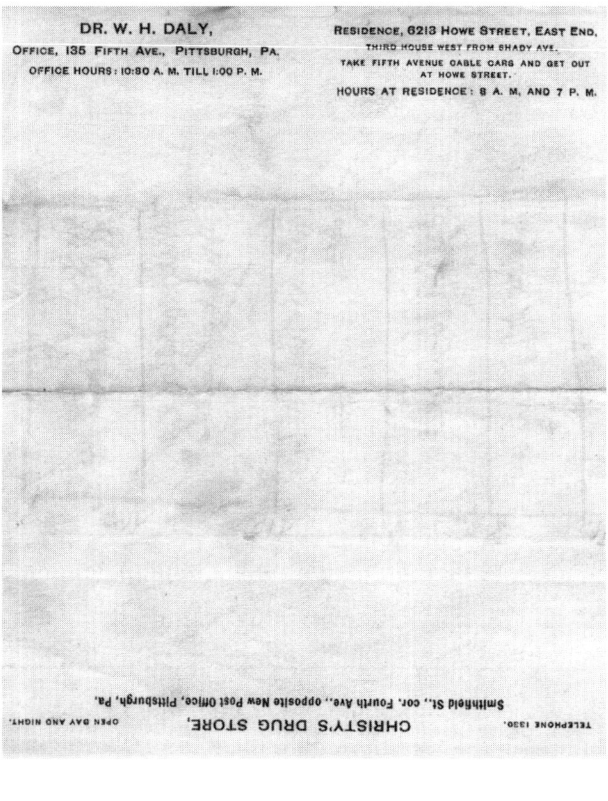

DR. W. H. DALY,
OFFICE, 135 FIFTH AVE., PITTSBURGH, PA.
OFFICE HOURS: 10:30 A. M. TILL 1:00 P. M.

RESIDENCE, 6213 HOWE STREET, EAST END.
THIRD HOUSE WEST FROM SHADY AVE.
TAKE FIFTH AVENUE CABLE CARS AND GET OUT AT HOWE STREET.
HOURS AT RESIDENCE: 8 A. M. AND 7 P. M.

Smithfield St., cor. Fourth Ave., opposite New Post Office, Pittsburgh, Pa.
TELEPHONE 1330. CHRISTY'S DRUG STORE, OPEN DAY AND NIGHT.

William H. Daly prescription pad.

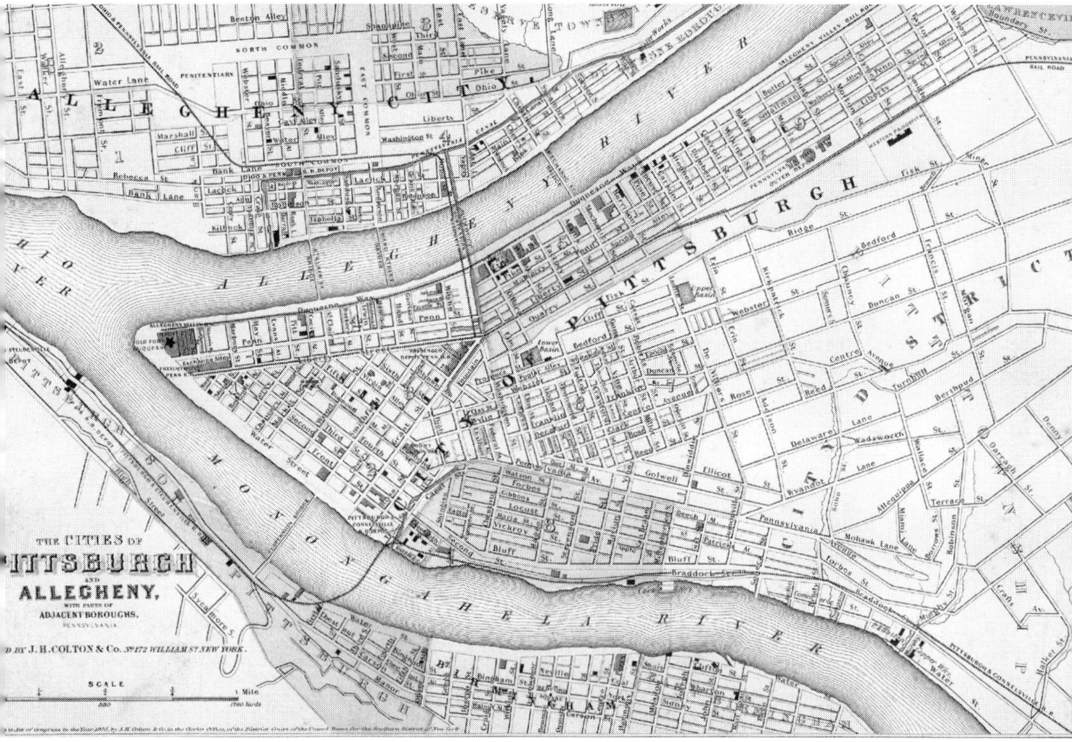

Cities of Pittsburgh and Allegheny map 1855. (*University of Pittsburgh Library Archives & Special Collections*)

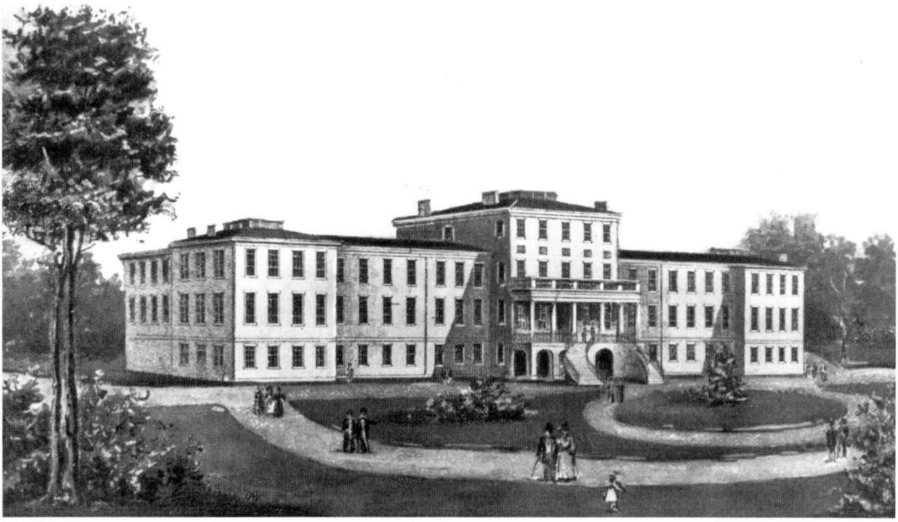

Western Pennsylvania Hospital, 1853. (*Annual Report of the Managers of the Western Pennsylvania Hospital for 1851–1853*)

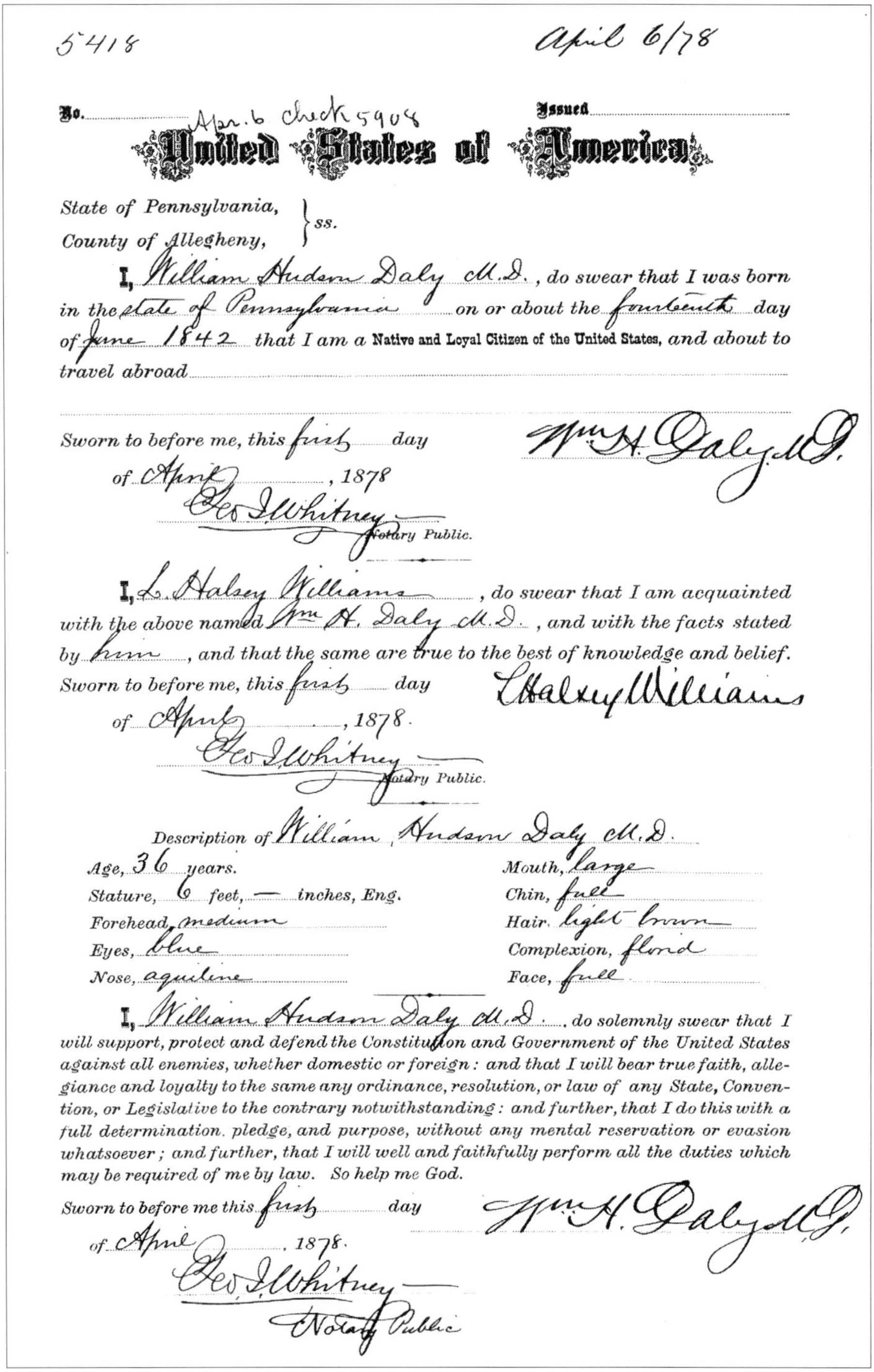

5418 April 6/78

No. Apr. 6 Check 5908 Issued

United States of America

State of Pennsylvania, }
County of Allegheny, } ss.

I, William Hudson Daly M.D., do swear that I was born in the state of Pennsylvania on or about the fourteenth day of June 1842 that I am a Native and Loyal Citizen of the United States, and about to travel abroad

Sworn to before me, this first day of April, 1878
Geo. I. Whitney
Notary Public.

Wm. H. Daly M.D.

I, L. Halsey Williams, do swear that I am acquainted with the above named Wm. H. Daly M.D., and with the facts stated by him, and that the same are true to the best of knowledge and belief.

Sworn to before me, this first day of April, 1878.
Geo. I. Whitney
Notary Public.

L. Halsey Williams

Description of William Hudson Daly M.D.

Age, 36 years.	Mouth, large
Stature, 6 feet, — inches, Eng.	Chin, full
Forehead, medium	Hair, light brown
Eyes, blue	Complexion, florid
Nose, aquiline	Face, full

I, William Hudson Daly M.D., do solemnly swear that I will support, protect and defend the Constitution and Government of the United States against all enemies, whether domestic or foreign: and that I will bear true faith, allegiance and loyalty to the same any ordinance, resolution, or law of any State, Convention, or Legislative to the contrary notwithstanding: and further, that I do this with a full determination, pledge, and purpose, without any mental reservation or evasion whatsoever; and further, that I will well and faithfully perform all the duties which may be required of me by law. So help me God.

Sworn to before me this first day of April, 1878.
Geo. I. Whitney
Notary Public

Wm. H. Daly M.D.

William H. Daly's passport application, 01 April 1878.

come from long use of this instrument. He is a man of strongly marked nervous temperament, and looks much more like an American than an Englishman.

He is of spare build, with rather large eyes, and long flowing moustache; of courteous but very decided manner; he is an artist of considerable merit as well as a great surgeon. I note these characteristic features of the man, as I presume that many Americans, like myself, who have read this distinguished man's writings, have formed ideas of his physical character that were as far out of the way as were my own.

At Guy's Hospital, to-day, I was shown, by Mr. Bryant and Mr. Forster, of the staff, a case of malignant pustule which was treated by excision; the former distinguished surgeon and author informed me he had never seen a case in his life until recently. In Mr. Calley's service there have been several cases, also, recently. In the wards of Guy's the successful cases have all been treated by excision of the pustule and surrounding cellular tissue as early as possible, under the antiseptic spray of Lister, with large doses of quiniae sulph. internally, and stimulants (vinous). All of the patients who have suffered from this disease were employed either in tanneries or along the docks, where it became part of their duty to handle the hides of cattle.

The carbolized spray was used by all the surgeons whom I saw operate to-day at Guy's hospital, excepting Mr. Bryant. A member remarked to me that he also would come to it soon.

Dr. J. Marion Sims, our distinguished countryman, now in Paris, whom I have had the pleasure of meeting frequently, and to whom I am deeply indebted for many courtesies, is now using the carbolized spray in his operations, in Paris and London. Dr. Weccer, the eminent ophthalmologist of Paris, whose clinics are immense, has also begun the antiseptic dressings after the extraction of cataracts. The gratuitous work done at hospitals and dispensaries, by the distinguished men in our profession, abroad, is something wonderful. I met Professor Wm. Pancoast, of the Jefferson Medical College, to-day, at the private operations of Sir Henry Thompson: he is en route for Paris.[15]

It appears Daly was in his element witnessing many new and novel operations and observing widespread use of antiseptic surgical techniques and anesthetics. The opportunity to watch and learn from leading surgeons was professionally fulfilling and would provide the impetus for Daly to subsequently apply the lessons he learned in his practice.

A month later, Daly attended the British Medical Association annual meeting held in Bath, England, on 05 August 1878. He once again chose to offer a report of the meeting to the *Medical and Surgical Reporter*. His observations about recent surgical discoveries and recognition of surgical pioneers are interesting to note. In the 26 October 1878 edition of the *Reporter*, he wrote, in part:

The British Medical Association held its meeting in Bath this year (Aug. 5th, 1878), with an attendance which I was informed was about an average one in numbers, and was about equal to an average meeting of the American Medical Association.

> The general business of the Association is transacted in the great body of the meeting; the professional and scientific papers are all read in the Sections, as with us.
>
> The delegation from the American Medical Association present consisted of Dr. J. Marion Sims, of N. Y., Professors Auger and Cleaver, of Iowa, Professor W. H. Pancoast, of Philadelphia, and your correspondent.
>
> Of the addresses before the Association, that of Mr. Wheelhouse, of Leeds, on Surgery, was probably the event of the meeting, and was characterized by its clear and able history of the progress in surgery, and the appliances and inventions which have been made in this branch of the healing art.
>
> There was possibly just a few oversights in giving credit to American surgery; for example, when the high tribute to the operation of ovariotomy was spoken, the name of Spencer Wells was mentioned, and deservedly too, but the illustrious name of McDowell, the father of the operation, was not mentioned. It seemed to me, as an American, that while names were being honored, it should be understood that medicine and surgery is broader than any mere country, and that in honoring the name of McDowell, as Spencer Wells himself does in his book, one can but do honor to his own manhood; and in failing to do so one commits an oversight, to say the least. Mr. Wheelhouse is well informed in surgery and its history.[16]

In the same report, Daly noted during his stay in London he had visited Guy's, St. Bartholomew's, and Royal London hospitals and witnessed a wide range of interesting procedures and innovative surgical interventions at the three teaching hospitals. Specific instances he mentioned in detail include, "extrophy of the bladder," "supra-pubic cystotomy," "numerous gastrotomy operations," and an operation for "straightening knock knees and curved thigh and leg bones, by means of artificial fracture." At Royal London Hospital, Daly was amazed by the number of patients treated. He remarked:

> The extent of the material is very great, this being probably one of the largest, if not the largest, eye clinics in the world, their in-patients last year numbering over two thousand, their new out-patients over twenty thousand, and the whole number of patients seen over one hundred thousand. It is a sight truly never to be forgotten, to see the vast throng of blind, half blind and weak-sighted poor that flock to Moorfields to avail themselves of the advice of such masters in the ophthalmological art as Mr. Solberg, Wells, Lawson, and their colleagues, some of whom, with their large corps of assistants, are to be found there every morning.[17]

While in England, Daly became aware of and observed the work of Sir Morell Mackenzie, who by then had become recognized for his innovative work in laryngology. By the time of Daly's visit, Mackenzie had long ago founded the Hospital for Diseases of the Throat—the first hospital in London dedicated to the specialty. As a result of his groundbreaking work, he had established himself internationally as the preeminent practitioner in the field. Of all the many new and inventive medical treatments and surgical procedures that Daly observed while in London, it was laryngology that captured his attention.

Upon his return to Pittsburgh in 1879, Daly began writing scientific articles and essays. His trip abroad seemingly energized him and imbued a sense of urgency in embracing the specialties of laryngology and rhinology, fields of practice in which he would soon become the preeminent practitioner in the city. As his proficiency grew, so did his interest in documenting and reporting on his clinical work and findings. He began in 1880 by authoring a series of papers, including "A Case of Syphilitic Stenosis of the Larynx, with Fibrous Adhesive Bands of the True Vocal Cords…" and "An Analysis of the Value of the Galvano-Cautery in the Treatment of Diseases and Growths of the Naso-Pharynx," which were published simultaneously in *The Transactions of the American Medical Association*.[18] Interestingly, the "Syphilitic Stenosis of the Larynx" essay is the first known instance in which Daly used illustrations to document his work.

During early 1880, Daly also had other articles published. His paper "Elongating Hypertrophy of the Femur and Tibia of Opposite Sides (The Osteitis Deformans of Paget)" was published in the *New York Medical Journal*, and a case review, "A Case of Luxation of the Left Cornua of the Hyoid Bone," was printed in the *Archives of Laryngology*.[19, 20]

As recognition of Daly's work grew, so too did his prestige and standing in the professional medical community of Pittsburgh. With his election as president of the

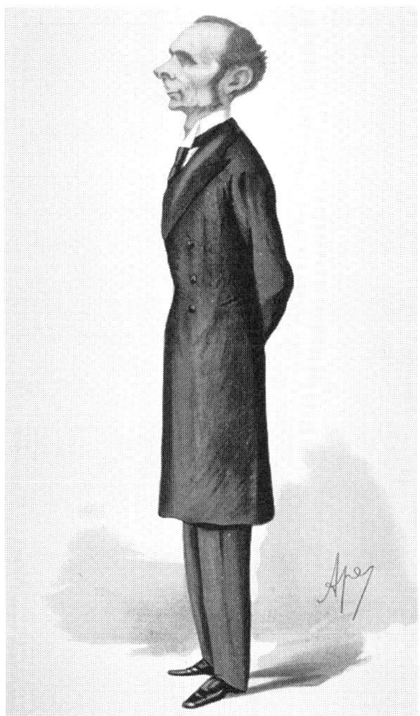

Caricature of Sir Morell MacKenzie. (*National Library of Medicine*)

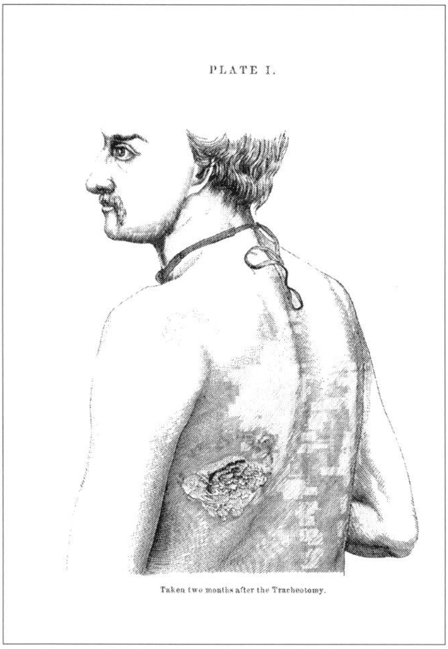

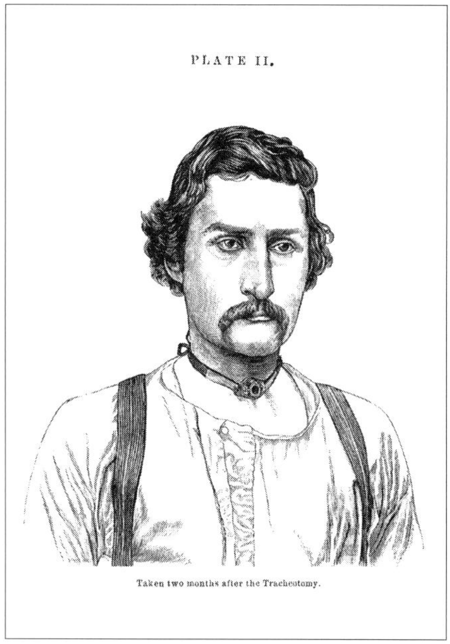

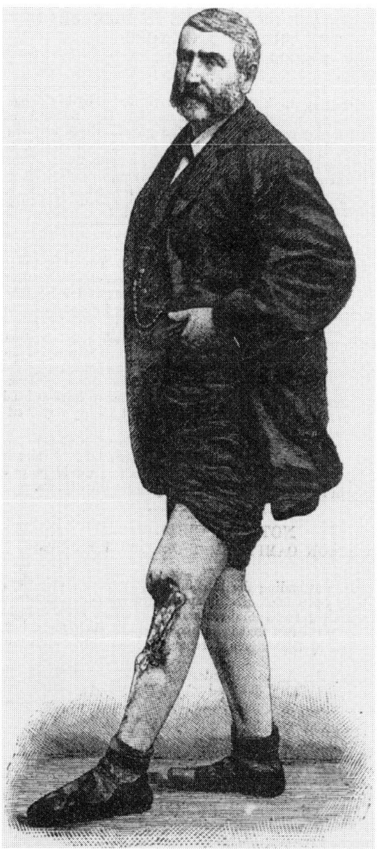

Above left: William H. Daly, "A Case of Syphilitic Stenosis of the Larynx with Fibrous Adhesive Bands of the True Vocal Cords," Plate 1, *Transactions of the American Medical Association*, Volume 31, 1880. (*American Medical Association Archives*)

Above right: William H. Daly, "A Case of Syphilitic Stenosis of the Larynx with Fibrous Adhesive Bands of the True Vocal Cords," Plate 2, *Transactions of the American Medical Association*, Volume 31, 1880. (*American Medical Association Archives*)

Left: William H. Daly's patient H. L. K., a locomotive engineer, who was burned during a railroad accident in October 1879. Twenty surgeons wished to amputate, Daly objected and the leg was saved. (*British Medical Journal, Volume 2, Number 1250, 13 December 1884*)

Allegheny County Medical Society in 1881, it would have been easy to assume he had reached the pinnacle of the local medical profession. However, that was not the case as he was just then hitting his stride. There was much more to accomplish medically—especially in his newly chosen fields of specialty—and even more to write.

Over the next several years, Daly continued to fill notebooks with case studies and clinical observations. He also began to test himself by writing down questions he encountered in his practice so he could later research the myriad subjects of importance that came to his attention. The notes would continue to provide fodder for his pen and words for use on the bully pulpit of his specialties in laryngology and rhinology. From shallow roots and humble beginnings in Pittsburgh's medical circles, he would soon rise to prominence nationally and internationally.

Between 1880 and 1900, it is estimated that Daly "contributed more than fifty essays on medical subjects to the current literature of the day."[21] Among his many presentations and published articles may be found the following:

DATE	SUBJECT	PUBLICATION OR VENUE
April 1881	"Nasal Polyps"	*Archives of Laryngology*
April 1882	"On the Relation of Hay Asthma and Chronic Naso-Pharyngeal Catarrh"	*Archives of Laryngology*
May 1882	"A Peculiar Injury to the Hip Joint"	*Philadelphia Medical News*
May 1882	"An address before the Pittsburgh College of Pharmacy"	Presented at the Pittsburgh College of Pharmacy
October 1882	"Naso-Antral Catarrh and its Treatment"	*Archives of Laryngology*
November 1883 December 1883	"A discussion of some questions relating to tonsillotomy of the nasal septum, with a presentation of two cases"	Presented at the Allegheny County Medical Society Reprinted in the *Medical and Surgical Reporter*
May 1884	"Gunshot wounds of the larynx: with the report of a case in which the vocal bands were involved"	*Transactions of the Sixth Annual meeting of the American Laryngological Association* Also reprinted in the *New York Medical Journal*
May 1884	"An Address in Medicine Before the State Medical Society of Pennsylvania: Some thoughts on scientific investigation and clinical observation. Conservatism in Medical Ethics. The Medical Profession and its specialties"	Presented at the 35th Annual Meeting of the Medical Society of Pennsylvania Reprinted in the *Transactions of the Medical Society of the State of Pennsylvania*

August 1884	"Laryngology and its Cognate Branches in America"	Presented at the Eighth International Medical Congress, Copenhagen, Denmark
December 1884	"Extensive Burn Involving the Cavity of the Knee-Joint"	*British Medical Journal*
May 1886	"The Simplest and Most Efficient Treatment of Diphtheria"	Presented at the American Laryngological Society Eighth Annual Congress, Philadelphia, Pennsylvania
September 1887	Inaugural Address of the President, Section of Laryngology	Presented at the Ninth International Medical Congress in Washington D.C.
June 1889	"An Address in Laryngology"	Presented at the Pennsylvania Medical Society 40th Annual Meeting
June 1889	"Marking an Era in Laryngology"	Presented at the 40th Annual Meeting of the American Medical Association
December 1889	"The Relation of Naso-Pharngeal Diseases to Deafness and Other Ear Affections"	Read before the New York Academy of Medicine
April 1890	"The Wakefulness of Neurasthenia as Affected by Seaside Residence: Its Successful Management and Cure"	*The Medical News*
February 1892 May 1892	"Leprosy" (in Cuba, Yucatan, and other parts of Mexico)	Read before the Allegheny County Medical Society Published in *American Lancet*
October 1892 January 1893	"A Clinical Study of Glanders in the Horse, with Special Reference to its Manifestations upon the Mucous Tissues of the Nose with Prophylaxis and Treatment"	Read before the Mississippi Valley Medical Association of Cincinnati Published in *The Medical Record*
May 1894	"Some Practical Observations on So-Called Malaria being a Water Borne Disease"	Read before the American Climatological Association

Daly's April 1883 article "Relation of Hay Asthma and Chronic Naso-Pharyngeal Catarrh" was well received in both the United States and Europe. A few years after its publication, Sir Morrell Mackenzie—Great Britain's internationally renowned dean of laryngology—singlehandedly promoted Daly's work to international prominence. In the August 1887 edition of the *London Journal of Laryngology and Rhinology*, Mackenzie wrote an editorial reply to a letter received from Pittsburgh physician D. N. Rankin. Rankin's letter is interesting to read in that it provides insight into Daly's work at the time:

> Allegheny, PA, July 5th, 1887.
> Dear Sirs,—In your obituary notice of the late Professor Hack, in the June number of your journal, you have erroneously accredited to him some honours which as a matter of correct medical history belong to Dr. W. H. Daly, of Pittsburgh, Pa., U.S.A. I believe the fact is generally known to laryngologists and the profession every where, that to Dr. Daly belongs the honour of making the original observations in 1878, 1879, and 1880, which demonstrated the intranasal causes of hay fever, and he gave the results to the profession in a paper entitled "Hay Asthma and Naso-Pharyngeal Catarrh" which he read before the Congress of the American Laryngological Association in New York, May, 1881. The paper was published in the Archives of Laryngology (vol. iii., No. 2, April, 1882). In that essay, Dr. Daly asked the pertinent question—"Whether we are warranted in believing any case of hay asthma purely a neurosis, without first eliminating the possible causation due to local structural or functional disease in the naso-pharynx?" Professor Hack's essay did not appear until 1884, three years after the reading of that paper, and after it had been quoted in medical journals, and reprints sent to laryngologists wherever known, Professor Hack among the number. I herewith transmit you also a copy of the reprint from the press of the Archives of Laryngology. This paper contains the gist and kernel of all that has been so ably observed and elaborated upon by Dr. Roe, of Rochester; the lamented Professor Hack; Dr. Mackenzie, of Baltimore; Professor Sajous, of Philadelphia; Professor Bosworth, of New York, and the increasing number of others who have been attracted to this field of observation, and who have so largely verified the original observations made by Dr. Daly. It may be said, with no little honour for him, that by the carrying out of injunctions so forcibly laid down by Dr. Daly in his original essay, Professor Hack and the many others have been enabled to do useful work in advancing this branch of medical science in a sure and lasting manner, and the comprehensive suggestions of Daly have been the means of not only curing more cases of asthma than was accomplished by any other method before known, but also of making a marked advance in the cure of other diseases of the upper air tract.[22]

Mackenzie's response to Rankin's letter provided additional background on the history of the matter. Among his comments, he stated: "We have much pleasure in publishing the above letter, and we are anxious to do full justice to Dr. Daly, as well as to all those who add to the sum of human knowledge." He further added: "Dr. Daly may justly be regarded as a founder of that surgical school of rhinology in America, which has at the present day so many distinguished representatives, by drawing forcible attention to the importance of intra-nasal surgical treatment."[23]

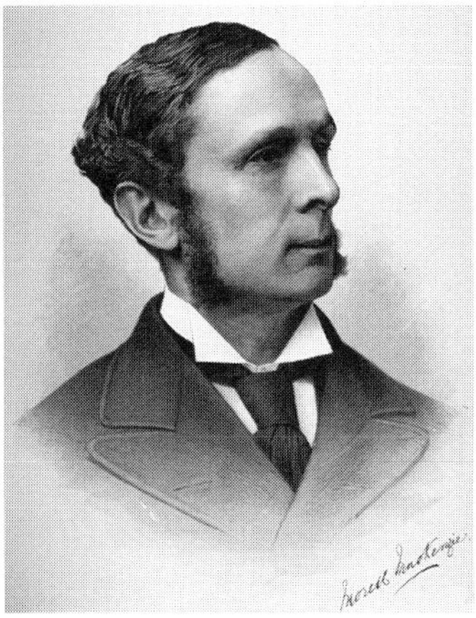

Sir Morell MacKenzie. (*National Library of Medicine*)

Daly's 1894 presentation of the "So-called Malaria Being a Waterborne Disease" essay likewise drew substantial national praise. While his thinking was moving in the right direction and well ahead of his peers in the United States, it was several years behind that of French military physician Dr. Alphonse Laveran. Nearly ten years prior, Laveran had already suggested it was the mosquito and not bad air or contaminated water as the cause of the disease.

Nevertheless, Daly was credited with advancing the research that elicited a fuller understanding of disease acquisition and treatment in the United States. In 1901, the *Michigan Alumnus* magazine reported:

> [Daly] was also several years in advance of the general trend of medical scientific thought, which is now becoming so strongly confirmatory of the theory that water instead of air is the medium by which malaria enters the human body. Drs. Patrick, Manson, Ronald Ross and other investigators upon the mosquito as a factor in infecting the water of springs and swamps on the one hand, and the blood of human beings on the other, have worked along the same line of thought as those made evident in the previous essays of Dr. Daly.[24]

By the late 1880s, Daly not only mastered the practice of medicine and his chosen specialties of laryngology and rhinology, but also the power of his pen. Each new article or presentation brought him more attention and acclaim. As his notoriety grew, so too did his stature in his chosen fields. He was now being asked to make presentations at meetings across the country and the world. Upon delivery, virtually all of his essays were included in the latest medical journals or printed as monographs, which were widely distributed. Other leading physicians extended his fame by reference to his research and findings. Such affirmation of his standing in professional medical ranks grew exponentially with each passing year. At this point in his life, Daly had indeed mastered the art of "writing things worth the reading."

6

Carriage Trade and High Society

The year 1869 was eventful as it marked yet another milestone in Daly's life. On 22 June, he married Athalia Cooper, the daughter of Mr. and Mrs. James M. Cooper. The marriage ceremony took place at Trinity Church in the heart of downtown Pittsburgh.

Athalia's father was a well-known banker and investor in the city. By virtue of his shrewd speculation in the firm of Hussey, Wells and Company of Pittsburgh in 1859, he also became recognized as an industrialist. The company, in which he became a partner, was the earliest in Pittsburgh to demonstrate iron could be converted to steel in a crucible. The discovery was important as it produced high-quality steel and offered substantial cost savings in the manufacturing process. The conversion to the crucible process now allowed a Pittsburgh company to compete aggressively with the finest steelmakers in England.[1] The firm was prominently located between 16th and 18th Streets and situated between Penn Avenue and the Allegheny Railroad.[2]

The Cooper family was affluent and influential in both industrial and political circles of Pittsburgh and Washington, D.C. Along with Athalia's parents, William and Athalia's names soon began appearing in Pittsburgh's social register. Daly's marriage to Athalia did much to propel him into high society, something that had previously eluded him. His career and marriage now brought him into a world that looked much different than the one he had emerged from little more than a quarter century before.

As was typical at the time of their marriage, Pittsburgh's gentry aggregated along Penn and Fifth Avenues. Between the end of the Civil War and the mid-1870s, however, many of the city's wealthiest citizens began moving to the East End of the city. William and Athalia followed the pattern and moved first from Fifth Avenue to Sixth Avenue, and then finally to Howe Street in Shadyside in 1887 where they stayed until the end of their lives. By the time of their move to

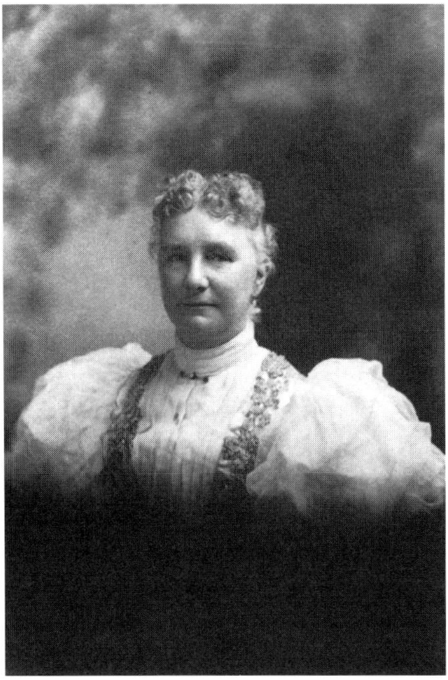

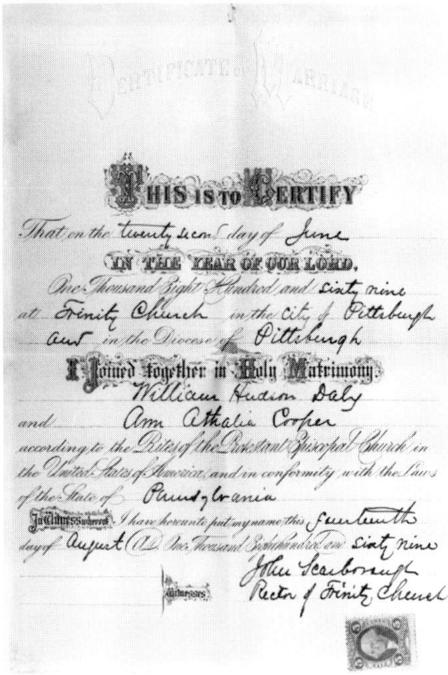

Certificate of Marriage

This is to Certify

That on the twenty second day of June

In the Year of Our Lord,

One Thousand Eight Hundred and sixty nine

at Trinity Church in the City of Pittsburgh

and in the Diocese of Pittsburgh

I Joined together in Holy Matrimony

William Hudson Daly

and Ann Athalia Cooper

according to the Rites of the Protestant Episcopal Church in the United States of America, and in conformity with the Laws of the State of Pennsylvania

In Witness whereof I have hereunto put my name this fourteenth day of August A.D. One Thousand Eight hundred and sixty nine

John Scarborough

Rector of Trinity Church

Witnesses

Above left: Athalia Cooper Daly, *c.* 1890s.

Above right: William H. Daly and Athalia Cooper marriage certificate, 22 June 1869.

Below: William H. Daly and Athalia Cooper wedding invitation, 22 June 1869.

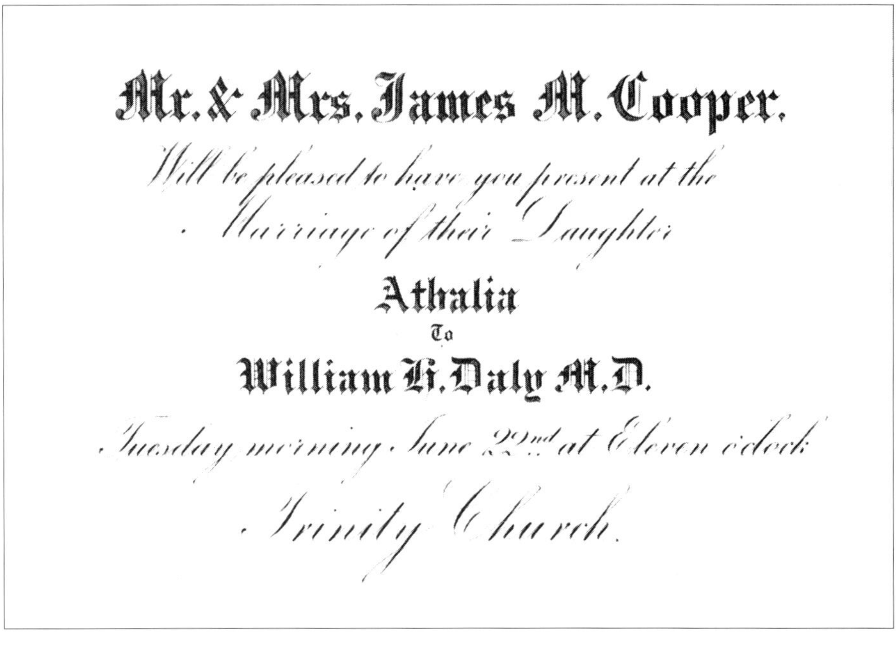

Mr. & Mrs. James M. Cooper.

Will be pleased to have you present at the

Marriage of their Daughter

Athalia

To

William H. Daly M.D.

Tuesday morning June 22nd at Eleven o'clock

Trinity Church.

Howe Street, the area had become the rural destination of choice for the city's most prosperous families as they sought to escape the din and dinginess of the inner city. As Samuel Hays noted in his book *City at the Point*, the opening of a streetcar line on Fifth Avenue did much to hasten the movement from the center of the city to the east.[3]

While they moved their day-to-day household to Shadyside, they also maintained their old home on Sixth Avenue. This situation complemented the couple's other investments in real estate throughout the city and its suburbs. Real estate was to become a major interest of William's from that point forward. By the time of his death in 1901, proceeds from real estate would comprise a significant source of annual income.

Marriage and family connections offered many new social opportunities for William. As Hays noted about the city's privileged families, "Like the elite in other American cities, these men and their wives used posh neighborhoods, social registers, luncheons and country clubs, and Presbyterian and Episcopalian parishes to define themselves as urban gentry." Athalia was well accustomed to such things, and while William had much to offer relative to his fast-growing professional stature, he still had much to learn. Together, they became an integral part of Pittsburgh's aristocracy and checked all of the "social" boxes that marked their arrival.

In October 1870, William and Athalia became the proud parents of their first child, James Cooper Daly, who was named in honor of Athalia's father. Everything Daly had worked for now seemed to come together. Life was indeed good for the young family. It seemed, however, perhaps there was one thing missing in Daly's life after his marriage and the birth of his first child—a connection to the military.

On November 1871, Daly was commissioned lieutenant colonel in the 18th Division of the Pennsylvania National Guard. Shortly afterward, he was promoted to surgeon-in-chief of the division. Unfortunately, the lure of the military and the luster of his advancement did not last long. In April 1874, his son, James, died unexpectedly from scarlet fever at the age of four. William and Athalia were devastated by the loss. After James' death, Daly seemed to become introverted and much more pensive. While he still enjoyed hunting trips and social influences, he resigned his position with the National Guard on 14 November 1874. On 12 December, he was officially discharged.[4]

Following the death of his child and discharge from the National Guard, Daly's brooding mood and quest for isolation seemingly provided impetus for his growing interest in traversing woodlands and streams in search of fish, game, and solitude. Around this time, he also started collecting weapons of varied nature, with older and odder guns preferred.

His hunting and fishing experiences appear to have had a positive effect on him and ostensibly served as a stimulus for igniting interest in writing for nature magazines in the mid-1870s. In 1893, Daly recalled: "The writer has for the past twenty or more years spent probably an average of two months annually in the recreative sports of the field, forest, and stream. The largest proportion of these holiday jaunts have been passed in the lowlands, or in the swamps of the lakesides, or seaside, in the pursuit of wild fowl shooting."[5] The correlation between the timing of his son's death and Daly's interest in taking long hunting trips is unmistakable.

Three years after the passing of their first son, William and Athalia were once again graced with the birth of another child, William Theodore Daly. Their joy, however, did not last a year. Young William died in 1877, four days before his first birthday. This child would be the last born to the couple.

With the passing of their second child, William and Athalia focused on other aspects of life. Athalia found consolation in spending increasing amounts of time with friends and relatives. She also found comfort in Pittsburgh's burgeoning social and artistic undertakings. Her influence in these activities had a profound effect on her husband, and together they became favorites of the city's social circuit.

Shortly after the loss of William Theodore, out-of-town relatives began visiting the Daly home. In July 1877 Athalia's sister, Virginia Cooper, arrived from Philadelphia and stayed for a few weeks to offer comfort and support. William appears to have enjoyed this social reawakening; he once again found pleasure in professional activities and ever more vigorous hunting and fishing activities. As noted in the previous chapter, in April 1878, he left for Europe to spend a year studying in London, Berlin, and Vienna. Upon his return from Europe, Mr. and Mrs. Thomas Dunaway arrived from Cass County, Illinois, for a prolonged visit at the Daly's Howe Street home. Mrs. Dunaway was William's sister.

Not long after the trip to Europe, William and Athalia began taking more frequent trips to the countryside of eastern Pennsylvania and the waterways of Maryland and Virginia. Their first trip after the death of William Theodore and their journey to Europe was in January 1888 to the Chesapeake Bay area of Maryland, where William engaged in duck hunting. The family visits and duck hunting trips appear to have had their immediate intended effect. While the couple could not stop mourning the loss of their children, they seem to have concluded that rigorous social, professional, and recreational activity could lessen the anguish.

It was around this time the Press Club of Pittsburgh began using the old Daly home on Sixth Avenue for its meetings.[6] The organization had formed in January 1881 to provide financial support for poverty-stricken newspapermen. It was the first such club to organize in the country. In March 1888, the Pittsburgh Duquesne Club considered using the Daly home for its meetings while the club's old building on Sixth Avenue, located not far from the Daly home, was being razed to make way for a new structure.[7] The club was founded as a "voluntary association to serve and cultivate some of the nation's greatest influencers," in 1873. Most of the city's most prominent businessmen, including William, were members.[8]

Over the years, Daly continued his long association with Western Pennsylvania Hospital and the Pittsburgh Free Dispensary. In 1879, he added another affiliation

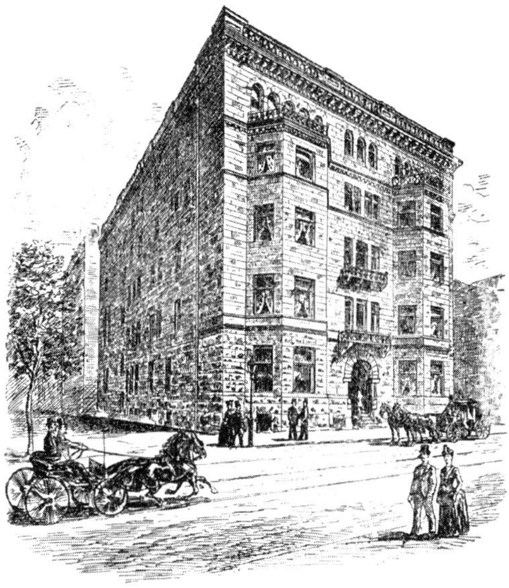

Duquesne Club (Pittsburgh), "Pittsburg and its Exposition." (*Press of Pittsburg Photo-Engraving Co., 1889*)

by becoming the general surgeon to the Pittsburgh and Lake Erie Railroad. The position was likely very challenging since railroad injuries were among the most prevalent industrial accidents occurring in the city during that period. Many of those accidents resulted in amputations. It was reported between January 1877 and October 1884, the surgical staff at Western Pennsylvania Hospital held the distinction of performing more amputations than any other hospital in the country.[9] Daly held the position with the railroad until 1887.

The first few years of the 1880s drew Daly into yet another professional medical endeavor and investment opportunity. In June 1883, the Western Pennsylvania Medical College was chartered. It was the first medical school in Pittsburgh and in Western Pennsylvania. Joining other prominent Pittsburgh physicians, many of whom had Civil War military backgrounds like Daly's, a small investor group was formed to fund the college through stock subscription. A total 250 shares of stock, valued at $100 per share, were sold. With the sale of the stock, funding was sufficient to construct a new building to house the college.

The facility was built near Western Pennsylvania Hospital on property located at 30th and Brereton Streets in the Polish Hill area of the city. Standing four-stories high and containing classrooms, a dissection room, laboratories, a medical museum, and a large two-story amphitheater, the building took a little more than two years to complete. The Medical College officially opened in September 1886 with an initial class of fifty-seven students.[10] While many of the other investors became faculty of the new institution, Daly elected to remain only an investor. The college became formally affiliated with the University of Pittsburgh in 1892

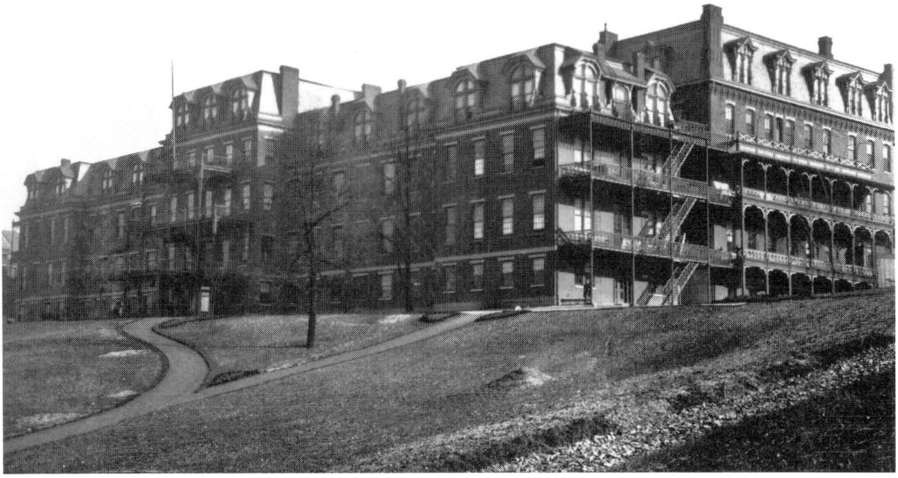

Western Pennsylvania Hospital, *c.* 1895. (*Western Pennsylvania Hospital*)

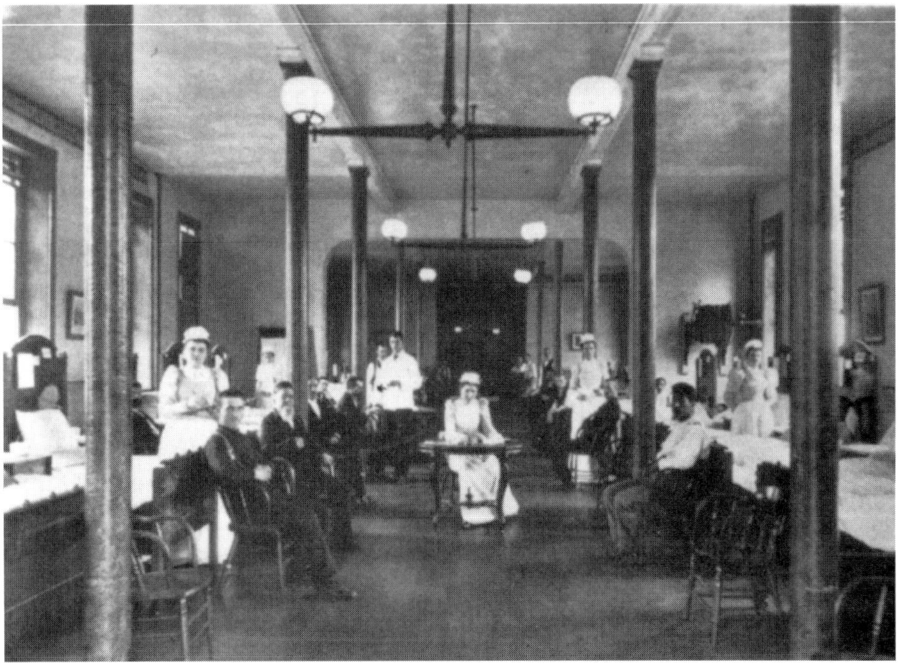

Western Pennsylvania Hospital Medical Department in the late 1880s. (*Western Pennsylvania Hospital*)

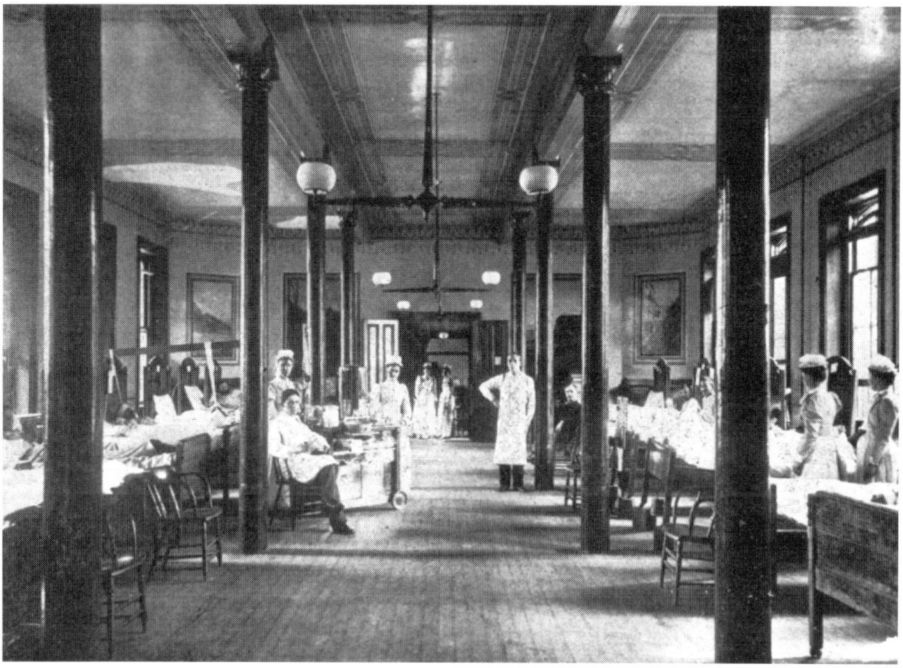

Above: Western Pennsylvania Hospital Surgical Department in the late 1880s. (*Western Pennsylvania Hospital*)

Right: William H. Daly, 1885. (*The New York Academy of Medicine*)

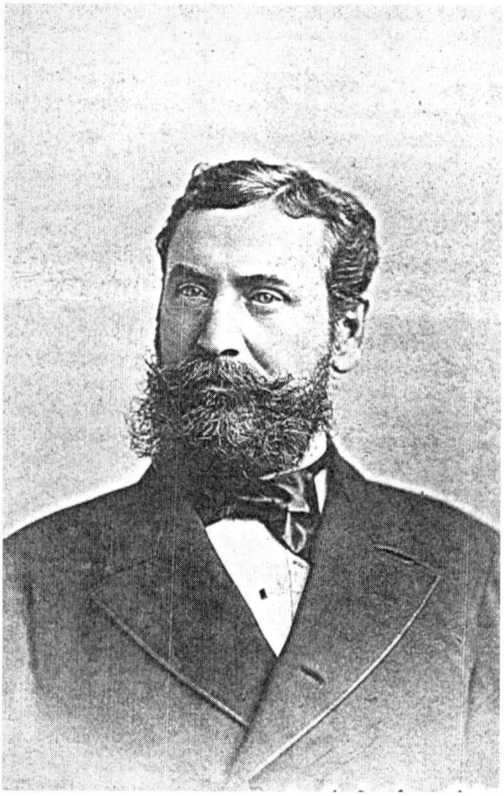

and was sold to the university in 1908. Today, it is known as the University of Pittsburgh Medical School.

During the month of August 1888, William and Athalia visited St. Clair Springs, Michigan, and stayed at the renowned Oakland Hotel. At the time, the area was a major tourist destination for those interested in the town's springs, baths, and wholesome air. The following month, the couple traveled to Berkeley Springs, West Virginia, to vacation and visit Athalia's sister and her husband. The spot was another favorite tourist attraction for those who, like the Dalys, were inclined to enjoy the area's mineral springs and spas. The town attracted many writers and artists, which was likewise very agreeable to them.

When the luster of regional trips began to wane or failed to adequately provide the stimulus they needed, William found a perfect way to merge Athalia's familial interests with his outdoor sporting pursuits. Together, they began taking trips to Garner, Iowa, to visit Athalia's relatives. It was during one of these trips that William became enamored with the thought of big game hunting. This subsequently led him to take extended hunting trips into the Bighorn Mountains of southern Montana and northern Wyoming. In the late 1880s, these trips would become an almost annual ritual.

On one of these trips, an attack by an enraged elk left him with a severe back injury that would plague him for the remainder of his life. His only consolation was the smiling glance he was afforded every time he passed the trophy elk rack hanging prominently in his home in Pittsburgh. On another trip, Daly met Buffalo Bill Cody and General Nelson Miles, two men who would later have a profound impact on his life.

The late 1880s were also a time when Daly began to embrace the social and professional value of deeper involvement in the work of numerous national and international professional medical associations. Writing about his research and clinical findings was one thing, effecting changes in everyday practices and elevating professional standards was another. He approached both with renewed vitality.

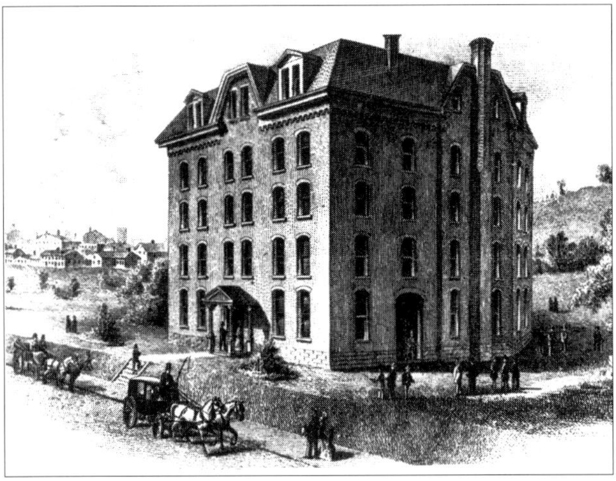

Western Pennsylvania Medical College, *c.* 1890. (*Western Pennsylvania Hospital*)

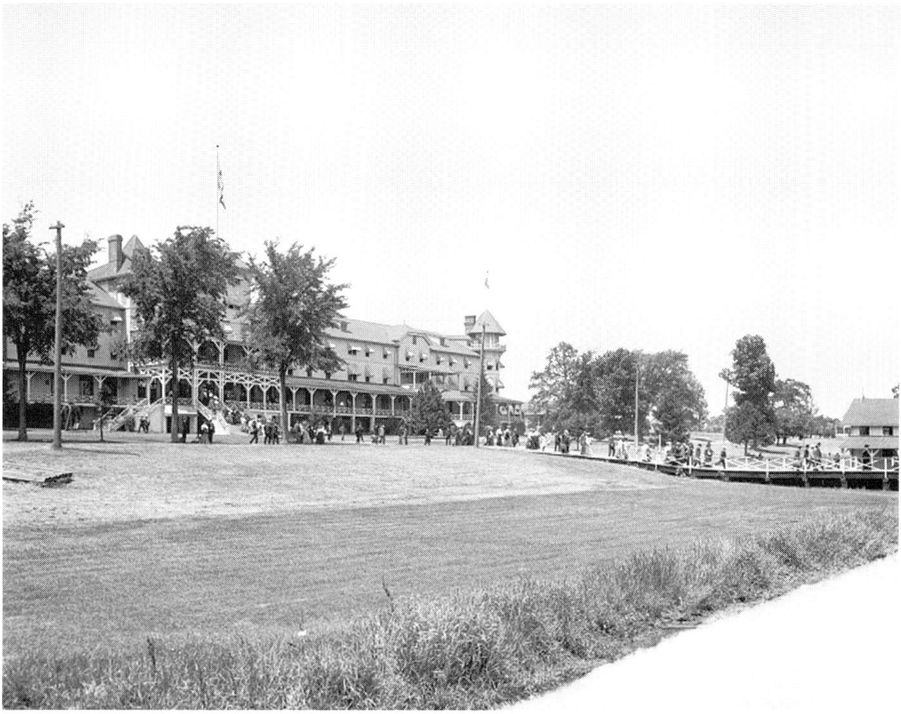

Oakland Hotel, St. Clair, Michigan. (*Library of Congress*)

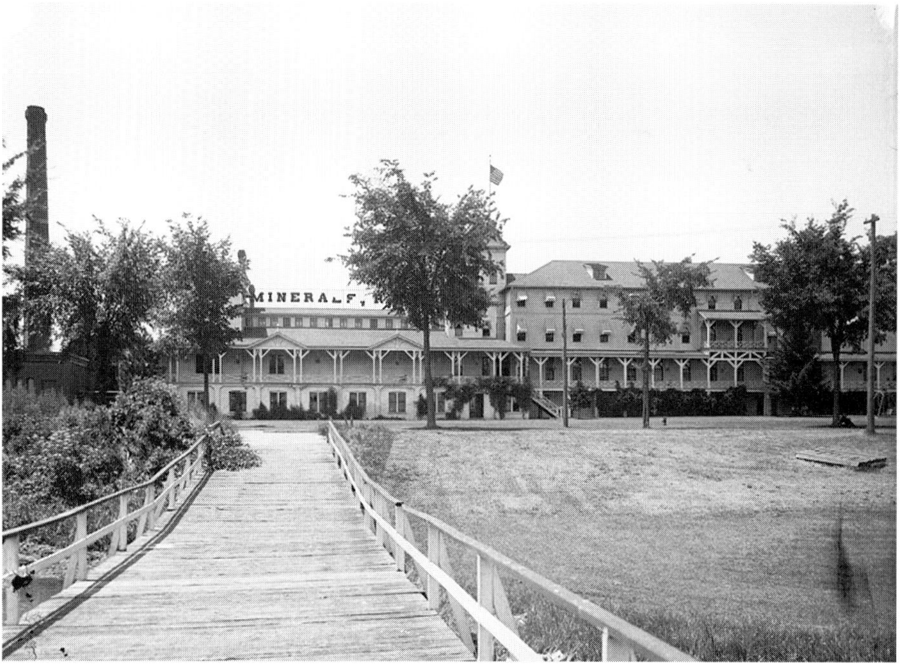

Oakland Hotel, St. Clair, Michigan. (*Library of Congress*)

In a presentation to the Medical Society of Pennsylvania in 1884, Daly took time to opine about the growing recognition of his chosen specialty of laryngology. At the meeting, he stated: "Laryngology is a special study that is fast claiming the respect of our profession, and justly so; it has grown up within a few years, and some of the most brilliant operations in surgery, notably extirpation of the larynx, has been performed repeatedly with success."[11] The rising prominence of the specialty—particularly in Western Pennsylvania—was in many ways attributable to his efforts in clinical practice and scientific writing.

In recognition of his growing national prominence among forward-thinking laryngologists in the country, Daly was elected president of the American Medical Association's newly formed Laryngology Section in May 1886.[12] The following year, in September 1887, he was selected to serve as chairman of the Laryngology Section of the Ninth International Medical Congress at its meeting in Washington, D.C.[13] His opening address to the Laryngology Section was the first for the specialty.

He also found it useful to join many of the most important professional medical organizations. Several of the most significant include the Allegheny County Medical Society; American Medical Association; British Laryngological, Rhinological, and Otological Association; British Medical Association; Pennsylvania Medical Society; and *La Société Française d'Otologie, de Laryngologie et de Rhinologie*.

With laryngology now his *métier*, his reputation continued to grow as did his influence on many professional medical organizations. As attested by his election to leadership roles in several associations, including the Allegheny County Medical Society (president in 1881); American Medical Association (official representative to the Eighth International Medical Congress, Copenhagen, Denmark, and on three occasions as its representative to the British Medical Association); American Laryngological Association (president in 1894); American Laryngological, Rhinological and Otological Society (president in 1897); and American Social Science Association (elected chairman of the Health Section in 1897), he seemingly had reached the pinnacle of his medical career. However, that would subsequently turn out not to be the case.

William and Athalia Daly's social and travel calendar was busy at the start of the last decade of the nineteenth century. In March 1890, a local society newspaper, the *Pittsburg Bulletin*, reported William's brother-in-law, Colonel Ransom, was visiting from Baltimore.[14] In June, Athalia's sister, Virginia Cooper, once again came to visit for several weeks. During her stay, the Dalys hosted a special reception in her honor. After Virginia's departure, the Dalys prepared for another trip to Europe. William once again managed to mix business with pleasure. From 04–09 August 1890, he attended the Tenth International Medical Congress in Berlin, Germany. The couple stayed in Europe for several weeks, returning home to Pittsburg on 22 October.

During late summer 1891, Daly was named to the Pennsylvania State Commission to Select Home for Chronic Insane. The commission was tasked with finding a suitable site for the erection of a new insane asylum in the eastern part of the state to serve those who required extended care. Daly was not an expert in mental illness; he was, however, one of Pittsburgh's most prominent physicians and well aware of prevalent best practices in providing care for the insane by way of his affiliation with Western Pennsylvania Hospital and its adjunct mental health facility, Dixmont Hospital for the Insane.

The committee selected property in Wernersville, Pennsylvania, located approximately 12 miles west of the City of Reading for the project. Once the site was chosen, the State General Assembly approved $500,000 for the purchase of land and erection of buildings. The Wernersville State Hospital buildings were modeled after Philadelphia's Independence Hall. The institution's grounds were designed without constraining walls and its buildings without window bars to allow patients to roam the grounds freely. At the time of the hospital's opening in June 1893, it was considered one of the country's most advanced facilities for long-term care of the non-criminal mentally ill.

At the end of 1891, the Dalys were once again appearing regularly in Pittsburgh society news. On 22 December 1891, the couple hosted a breakfast for well-known actor and comedian Joseph Jefferson, his wife, and son. Jefferson was nationally recognized for many of his stage works, including his most famous long-term role depicting Rip Van Winkle. He was also one of the country's earliest film actors who counted among his friends many leading politicians, writers, and artists.

Other guests who attended the breakfast included Mr. and Mrs. Dewees Woods and Mrs. E. Moorewood Ferguson. Dewees Woods was a prominent iron and steel manufacturer, who had established a plant in McKeesport in 1851. He was credited with inventing and patenting a process to manufacture "American Russia sheet iron." Mrs. Ferguson's husband was the president of Merchants and Manufacturers National Bank.

Jefferson was in Pittsburgh to perform his play, *The Rivals*, which began on 21 December 1891, at the new Alvin Theatre. The theatre had opened three months earlier, on 21 September 1891. It took very little time for the theatre to become one of the city's prime venues. On the opening evening of the play, William and Athalia were in attendance and participated in a special theatre party.

On the day after Jefferson's play opened, the same day of the Daly breakfast, the *Pittsburg Dispatch* newspaper reported: "*The Rivals* was played splendidly by Joseph Jefferson and his company last night. The play was exquisitely staged. The audience contained many distinguished citizens and was cordial. The new conservatory was thrown open last night, adding a large room prettily decorated and lit to the foyer, where the audience could enjoy a walk among palms and fountains."[15]

Extending their day of cultural activity in the city, the Dalys dined with another celebrated comedian and actor, Stuart Robson, at the Duquesne Club that same evening. Robson was in the city playing a leading role in *The Henrietta* at the Pittsburgh Grand Opera House.

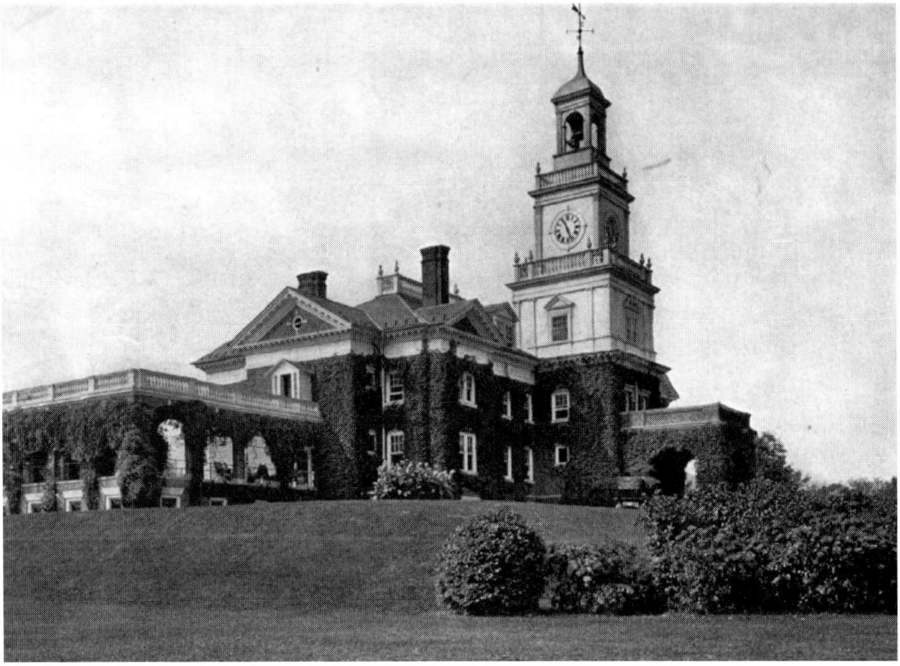

Main building, Wernersville State Hospital, Wernersville, Pennsylvania. (*The American Architect Magazine*, *May 1911*)

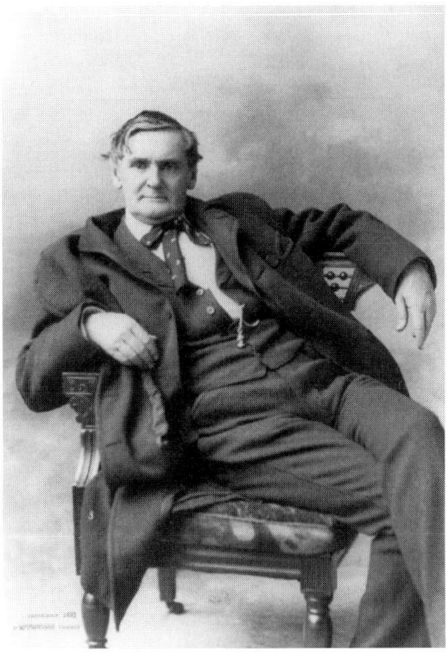

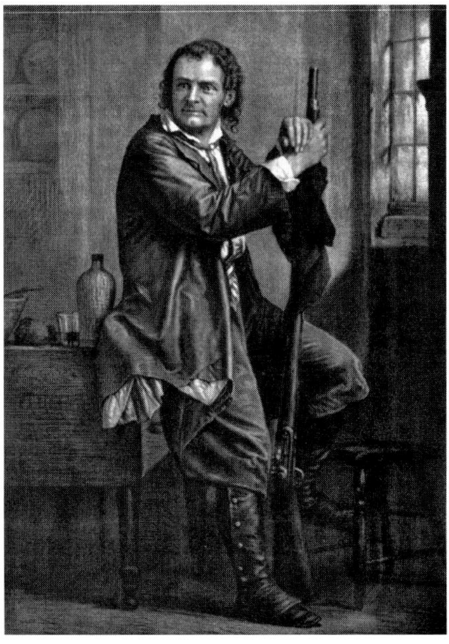

Above left: Actor Joe Jefferson, 1893. (*Library of Congress*)

Above right: Actor Joe Jefferson as Rip Van Winkle. (*Library of Congress*)

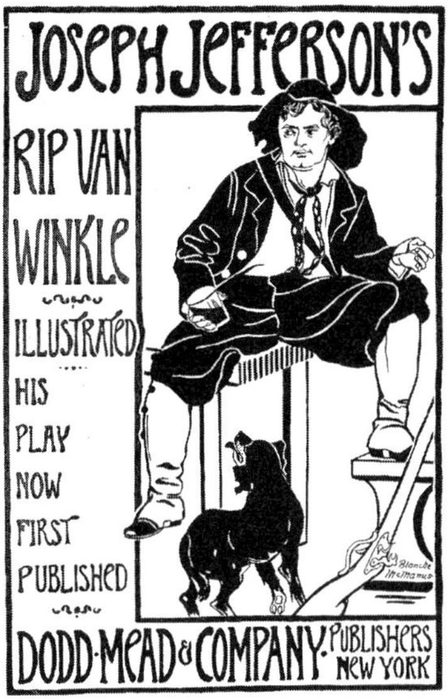

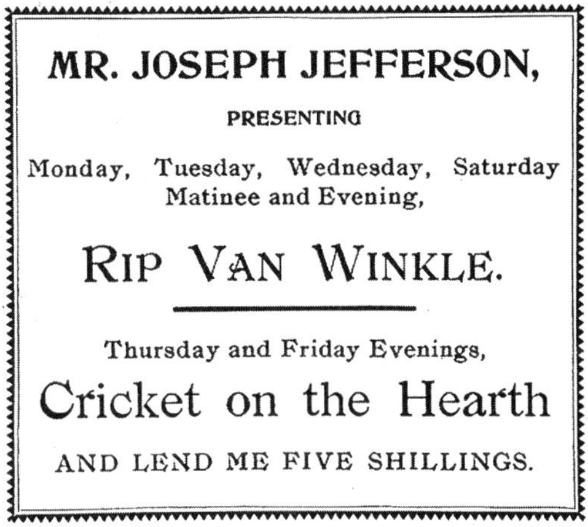
MR. JOSEPH JEFFERSON,
PRESENTING
Monday, Tuesday, Wednesday, Saturday
Matinee and Evening,
RIP VAN WINKLE.
Thursday and Friday Evenings,
Cricket on the Hearth
AND LEND ME FIVE SHILLINGS.

Above left: Joseph Jefferson's Rip Van Winkle play illustrated. (*Library of Congress*)

Above right: Mr. Joseph Jefferson, Rip Van Winkle advertisement, Alvin Theatre, 09 November 1896. (*Library of Congress*)

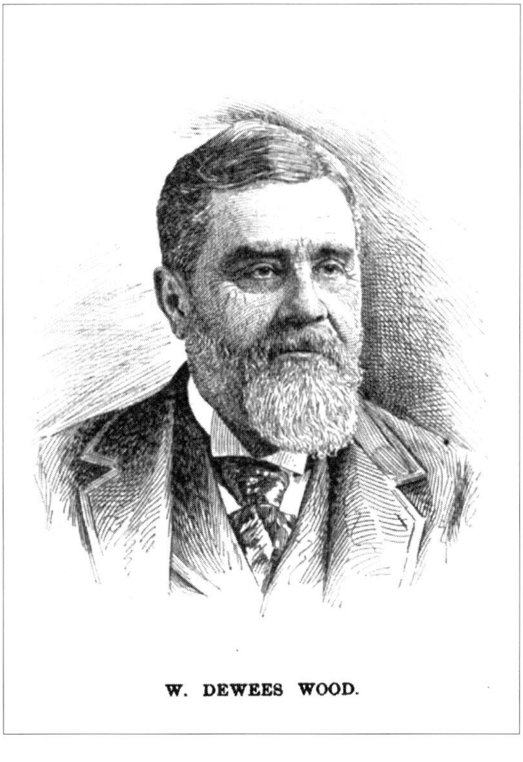

Right: Dewees Woods. (*Sanitary and Heating Age magazine, 14 January 1899*)

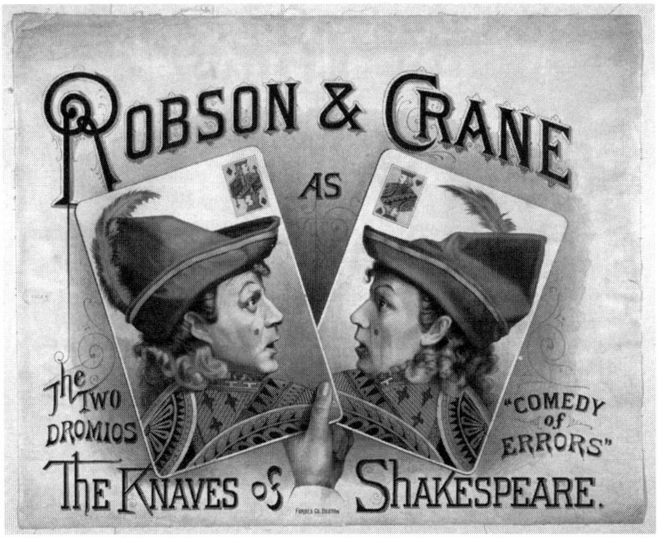

Robson and Crane as the Knaves of Shakespeare, theatrical poster, 1879. (*Library of Congress*)

In February 1892, Daly took a long trip to Cuba, Yucatan, and other areas around the Mexican peninsula. As previously noted, Daly used this trip to study leprosy. Upon his return, he presented his findings to the Allegheny County Medical Society. In May 1892, his paper on the subject was published in the *American Lancet* journal.

March 1992 was filled with wedding preparations for William's niece, Miss Nellie Johnstone. Nellie married Samuel Bowman Hubley at a ceremony held at the home of Nellie's mother and William's sister, Agnes Daly Johnstone, on Dinwiddie Street. The bride was given away by William's older brother, Thomas L. Daly, from Gibsonton, Westmoreland County. Thomas's daughter, Athalia, (named after her aunt) served as one of the bridesmaids.

Daly also traveled to Kentucky in early 1892. Little is known about the trip other than he used the occasion to purchase a thoroughbred horse. His return to Pittsburgh with the horse was noted in the society pages of the *Pittsburg Bulletin* in May.[16] The newspaper commented that horseback riding was "now quite the thing," and reported when the weather was cooperative, many riders could be seen on East End roads and in Schenley Park in the evenings. Daly's purchase coincided with the creation of his essay "A Clinical Study of Glanders in the Horse," which he presented at the Mississippi Valley Medical Association of Cincinnati on 12 October 1892 and was reprinted in the *Medical Record* journal of January 1893.[17]

Achieving medical and social prominence would be achievement enough for many people, but for Daly, it was simply an invitation to accomplish more. Over the next several years, Daly would continue to engage in even more arduous professional and recreational activities. By the close of the decade, his name would appear regularly in newspapers across the country.

7

Hunting With Buffalo Bill and General Nelson A. Miles

As Daly's interest in hunting grew, he found pleasure in taking more frequent and much longer periods away from his medical practice to engage in the sport. Initially, he had a salaried assistant look after his patients while he was away. That association soon soured, however, after Daly received repeated reports of unhappiness with the arrangement from his patients. His relationship with the assistant eroded once the assistant resigned and struck out on his own to establish a competing practice not far away from Daly's office. While perturbing, the situation did little to impede Daly's practice or travel plans. As had frequently happened in Daly's life up to this point, Lady Luck once again placed her hand on his shoulder. He would soon meet a young new physician who would help him resolve his office issues while traveling.

After graduating from Philadelphia's Jefferson Medical College in April 1886, Chevalier Q. Jackson arrived in Pittsburgh to establish a medical practice. He was born to William S. and Katherine Ann (Morange) Jackson on 04 November 1865 at their home on Fourth Avenue in downtown Pittsburgh. His birth occurred just as Daly was entering the University of Michigan Medical School. While born twenty-three years apart, their professional medical careers and interest in laryngology would soon become intertwined and remain so for years.

While in medical school, Jackson became interested in the newly recognized medical specialty of laryngology. After graduation, he visited Europe to study medicine. In London, just as Daly had done in 1878–79, but independent of any connection to him, Jackson also elected to study the work of Sir Morrell Mackenzie, the world's foremost expert in the field. Like Daly, he was captivated with the new specialty and decided to make laryngology his primary practice area upon his return to Pittsburgh. Jackson later referred to his trip to London as a visit to "the cradle of laryngology."[1]

Jackson's decision on where to locate his practice in Pittsburgh was not a hard choice; finding office space, however, proved more challenging. During that period, most of Pittsburgh's specialists had their offices in the heart of the city on either Penn or Sixth Avenues. The entire medical specialty field was thriving at the time and office space was at a premium. Timing and good fortune, however, allowed Jackson to secure two rooms in a recently vacated tailor shop on Sixth Avenue. To his delight, he found the location to be near Daly's office as he noted in his autobiography:

> The location had the advantage of nearness to Doctor William H. Daly, who was a pioneer throat specialist in Pittsburgh; he was quoted in the literature. He was always helpful to me. He subscribed for the leading medical magazines, and he had a copy of almost every laryngeal book published; these he generously loaned to me, and his aid in those lean years was invaluable.[2]

Jackson went on to report that patients who were displeased with Daly's assistant soon started coming to him for care. Out of respect, and in repayment for Daly's many kindnesses, Jackson would send the patients back to Daly immediately upon his return. If they decided they did not wish to return to Daly, Jackson would dismiss them entirely. The result, he said, "was that on departure for the next voyage Doctor Daly left the instructions: 'Send patients to young Doctor Jackson if they cannot wait till I get home.'"[3]

To state that Daly inspired Jackson in his early years of practice is an understatement. In 1884, Daly had already received international recognition for his presentation "Laryngology and its Cognate Branches in America" at the Eighth International Medical Congress, in Copenhagen, Denmark. He had also been named the president of the American Medical Association's Laryngology Section in 1886, and in 1887, he would represent the organization as chairman of the Laryngology Section of the Ninth International Medical Congress in Washington, D.C. Also in June 1887, Jackson's idol, Sir Morrell Mackenzie recognized Daly "as a founder of that surgical school of rhinology in America."[4] Thus, Daly was well recognized as an expert in the diagnosis and treatment of diseases of the ear, nose, and throat. Jackson, therefore, saw a relationship with Daly as an advantage.

Despite, or perhaps as a result of, Daly's prominence, Jackson was eager to make his mark on the specialty. He would go on to become famous in his own right for inventing the esophagoscope and perfecting the bronchoscope, instruments that saved countless lives over the decades and remain in use today.[5] Like Daly, Jackson would later become involved in a national debate on public health. In Daly's case, his work would serve as a precursor to the passage of the Pure Food and Drug Act of 1906. In Jackson's case, his efforts would lead to the passage of the 1927 Federal Caustic Poison Act.

For Daly, the symbiotic relationship he nurtured with young Dr. Jackson proved an immense personal benefit. It freed him from the encumbrance of day-to-day practice and worries about losing patients. More importantly, perhaps, it afforded him the time he sought to pursue travel and sports hunting.

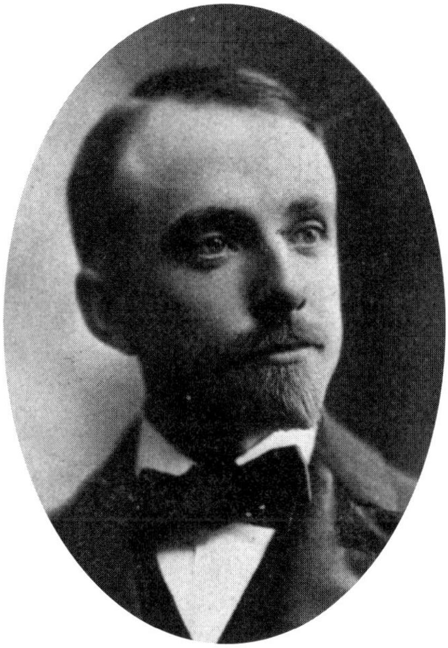

Dr. Chevalier Q. Jackson (*Carnegie Library of Pittsburgh*)

It was on one of his long hunting trips to the Bighorn Mountains in the late 1880s that Daly first encountered William F. (Buffalo Bill) Cody, and General Nelson A. Miles. As the story goes:

> Daly was in his camp one evening when a man on horseback "came tearing over the range," asking for a doctor to accompany him to examine a sick patient in a nearby camp. Daly agreed to go with him and successfully treated a young girl. The courier, as it turned out, was Buffalo Bill, and the grateful father of the young girl was General Miles. The three men became close friends and hunting companions over the next several years, and General Miles figured prominently in Daly's last term of military service.[6]

Little is known about the exact nature of Daly's subsequent hunting trips other than he went on several such excursions with General Miles and Bill Cody. While no first-hand descriptions of what transpired on these trips have been discovered, there are a few newspaper accounts that document when some of the trips occurred.

On 24 August 1892, the *Pittsburg Dispatch* noted in its "Social Chatter" column, "Dr. William H. Daly, contemplates six weeks' shooting in the West in the autumn."[7] Two months later, on 09 October 1892, the newspaper reported:

> The neighbors of Dr. Daly in the East End have been enjoying the luxury of prairie chicken the past few days. The doctor is just back from a flying trip of 1,200 miles to the prairies of the West. He made the trip in exactly one week and had four days of splendid shooting. General Miles, U.S.A. who in spite of his weakness for hunting Indians, descends once

> in a while to the more prosaic divertissement of hunting prairie chickens, was one of the sports, and the doctor's brother a third member. "It was an ideal trip," said doctor yesterday. The party got all the game it could get home and had a splendid time generally.[8]

Without the benefit of an actual written account from Daly, it is still easy to surmise what transpired using written descriptions of similar hunting trips left by Miles and others. Miles, in his "Hunting Large Game" account published in the *North American Review* in 1895, described some of his early hunting experiences in the region:

> My personal experience with game and hunting has been somewhat limited. During the years that I was in that wild country of the West, much of my time was devoted to hunting hostile Indians. In Kansas in the early part of 1870, I found some leisure, however, to devote to hunting buffalo with General Custer, who had a cavalry command near mine, and who was well equipped with horses and had a large pack of dogs. I also found much healthful exercise and recreation in hunting wild turkey, prairie chicken and quail, over the rolling prairies of Kansas, where there was plenty of cover in the wild grass, which yet was not so high but that we could see the intelligent and well-trained setters and pointers work to perfection. I preferred the prairie chicken to the quail as being a much better mark as well as a finer bird. The wild duck could be found in considerable numbers at that time in Western Kansas. In the timbered reaches of the "Rockies," the blue grouse were and are quite abundant.[9]

In the same account, Miles wrote about an early encounter with Buffalo Bill:

> During the construction of the transcontinental railroads, a large amount of game was killed for the use of the men employed in that work. In this way, William F. Cody made his reputation as a buffalo hunter. He was at that time a young man in his twenties, tall, stalwart and of magnificent physique—one of the handsomest and most powerful men I have ever known, with auburn locks of a golden hue, large, brilliant, dark eyes, and perfect features. He was a daring rider and a most expert rifleman. He excelled in the rush after game, and could kill more buffalo during a single run than any other man I have ever known.[10]

He later described his interest in hunting bighorn mountain sheep, a passion he most assuredly shared with Daly. Miles wrote:

> I regard the meat of the mountain sheep or big-horn, as the finest of all large game. The pursuit of this animal requires great skill, hard work, and dangerous climbing. They frequent the little mesas and ledges at the foot of precipitous cliffs. They are very keen-sighted and difficult to approach. When in repose they are usually found on little ledges where they can survey the country below. For this reason, the hunter aims to get above them, and is prepared to shoot at first sight.[11]

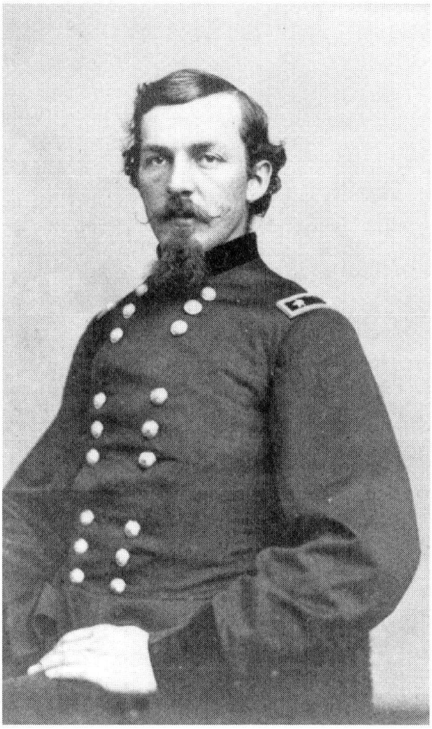

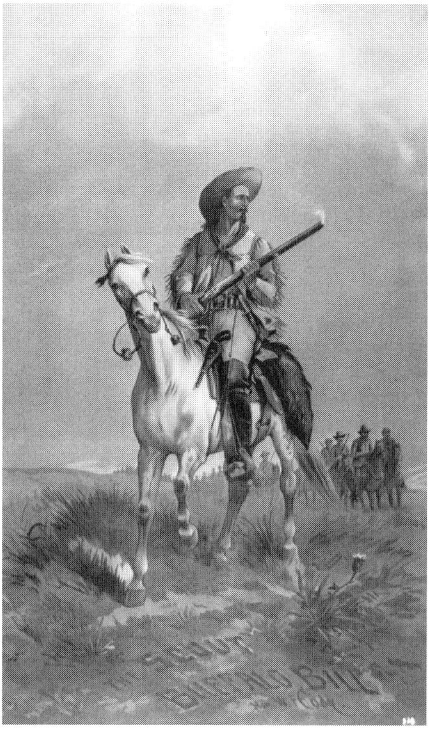

Above left: Nelson Appleton Miles, photograph taken between 1861 and 1870. (*Library of Congress*)

Above right: The scout Buffalo Bill Hon. W. F. Cody, 1872. (*Library of Congress*)

He also took great delight in hunting gray wolves.

One area of hunting that both Daly and Miles always agreed upon and is well documented is the breeding and use of hunting dogs. Miles stated: "There is, however, rarer sport than this to me in hunting the bear with a well-trained pack of dogs. Bear hunting is the most dangerous of all kinds of sport, and is uninteresting unless one is equipped with a well-trained pack of dogs."[12] William H. Daly and his brother, Thomas L. Daly, were both dog breeders. William preferred breeds best suited for waterfowl hunting. Thomas, on the other hand, fancied English Setters, which were better suited for big game hunting. In 1892, Thomas' gave one of his prize dogs to Nelson Miles. It was a black, white, and tan English Setter whelped on 28 April 1892.[13]

C. H. Morrill left another account of hunting trips with Cody and Miles. Morrill was a cattle baron, banker, and land speculator known for the important role he played in the development and early history of Nebraska. In his autobiography, Morrill wrote:

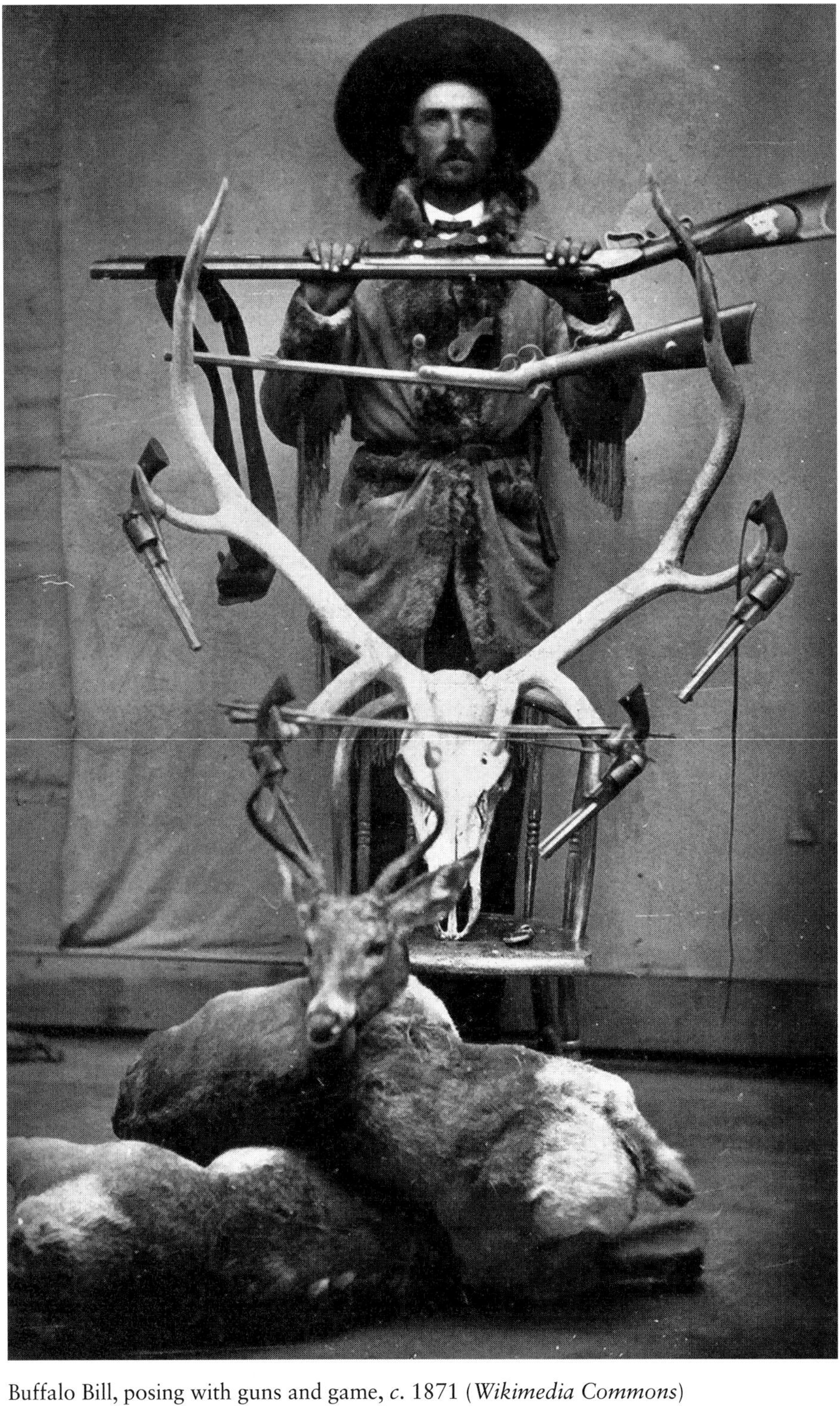

Buffalo Bill, posing with guns and game, *c.* 1871 (*Wikimedia Commons*)

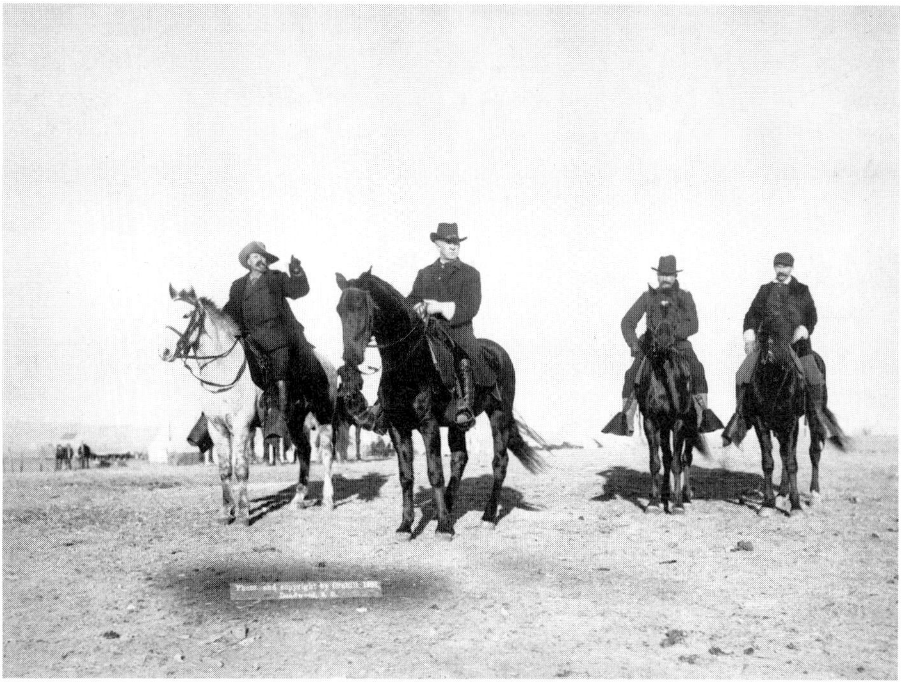

Buffalo Bill, Nelson A. Miles, Captain Frank Baldwin, and Captain Marion P. Maus on horseback viewing hostile Indian camp, 1891. (*Library of Congress*)

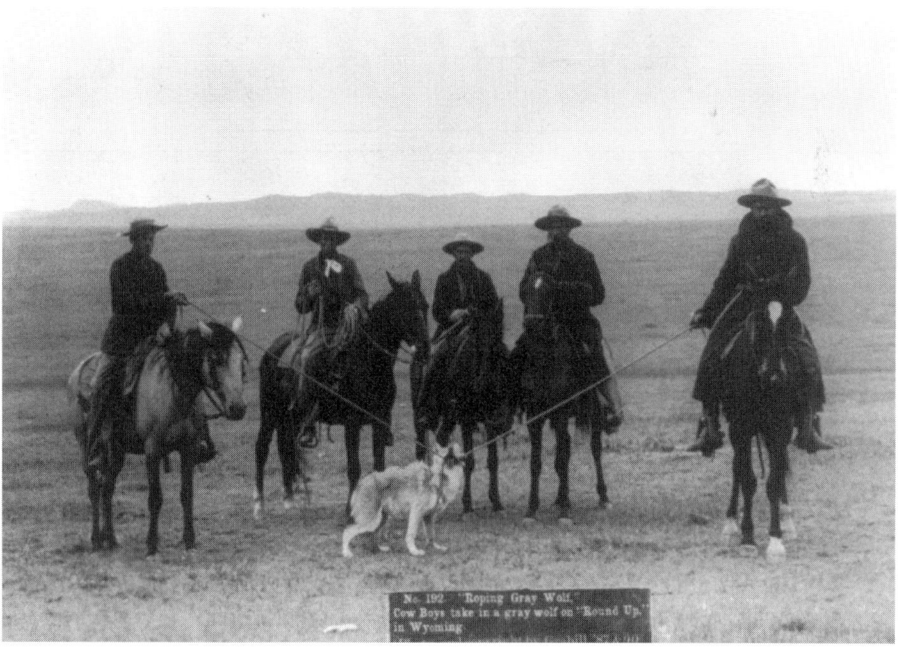

Cowboys take in a gray wolf on round up in Wyoming, 1887. (*Library of Congress*)

> On one of my trips to the Big Horn Basin in company with Mr. T. E. Calvert, we met General Nelson A. Miles of the United States army, and Colonel W. F. Cody (Buffalo Bill). They had just returned to Cody, Wyoming, from a trip up the southern fork of the Shoshone River, where they had been spending a vacation at Colonel Cody's hunting preserves, known as the T. E. ranch. This ranch was located about fifty miles west of the town of Cody, very near the borderline of Yellowstone Park. The mountains on either side of the Shoshone River are lofty and come close together, and it is a rugged and wonderfully picturesque place. To see the sky one must look almost straight up. In all my travels I have never seen a mountain ranch with so many attractions. General Miles had, during different Indian wars, traversed this entire country many times.[14]

On 09 November 1899, another news article highlighting a Daly hunting trip was printed in *The Billings Gazette*: "M. B. Cooper of Garner, Iowa, Major I. D. Black of Valley City, N.D., and Dr. W. H. Daly of Pittsburg, Pa., were in the city yesterday, returning from a hunting trip in Wyoming, south of Red Lodge."[15] Red Lodge was a prime big game hunting locale in southern Montana nestled in the Beartooth Mountains. It was close to Billings, Montana; Cody, Wyoming; and Yellowstone National Park. While in Billings, Montana, the trio stayed at the Grand Hotel.

Little is known about Major Black; however, it is likely he was a military officer associated with General Miles. At the time, evidence suggests Bill Cody was encouraging Miles to become an investor in his Shoshone Irrigation Company, which he hoped would allow him and his partners to develop Cody, Wyoming, Buffalo Bill's new namesake town located approximately 100 miles southeast of Sheridan, Wyoming. Whether or not Miles knew about the land speculation scheme of Cody and his partners, there was little doubt the Shoshone project was in financial trouble. Miles was nevertheless interested because the Burlington Railroad was expected to make a decision soon about bringing a spur line to the town. Assuming the irrigation project could be finished, and the railroad line added, there was no doubt the planned town would be a huge financial success.

With Cody's encouragement, Miles agreed to invite other potential investors to the area. As author Robert E. Bonner noted, hunting season was Cody's favorite time of year, and in fall 1899, "There was other big game on his mind as well. Early in October, he wrote that General Nelson Miles would surely be coming this year, with a party of nine around the 26th. Some of these men were wealthy enough that he did not want it generally known that they were coming; he expected that Miles and some of the others would want to invest."[16]

The Daly brothers and William's brother-in-law, M. B. Cooper, were considered good candidates and the timing of their trip was fortuitous. While the trip is well documented, and all three are known to have made numerous real estate investments, there is no evidence that Cooper or the Daly brothers invested in Cody's venture.

M. B. Cooper was Athalia's brother who owned farmlands and raised cattle in Garner, Iowa. William and Athalia would visit him and his family on many

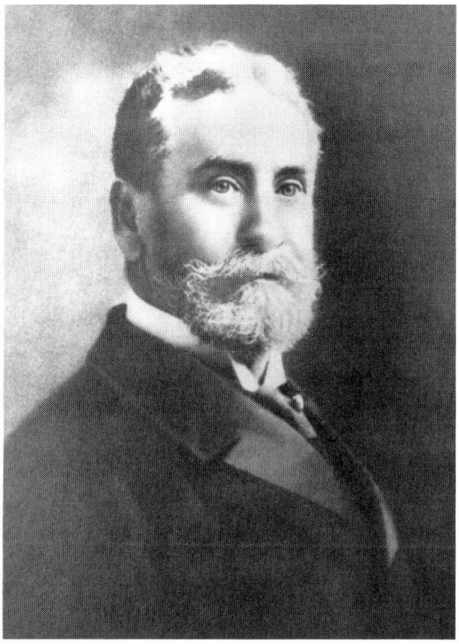

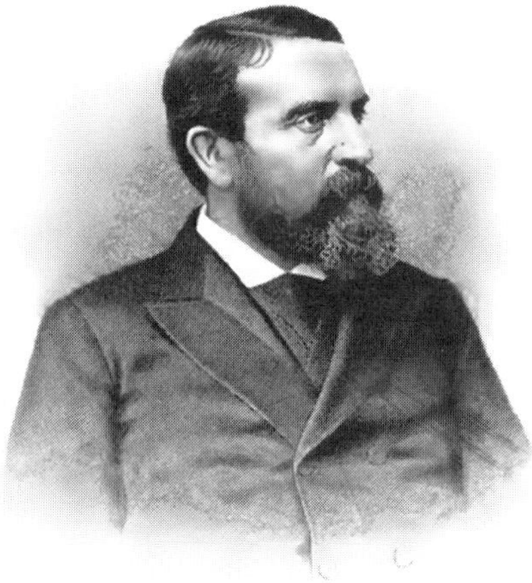

Above left: William H. Daly, president of the Allegheny County Medical Society, 1881. (*Allegheny County Medical Society*)

Above right: Thomas Lafayette Daly. (*History of the County of Westmoreland, Pennsylvania.* (*Philadelphia: L. H. Everts & Co., 1882*)

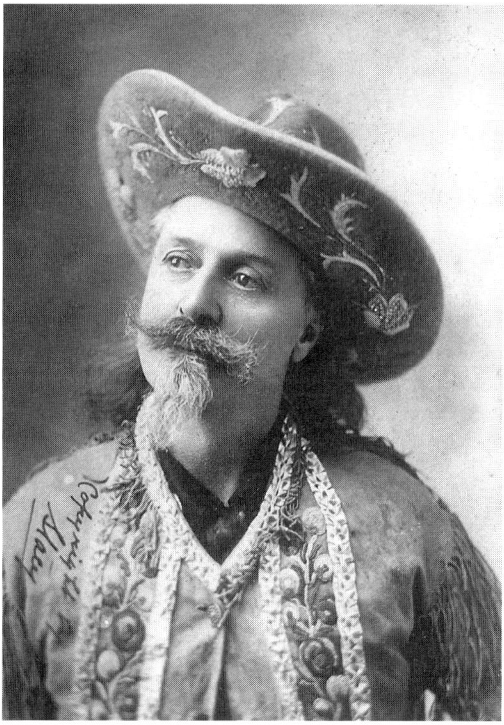

Cabinet card of Buffalo Bill Cody by Stacy, *c.* 1890. (*Wikimedia Commons*)

of their trips to the west. Cooper participated in only a few of Daly's hunting trips; however, the November 1899 trip was one in which he did. The occasion was memorable, but not for the prospect of land speculation or hunting. Several days after their return, on 22 November 1899, Athalia Daly died at her brother's home.

Athalia typically accompanied William on his hunting trips to the west, but she did not participate in the sport. Instead, she preferred to stay with her relatives in Iowa where she often found interest in working with American Indian women. In this regard, she is recorded as expressing "her own deep concern for elevating the station of Indian women on reservations. She helped to establish schools on the reservations and, from her home in Pittsburgh, regularly sold American Indian-made lace to Pittsburgh matrons."[17]

Athalia's death resulted from acute Bright's disease (chronic inflammation of the kidneys). Her sudden death had a profound dilatory effect on Daly's mental health and left him in a deep state of melancholic depression. After her passing, William temporarily lost interest in big game hunting and expansion of his medical practice. He did, however, continue to enjoy short hunting trips with family members, but restricted his practice primarily to routine office and hospital work.

Notwithstanding his bereavement and concomitant emotional anguish, military matters also still seemed to hold his attention. On 15 May 1894, some months after returning from one of his hunting trips with General Miles, Daly received a letter from the U.S. Surgeon General George Miller Sternberg's office. The letter inquired:

> ... are you identical with Dr. W. H. Daly late Acting Assistant Surgeon who has been reported as serving on duty as AAS (Acting Assistant Surgeon) at White Hall U.S.A. General Hospital from about May or June 1864 until February 1865 then on duty at Jacksonville Fla. and Hilton Head, S.C., Savannah, GA, during Summer of 1865 (the summer the war ended) at time war closed was Post Surgeon at Hilton Head, S.C.[18]

The inquiry appears to have been received quite unexpectedly, as Daly responded affirmatively but questioned "may I ask what this information is for?"[19] No response to his question has been discovered. It is likely the request for background information on Daly was initiated by General Miles, who was contemplating yet another military engagement for his friend and hunting companion.

Miles and Daly had many opportunities to talk about their military careers while hunting and socializing. Both men had extraordinary prior military experiences. Whether or not they discussed a new military role for Daly between 1894 and 1897 is unknown, but an answer may be found in the fact that Daly was once again called into military service by Miles in early 1898 as the country moved ever closer to war with Spain.

8

Carvin' Spaniards in the Mornin'

Elected president of the American Laryngological, Rhinological, and Otological Society in 1897, it was William H. Daly's responsibility to deliver opening remarks at the society's fourth annual meeting in Pittsburgh on Wednesday 11 May 1898. It was the first day of a two-day meeting being held in the parlors of Pittsburgh's Hotel Lincoln.

It was a magnificent morning in the city and Daly could not have been happier. He had risen rapidly to a leadership role in the young society; his clinical reputation, research, and writing provided prominence in the specialty that could only be matched by a handful of others in the country at the time. He was likewise thrilled to be in a position to attract so many of his illustrious colleagues to the city as he noted in his opening remarks:

> I have much honor and pleasure in bidding you a hearty welcome to our city. I am sure you will all experience an agreeable surprise, on this your first visit here, since the just reputation of Pittsburg being a vast manufacturing center, has also made it to be regarded, as only remarkable for that distinction; but you will, notwithstanding, also find other things of vast proportions, that will appeal to your higher and esthetic senses.
>
> Here we have hundreds of acres of public parks, just now presenting an unexcelled beauty of hill, and dale, and vista. The public conservatory of plants, a present from a generous citizen, Henry Phipps, is equal to the best in the country; and Carnegie Music Hall, Library, and Museum, a gift of the noble Pittsburger whose name it bears, is in keeping with the most liberal expenditure, and advanced taste of this wonderful age. Without over stepping the bounds of modesty, we may say Pittsburg, therefore, like good, old wine, "needs no bush," and, while you have brought us rich presents of scientific value in learned lore, as indicated in the charming programme before us, reaching, as it does, from our distinguished *confrère*, Lennox Browne

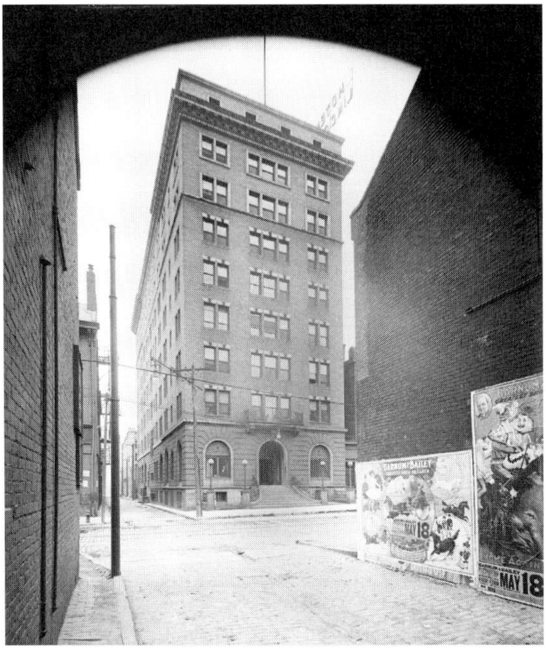

Hotel Lincoln, Pittsburgh, *c.* 1900. (*Library of Congress*)

> of London, to Massei of Naples, with other learned lights in our profession from the great cities of our own land. We, with grateful hearts, your Pittsburg members, through me, thank you deeply for having honored us. We are twice honored, in fact as well as in sentiment, for it was in this city, two years ago, that the older national organization of laryngologists, which we all revere, for its high scientific work, met, with just the same number of papers to be read and discussed, *viz.*: thirty-four, and, also, with your present speaker as its President. Truly, Pittsburg has been honored, and your speaker placed under a debt of gratitude, for the kindliest partiality, and consideration, that any man can ever receive from distinguished *confréres*, whose names are as house hold words, in all the higher planes of thought, in laryngology, rhinology, and otology. What more can I say, than to express a personal pride to you in being, as you are well aware of, unsolicited on my part, called to the office of your President? This honor is all the more touching, since the membership is largely made up of the young men, whose names are not only the glory and pride of laryngology, but men whose writings and discussions are read with avidity, that speaks without saying it, that they are of the highest scientific and analytical value.[1]

Daly was little more than midway through his opening comments when an urgent telegram arrived shortly after 10 a.m. Momentarily distracted, he anxiously read the message.[2] He was being called to military service. On 09 May, his friend, General Nelson A. Miles, was given orders to assemble an army of 70,000 men for the invasion of Cuba. Daly was to be a part of this deployment. The message stated Daly was to report for immediate active duty.

It was a moment he had thought possible, but not fully anticipated once Congress declared war on Spain on 20 April 1898. War fever had been rampant since the U.S. battleship *Maine* exploded in Havana harbor on 15 February 1898 with more than 250 officers and enlisted men killed, and things were moving fast. Nevertheless, the telegram was still a surprise. As Miles later commented: "The feeling at that time in the country was one of impatience, amounting almost to impetuosity, and the cry of 'On to Havana' was similar to that of 'On to Richmond' in June of 1861."[3]

During his hunting trips with General Miles and Buffalo Bill, they had often spoken about their military service and Daly had frequently mused about a return to military life. Talk over a campfire was one thing; actual orders in hand another. As he read the message, it took time for reality to fully register. The telegram contained orders for him to arrive in Washington, D.C., by mid-May to join the personal staff of General Miles, Commanding General of the U.S. Army. Upon concluding his opening remarks, Daly quickly made arrangements to turn chairmanship of the meeting over to Dr. S. E. Solly so he could leave the session to respond to the telegram.[4]

Daly later returned to the meeting. He reported to the group—with pride and patriotic fervor—he was to be commissioned major and chief surgeon, U.S. Volunteers, and he would depart for Washington, D.C., on 15 May. From Washington, he informed society members, he would leave by train with General Miles and other staff to travel to Tampa, Florida, where they would establish headquarters to begin preparations for a planned invasion of Cuba.

Members of the Society rushed to organize a banquet to honor the soon-to-be-deployed president. On 12 May, a dinner was held at the Duquesne Club, during which Daly offered his farewell. Members responded with a long goodbye and a song:

> This song written impromptu by a member of the American Laryngological, Rhinological, and Otological Association, Dr. Frank Harcourt Koyle, of Hornellsville, N.Y. and sung by members at their banquet to the tune of "Off to Philadelphia in the Morning," at their annual meeting at the Duquesne Club, Pittsburg, Pa., the evening of May 12, 1898, humorously celebrating the then sudden departure, and the goodbyes to Dr. W. H. Daly their President, just leaving the Banquet Hall, under orders of General Miles, Commander in chief of the U. S. Armies for the War in Cuba. And although the song is written impromptu in a humorous vein for, and at the wish of the American Laryngological, Rhinological and Otological Association, in the mellow haze of Pittsburg smoke, and under a somewhat similar condition of mind, suggesting the unique and unerring hospitality of Dr. Daly which they were then enjoying. It is affectionately dedicated to him, "The Grand Old Man" of the Association, who only a few short hours before to our infinite surprise notified us

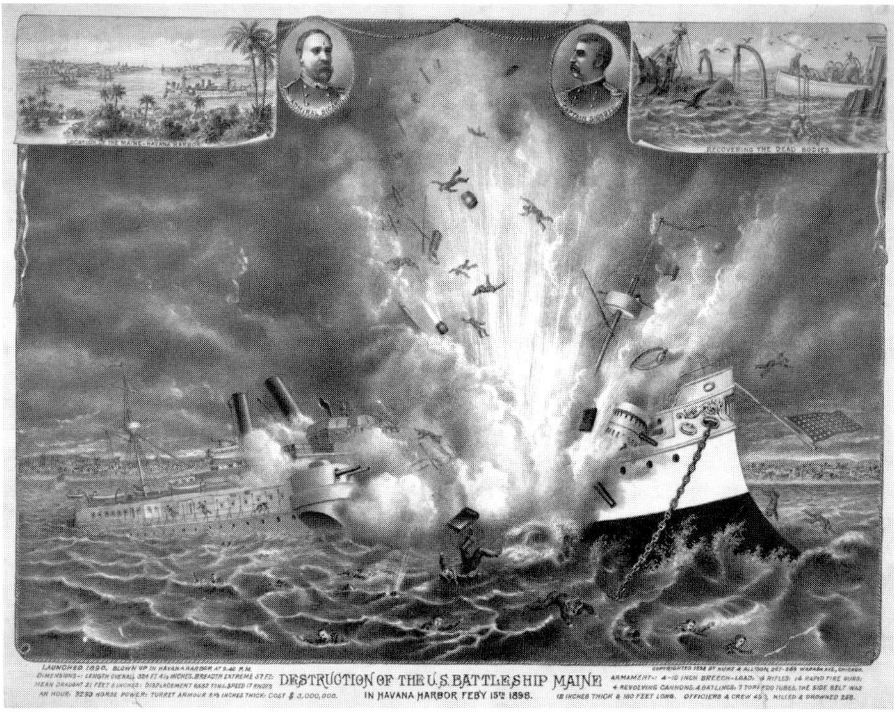

Destruction of the U.S. battleship *Maine* in Havana Harbor, 15 February 1898. (*Library of Congress*)

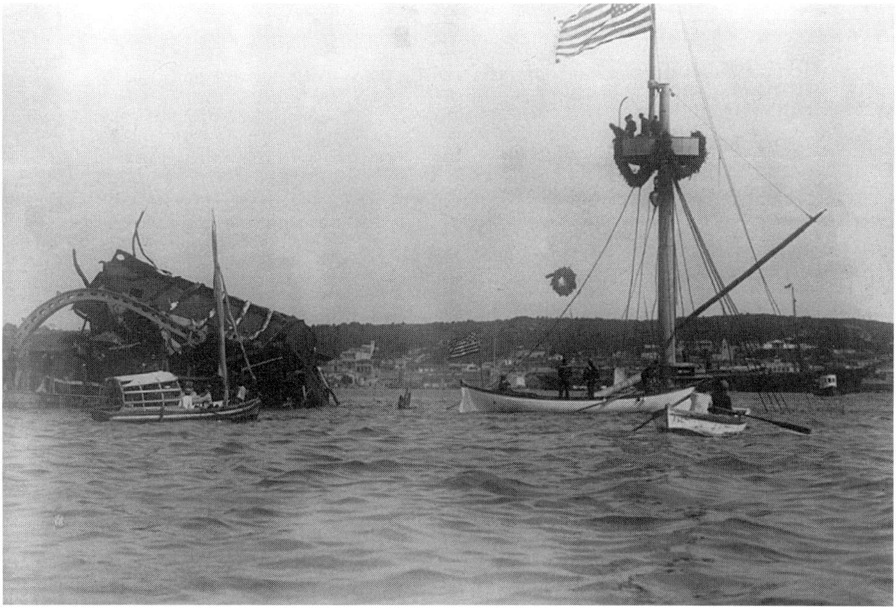

Destruction of *Maine*, Havana Harbor, Cuba, 1898. (*Library of Congress*)

that he leaves tonight to serve our flag and our country in the War against Spain, for the freedom of Cuba. No one more noble, brave, nor skillful, could have been chosen from the profession of which he is a beloved and distinguished representative, and as a national medical body we feel honored to have had one of ours selected to fill the high position to which he has been called, upon the staff of the General Commanding the Armies of the U.S. as Chief Surgeon with rank of Major U.S. Vols. and no more affectionate goodwill goes with him, our dear president and friend, Major William H. Daly, Chief Surgeon U.S. Vols., than that of Frank Harcourt Koyle, the author.

The song was called "I Shtart to free ould Cuba in the Mornin'"

(1) Oh, me name is William H. Daly,
And a scalpel and a shillaleh
I can handle any minute widout warnin',
Wid a good black thorn forninst me,
He'll get hurt who runs ag'inst me
When I shtart to free ould Cuba in the mornin'.

CHORUS: But tho' me black thorn's on me shoulder
Faith there's no man could be boulder;
Though I'm lavin' now the shpot that I was born in,
For I lately tak the notion for to cross the briny ocean,
And I shtart to free ould Cuba in the mornin'.

(2) Whin Miles tould me I must lave this place
I tried to kape a cheerful face,
For a bottle and a hot bird I'm not scornin';
But I trust yez will not mind me,
If I lave yez dhrunk behind me,
And I hope yez'll have no headache in the mornin'.

CHORUS: For 'tis dhrunk yez will be gettin'
If yez keep your t(h)roats a wettin'
Iv'ry toime yez drink a liquor widout corn in,
Shtick to high-balls of good whiskey,
Tho' they make yez somewhat frisky,
And the hat of aich will fit yez in the mornin'.

(3) And I hope that iv'ry sinner
Who is prisint at this dinner,
Will forget he has a shpot that has a thorn in;
And we'll drink to our President Daly, who wid scalpel and shillaleh,
Makes his start for carvin' Spaniards in the mornin'.

CHORUS: For me black thorn's on me shoulder,
And there's no man could be boulder
Tho' I'm lavin' now the shpot that I was born in;
Miles and me has tuk the notion for to cross the briny ocean,
And we shtart out to free ould Cuba in the mornin'.

(4) There's a place that I'll not mintion,
Paved wid many a good intintion;
'Tis the place the Spanish Dons will be adornin',
For I've just got my Commission,
And me bhoys wid your permission,
Wid the Dons I'll raise hell's blazes in the mornin'.

CHORUS: Wid me shtraps upon me shoulder,
And me courage niver boulder,
We will carve the bloody Dons as sure as thunder;
And the pleasure will be mine
Whin I luk upon thim dyin;
For at carvin' yez all know byes I'm a wonder.

(5) And whin the War is over,
Won't the Cubans be in clover,
As they see their bloody inimies lave for Cadiz,
We will tell thim our idea(r)
Was to come and make thim freer,
And to give them haughty Dons a taste of Hades.

CHORUS: For 'tis surely up ag'inst us
To defeat the foe forninist us,
And yez know me byes a bullet cannot harm me
So wid Miles and me a-leadin'
Shure the Dons will soon be pleadin'
Before us two who lead the mighty Army.[5]

During the dinner, Daly was also presented with a special sword as a sign of affection and respect. In August 1898, he wrote an acknowledgment in the *Pennsylvania Medical Journal* thanking members of the Society for "the handsome presentation sword ... an attention I appreciate and value most highly"[6]

Daly left Pittsburg by train as planned on the morning of 15 May 1898. Several days later, on 28 May, he received his commission signed by President William McKinley.[7] Late on the evening of 30 May, Daly accompanied General Miles, the General's family, and a host of other command staff as they departed Washington,

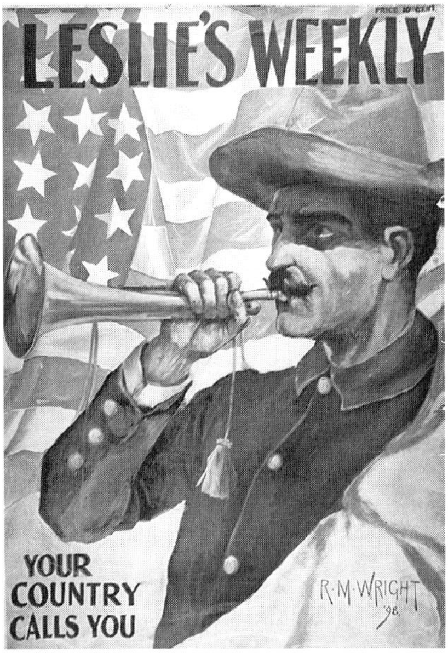

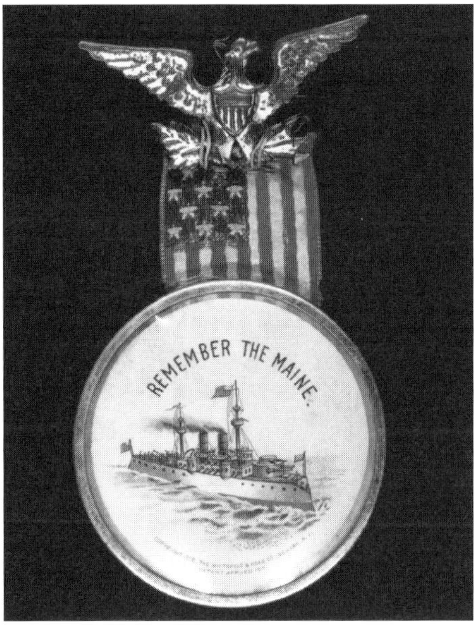

Above left: Your Country Calls You. Cover of *Leslie's Weekly* magazine, June 30, 1898. (*National Archives and Records Administration*)

Above right: Remember the *Maine* badge, 1898.

Below: Puck Magazine centerfold "Save me from my friends." Uncle Sam wearing a sword and using the American flag to shield a woman labeled "Cuba Libre" from three men wearing hats labeled "Insurgent Leader;" they are standing on soil labeled "Cuba" and shows the "U.S." as just across a narrow body of water. Puck, Volume 44, Number 1122, 07 September 1898. (*Library of Congress*)

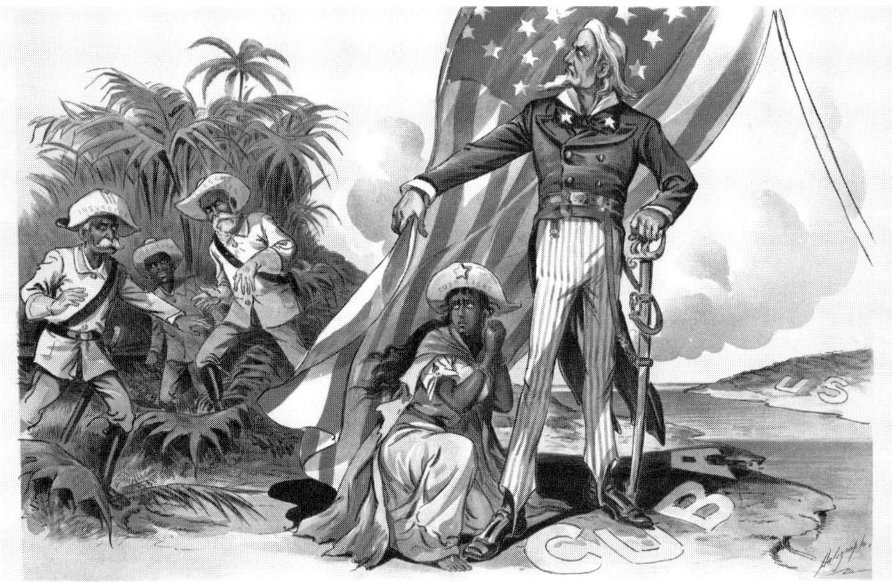

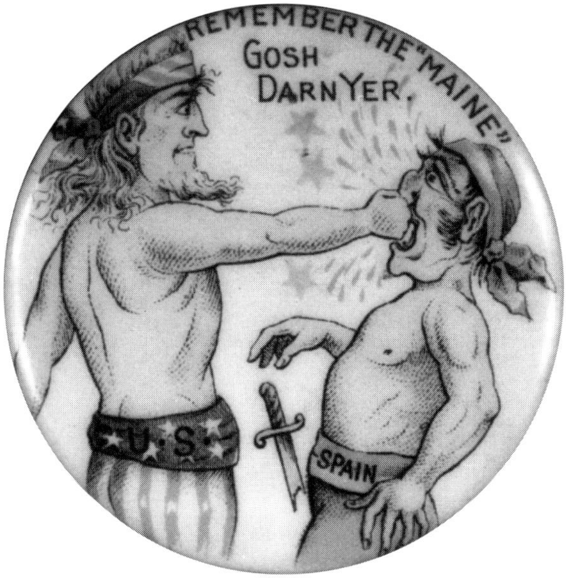

Remember the "Maine" Gosh Darn Yer pinback button manufactured by Whitehead and Hoag Company, 1898.

D.C., *en route* to Tampa, Florida. The next morning, a newspaper article made a note of the departure:

> Major General Nelson A. Miles, commanding the United States army, accompanied by the members of his family and his personal and official staff, left at 11 o'clock last night for Tampa, Fla. The party comprising the 64 persons occupied a special train on the Southern railway, consisting of one Pullman sleeping car, one special car, one combination baggage and day coach, and one baggage car. Secretary (Secretary of War Russell A. Alger) and Mrs. Alger were at the Sixth street station to see the party off, as were also about a hundred other persons, friends, and relatives of the officers. No demonstration of any kind occurred as the distinguished party took its leave.
>
> Gen. Miles will proceed directly to Tampa, where he will establish temporarily the headquarters of the army. He will personally direct the movements of the troops and the invasion of Cuba.
>
> Following is the personnel of the party which left last night: General Miles, Mrs. Miles, Miss Miles, and A. Herman Miles; General Rodgers, General Stone, Colonel Maus, Colonel Michler. Colonel Osgood, Major Daly, Chief Surgeon, Major Sayburn, Major Davis, Captain Alger, Lieutenant Rowan, Lieutenant Parker, and Lieutenant Townsley.
>
> General Collaze and Colonel Herandez, of the Cuban army, were of the party as were also privates of the Sixth cavalry who will act as orderlies and eleven secretaries and clerks.[8]

Nothing is known about what occurred on the train ride to Tampa, which arrived on 01 June. In his 31 July 1898 report to George Miller Sternberg, Surgeon General

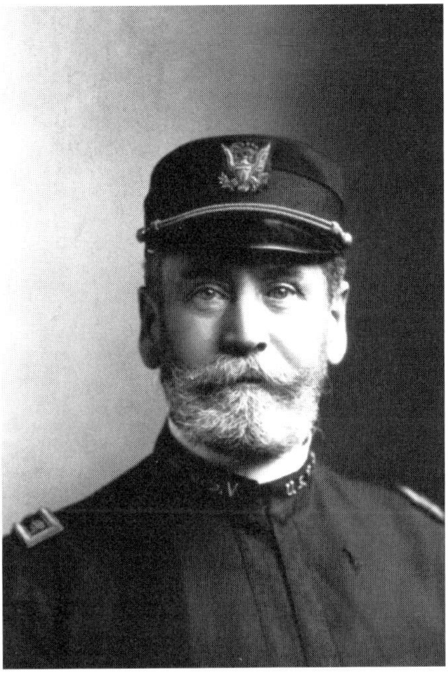

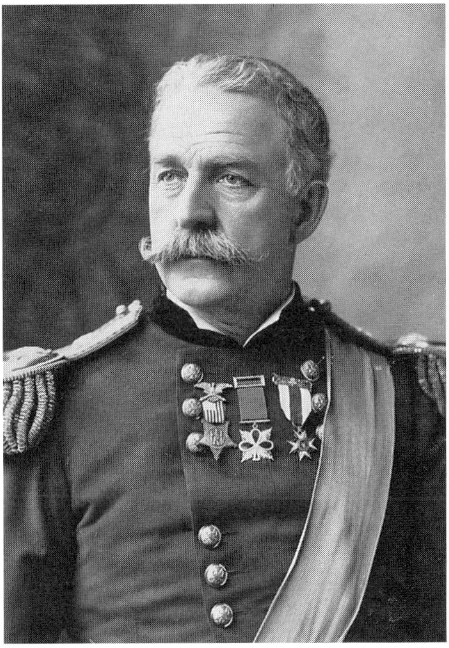

Above left: William Hudson Daly in military uniform, *c*. 1899. (*National Library of Medicine*)

Above right: General Nelson A. Miles by Brands Studios, 1898. (*Wikimedia Commons*)

of the U.S. Army, Daly indicated he was already in Ponce, Porto Rico (present-day Puerto Rico). At the time the report was written, he noted he was stationed there at Headquarters of the Army under the War Department's Standing Order 125, dated 28 May 1898. He also specified he had been *en route* to Porto Rico from 9–26 July and on duty at Headquarters in Porto Rico between 26 and 31 July.[9]

By the time Daly wrote his report, the Spanish-American War was already well underway. On 28 May, Major General William Rufus Shafter received orders to mobilize troops in Tampa for an attack on Cuba. By 06 June, Santiago de Cuba was under siege by the U.S. Navy in an attempt to soften Spanish coastal defenses. On the same day, General Miles received final plans from the War Department for a joint U.S.–Cuban Liberation Army attack.

After delays caused by concern over a reported Spanish war armada assembling along the northern coast of Cuba, the invasion expedition finally set sail from Tampa on 14 June. On 22 June, Shafter's troops, including Theodore Roosevelt's Rough Riders, landed on shore and began their march toward Santiago. Miles later lamented: "As most of the regular Army was included in this expedition, and on account of the importance of the enterprise, I desired to go with it but was directed to return to Washington."[10]

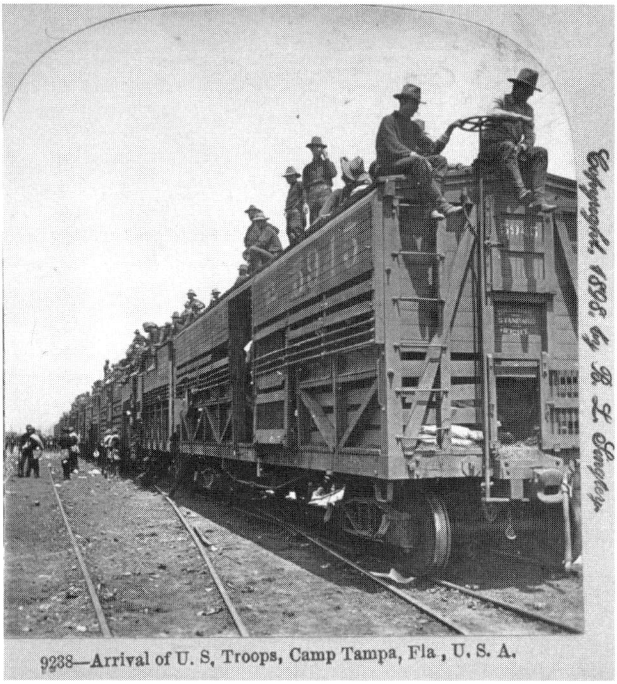

Arrival of U.S. troops at Camp Tampa, Florida, 1898. (*Library of Congress*)

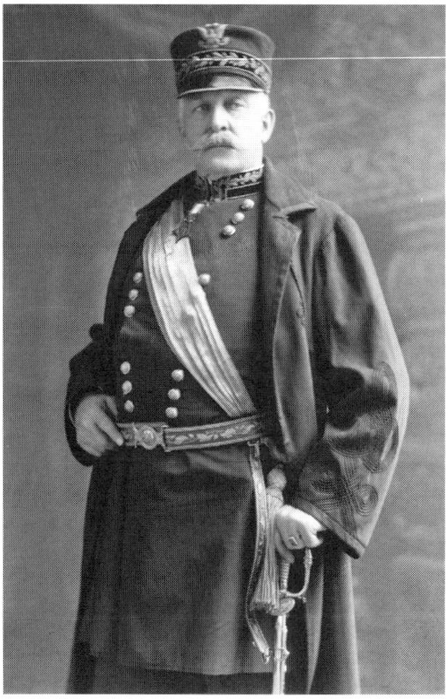

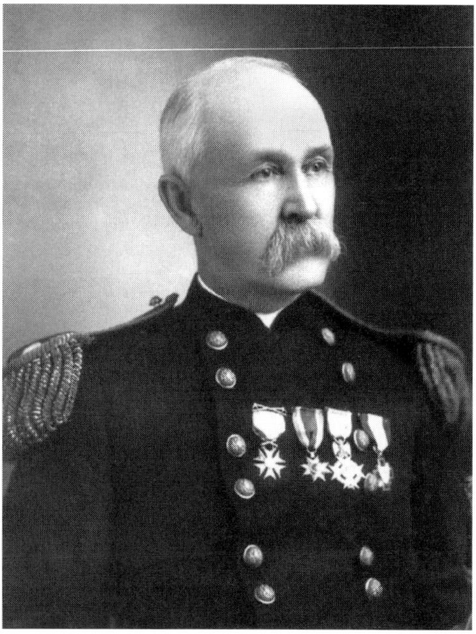

Above left: General Nelson A. Miles, 1894. (*Library of Congress*)

Above right: General George Miller Sternberg, U.S. Army Surgeon General, 1893–1902. (*Wikimedia Commons*)

In Washington, Miles expressed concern about the proposed timing of the invasion. He later wrote:

> I sent the necessary orders for the movement of the advance corps, and instructions as to its landing on the north coast of Cuba; and supplies for ninety days for the men and thirty days for the animals were ordered concentrated at Tampa, Florida. It is with great reluctance that one hesitates to accept the command of an army of that magnitude in the field; yet, knowing the condition of the troops, the strength of the enemy, and the near approach of the sickly season in a district infested with yellow fever, I considered it my duty not only to the troops, whose lives must necessarily be sacrificed, but to the country, to explain fully to the highest authority the serious objections to such a movement at that time, and also to express my regret that I felt called upon to state such objections.[11]

The concerns the general expressed to Secretary of War Alger about yellow fever and other infectious diseases were well founded. Such diseases would later prove to the cause of more fatalities than injuries resulting from wounds received in battle. At the time, Miles also communicated apprehension about the lack of adequate food supplies and the ability of the Commissary General to overcome logistical and food quality issues in supplying the Army. By the end of the war, his angst in all the above regards proved prophetic. The same concerns would soon consume the remainder of Daly's military career and life.

Miles left Washington for Santiago on 07 July. In an article published in the *North American Review*, he recalled:

> At a council of war held at the White House on the next day (06 July), the subject was seriously considered, and it was then decided that the garrison at Santiago must be destroyed or captured; and it was also decided that I should proceed immediately to Santiago and take such measures as would accomplish that object. It was my purpose to land the troops that were then en route to Santiago on the west side of the harbor, within two and a half miles of Morro Castle, and I left with the assurance that I would have all necessary assistance from Admiral Sampson's fleet.
>
> I left Washington on the 7th of July and reached Columbia, South Carolina, on the 8th, and thence proceeded by special train to Charleston, at which place I arrived on the evening of the same day and immediately boarded the swift steamer *Yale*, the Atlantic liner, better known as the *Paris*, which was already loaded with troops, ready to heave anchor, off the harbor and city of Charleston. She was accompanied and convoyed by the U.S.S. *Columbia*, also carrying troops. At midnight these two fleet steamers headed for the south with all possible speed and arrived off the harbor of Santiago on the morning of July 11th, while the fleet there gathered was still bombarding the works near Santiago harbor. I immediately communicated with

> Admiral Sampson, apprising him of my purpose, and he promptly came on board the *Yale*. I at once acquainted him with my plan of operation, in which he cordially acquiesced and signified his readiness to support me heartily in carrying it out. As soon as the necessary arrangements could be made for that purpose, I landed on July 12th, and proceeded to General Shafter's headquarters.[12]

Nine days later, on 15 July 1898, forces under Spanish commander José Torál surrendered with approximately 12,000 troops taken prisoner. By 17 July, the Battle for Santiago was over, and control of the island certain.

Based on Daly's 31 July report, the 07 July date of Miles's departure from Washington, D.C., for Santiago, Cuba, and the 20 July date when General Miles departed Guantánamo, Cuba, for Porto Rico, it is reasonable to conclude that Daly joined Miles before he sailed to Cuba. This sequence of dates also makes it probable that Daly was among the 3,300 troops that left Guantánamo on nine transport ships on 20 July. Since the convoy is known to have arrived at Guánica, Porto Rico, on 25 July, the date also aligns with Daly's report of being on duty at Headquarters in (Ponce) Porto Rico (Guánica lies approximately 20 miles east of Ponce) beginning on the 26 July.

The capture of the city of Ponce was an important action supporting the U.S. invasion of Porto Rico. As the island's largest city, it had a good port, excellent roads, and important communication infrastructure that allowed easy movement of troops and supplies. American troops began landing at Ponce on 27 July; the next morning, General Miles and a large contingent of reinforcements arrived from Guánica. Upon arrival, and as indicated by Daly's report, Miles established headquarters in Ponce from which he directed further military action against Spanish troops who had retreated from the city and taken up positions in the surrounding mountains.

Daly's next "Personal Report" to Surgeon General Sternberg was sent from Ponce on 31 August 1898. He reported that from 01–28 August 1898 he was on duty with Headquarters of the Army, "inspecting, cleansing and organizing hospitals and barracks, attending sick and etc." This communication also offered details of a new responsibility he had been assigned. His report stated from 28–31 August 1898, under Special Field Order No. 37, Headquarters of the Army, he was on duty "in command of transport Steamer *Panama*, preparing same for use for transporting convalescents to the United States."[13]

Compared to the Civil War, the level of wounds and disease encountered during the Spanish-American War was substantially less. However, similar to what occurred during the Civil War and as previously noted, the percentage of deaths caused by disease was much higher than those caused by wounds. Vincent Cirillo, in his study of military medicine during the Spanish-American War, notes: "Hostilities lasted only four months, and the number of dead (345 from combat, 2,565 from disease) paled in comparison to those in the U.S. Civil War (204,070 from combat, 388,586 from disease)."[14]

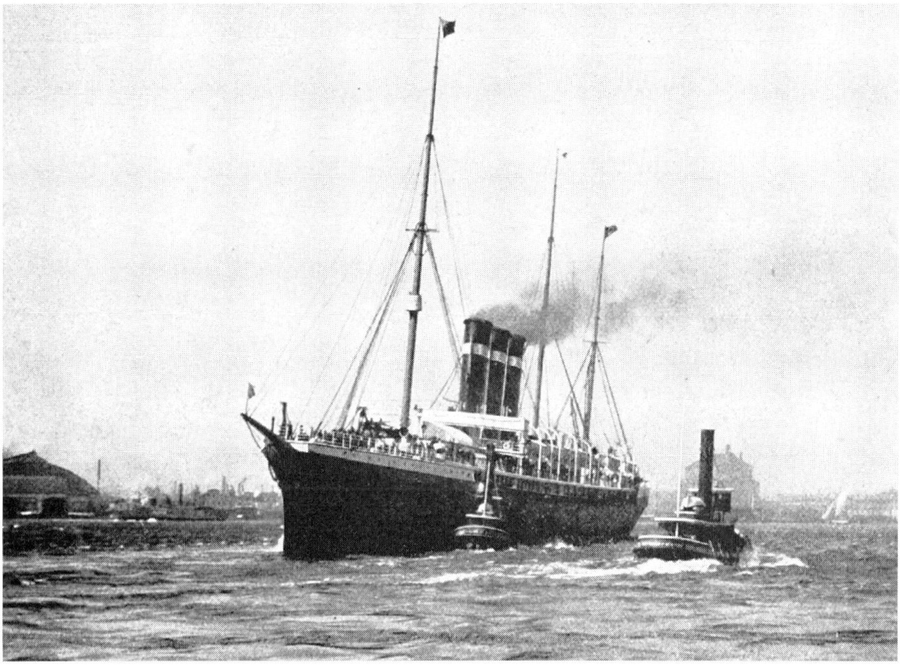

U.S.S. *Yale*. Photographs of the Great Spanish-American War, L. Nichols & Co., 1898. (*Library of Congress*)

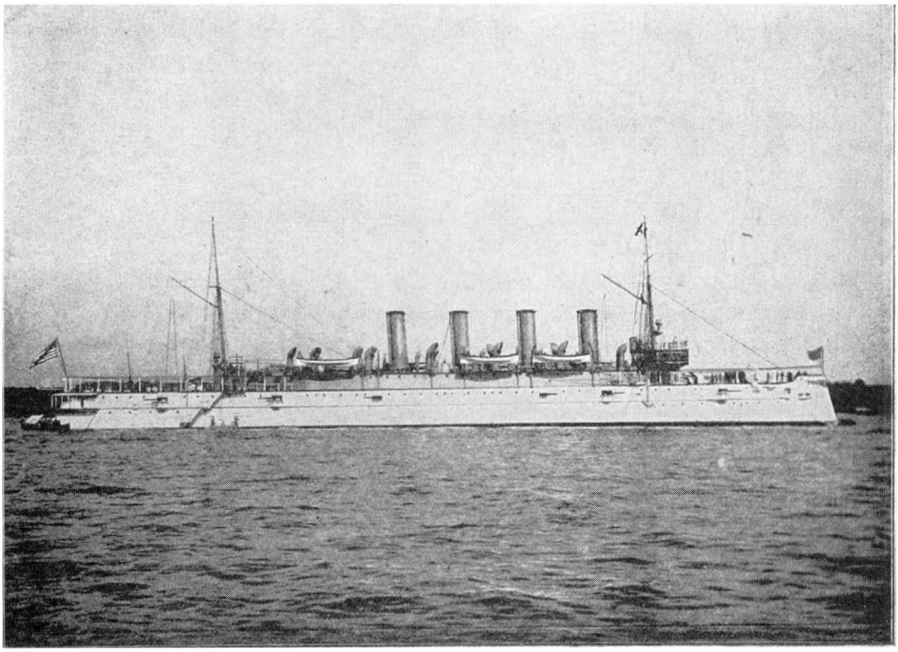

U.S.S. *Columbia*. Photographs of the Great Spanish-American War, L. Nichols & Co., 1898. (*Library of Congress*)

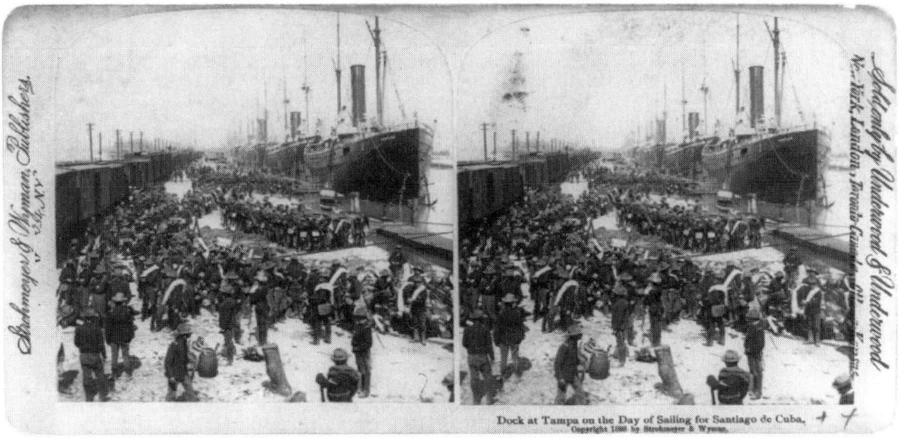

Soldiers on dock between railroad cars and ships at Tampa on the day of sailing for Santiago de Cuba, 1898. (*Library of Congress*)

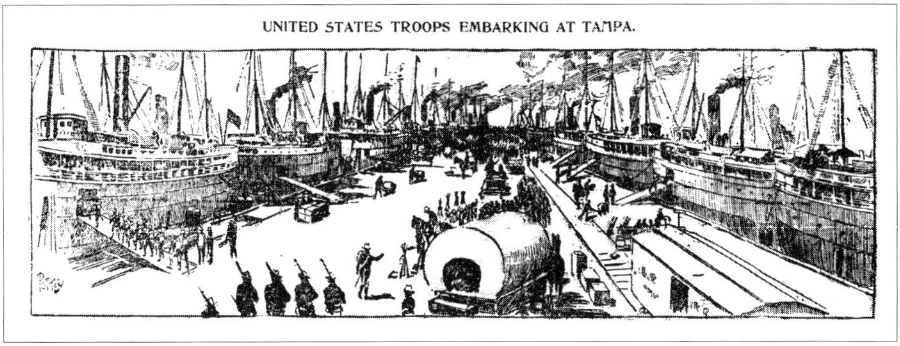

Troops embarking at Tampa. (*The Salt Lake Herald*, 31 May 1898)

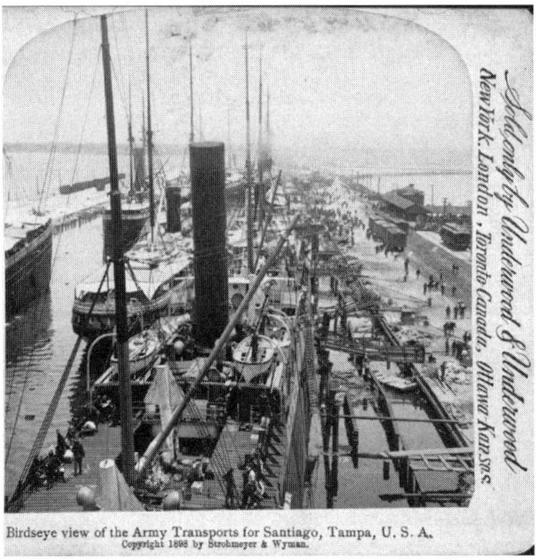

Birdseye view of the Army transports for Santiago, Tampa, U.S.A. (*Library of Congress*)

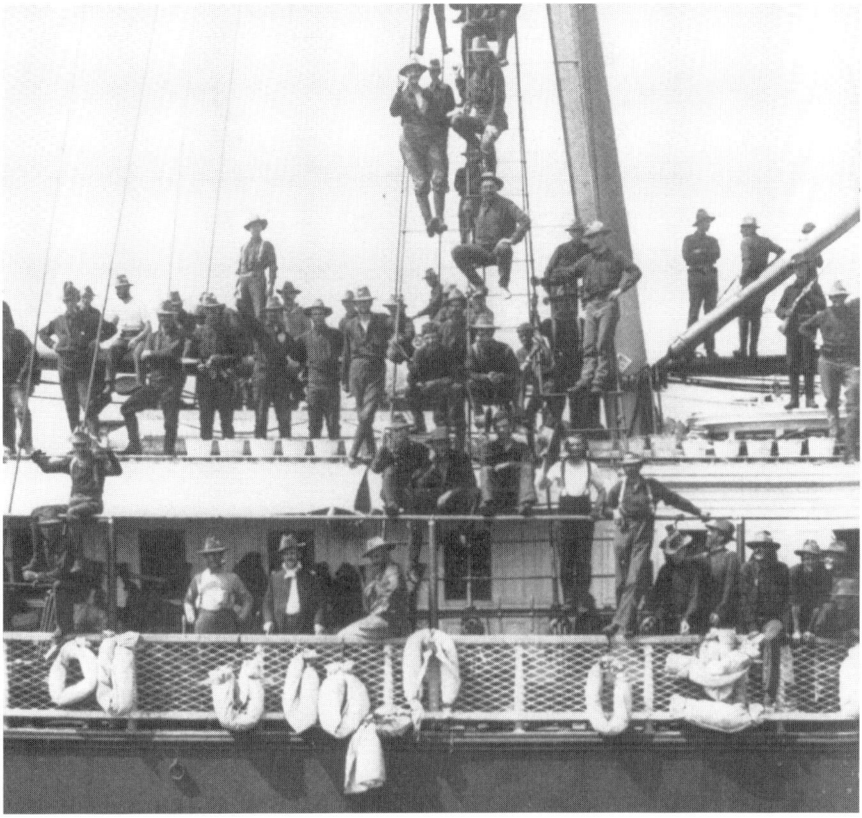

U.S.S. *Yucatan* carrying the Teddy Roosevelt's "Rough Riders" to Cuba, 1898. (*Library of Congress*)

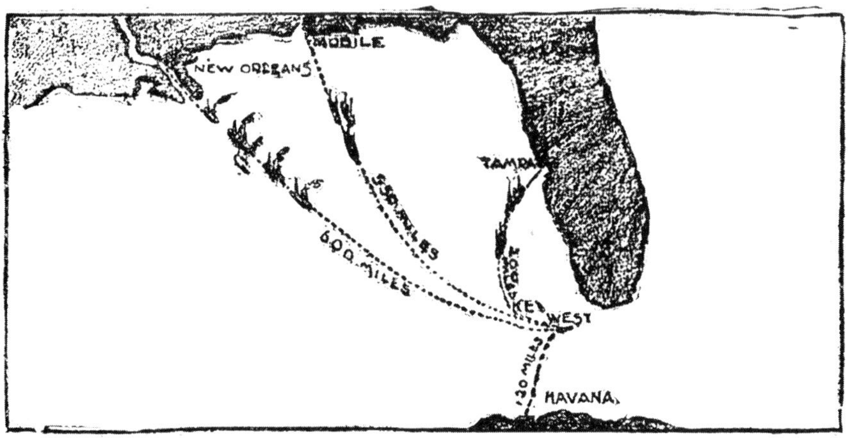

ROUTES OF THE INVADING EXPEDITIONS.

Routes of the invading expedition. *The Salt Lake Herald*, 31 May 1898. (*Library of Congress*)

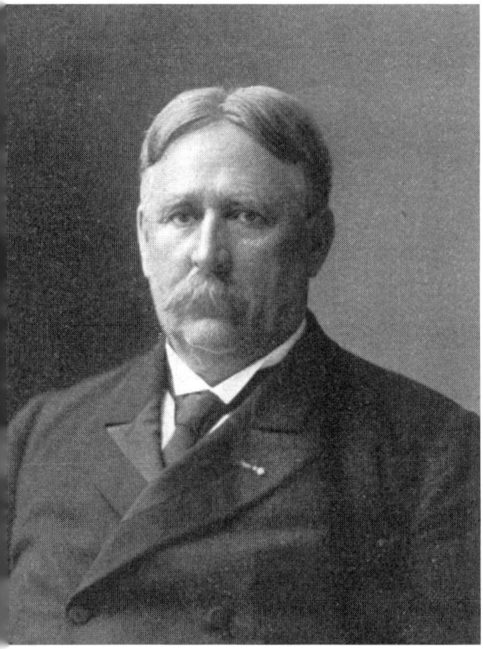

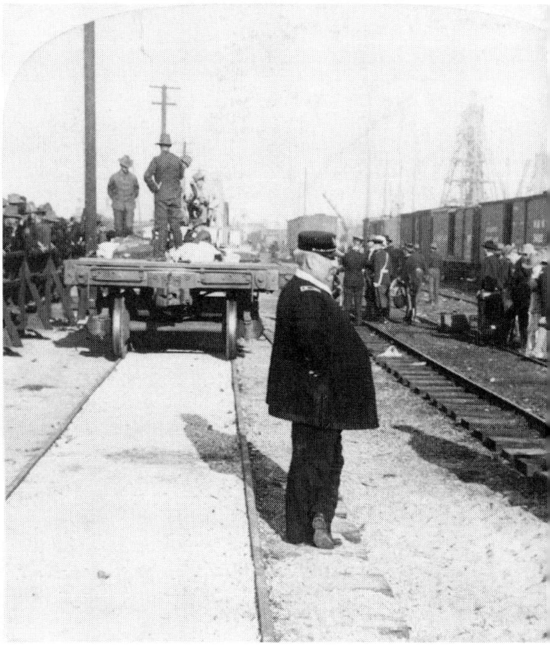

Above left: Maj. Gen. William Rufus Shafter. (*Library of Congress*)

Above right: Maj. Gen. Shafter commanding the first expedition to Cuba. (*Library of Congress*)

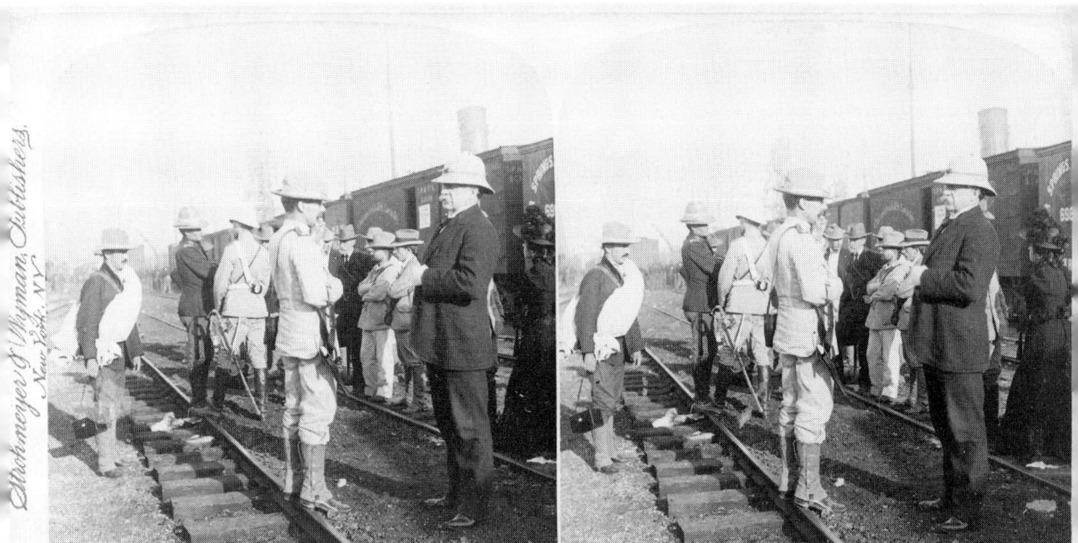

Maj. Gen. Nelson A Miles, Commander of the United States speaking with a soldier. (*Library of Congress*)

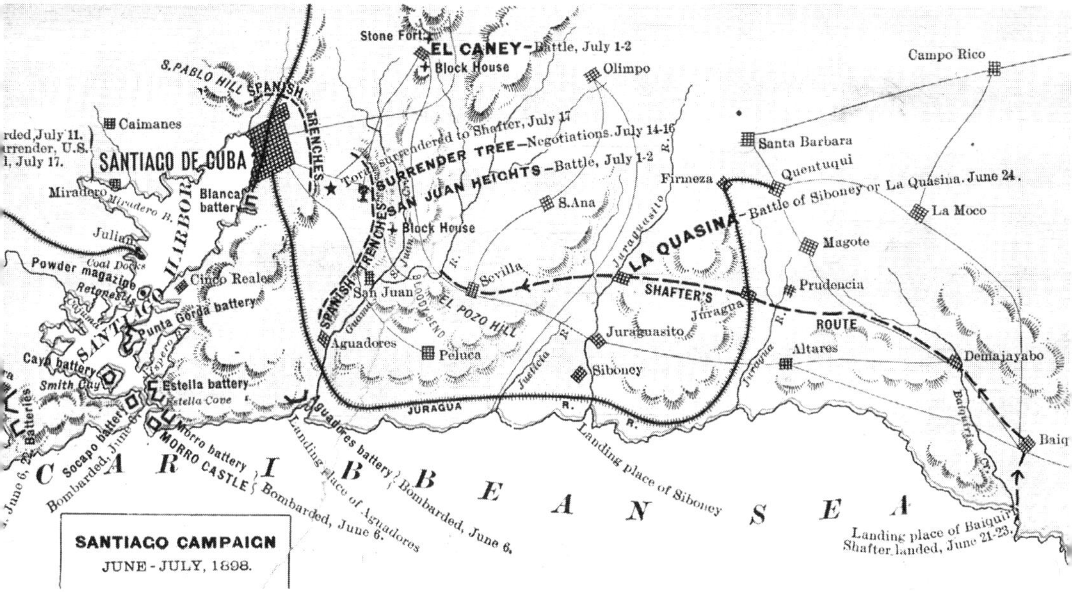

Santiago Campaign map from Goff's historical map of the Spanish-American War in the West Indies 1898. (*Library of Congress*)

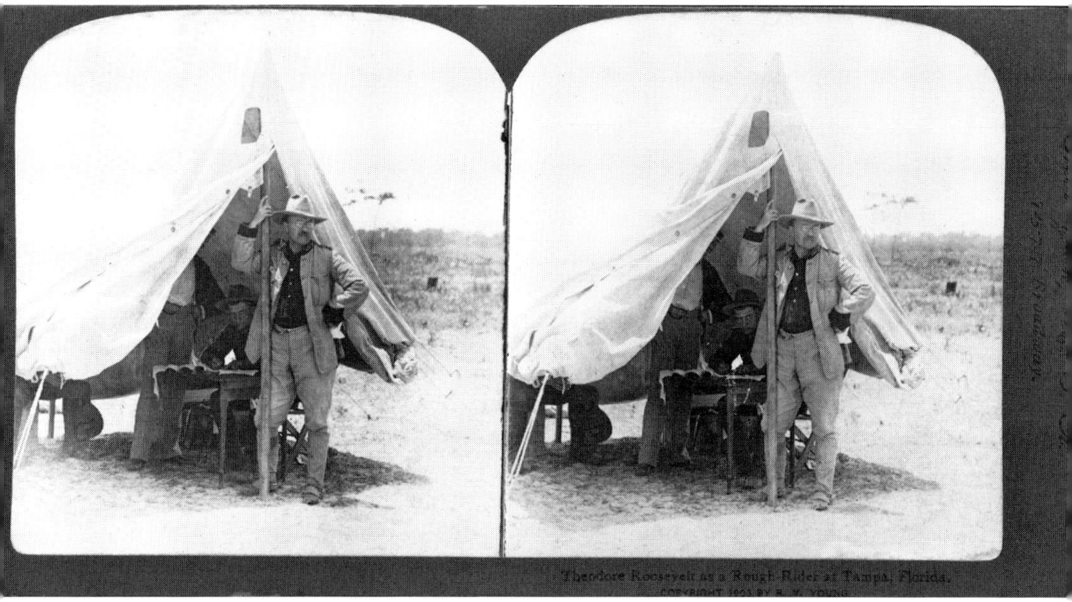

Stereograph showing Theodore Roosevelt as a Rough Rider at Tampa, Florida. (*Library of Congress*)

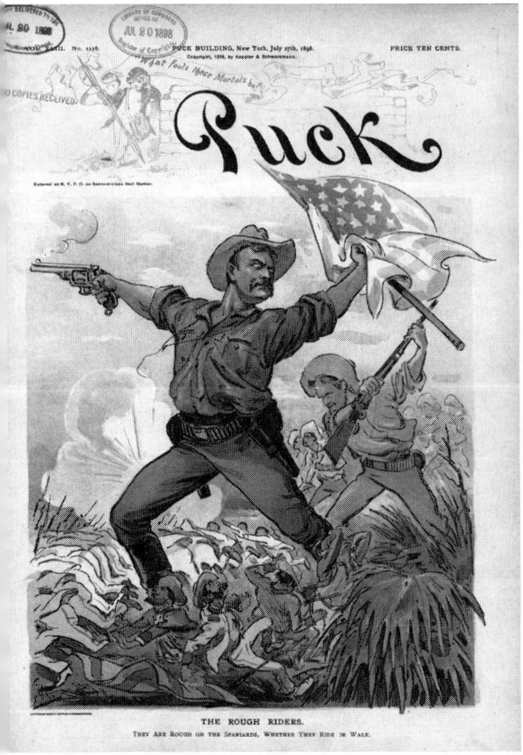

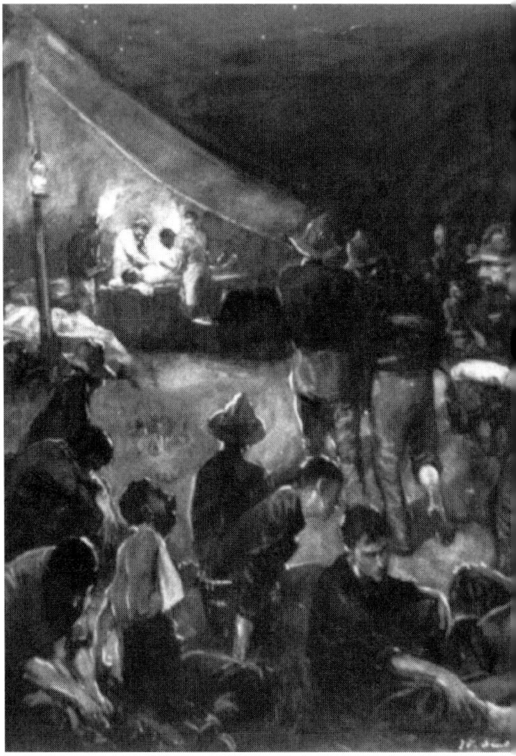

Above left: Puck magazine cover showing Theodore Roosevelt leading the Rough Riders into battle against the Spanish in Cuba during the Spanish-American War. (*Library of Congress*)

Above right: "The Night after San Juan," showing a field hospital, 1898. (*Library of Congress*)

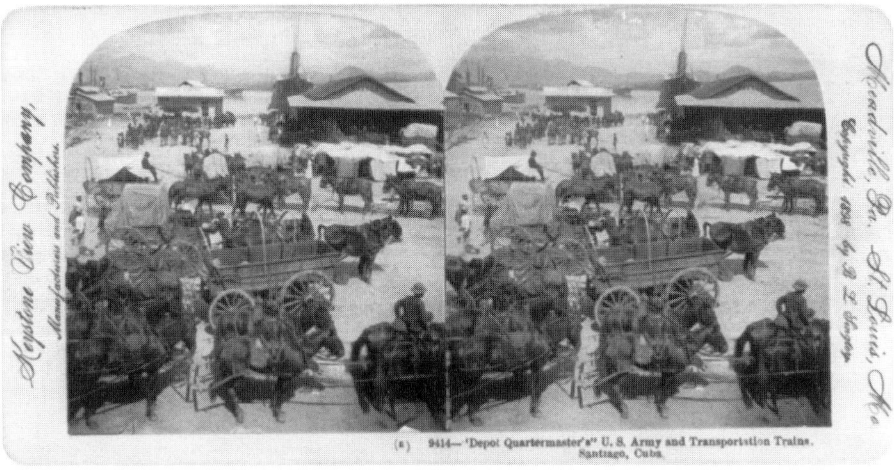

U.S. Army and Transportation Trains at Quartermaster depot Santiago Cuba. (*Library of Congress*)

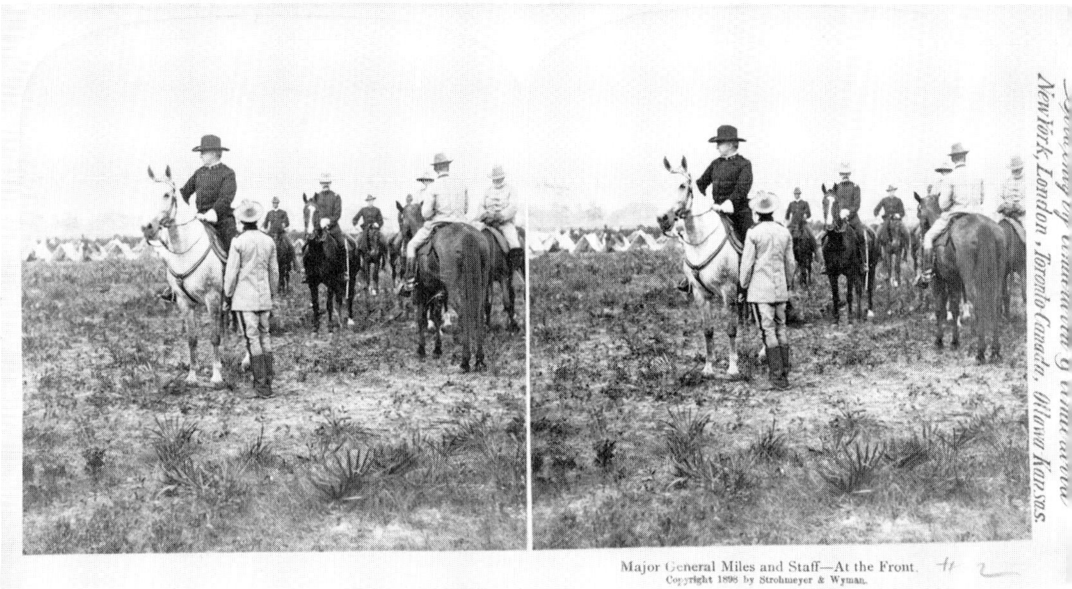

Stereograph showing Maj. Gen. Miles and staff at the front. (*Library of Congress*)

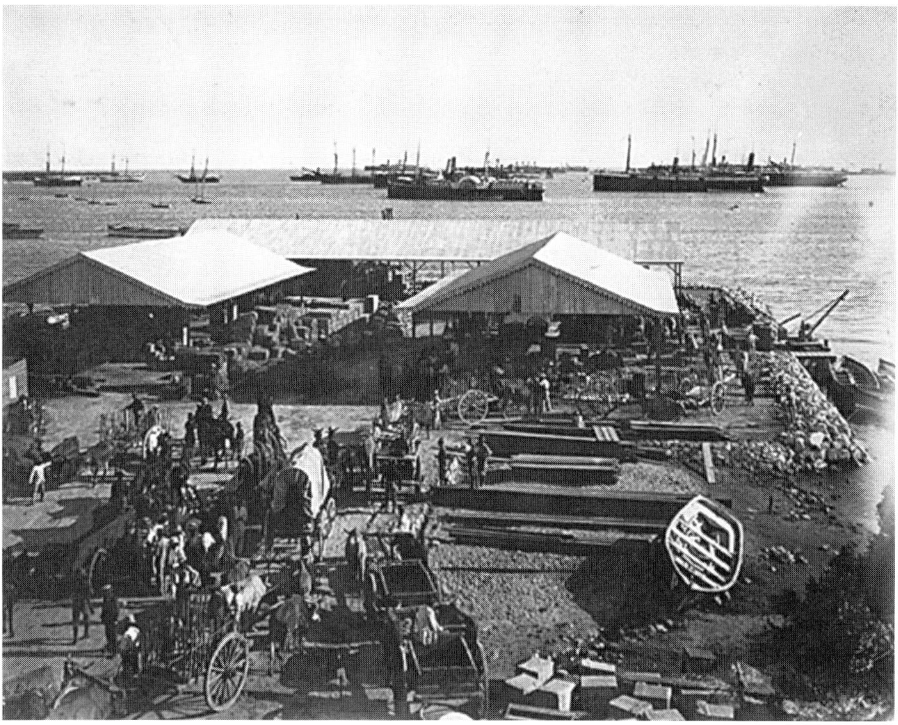

Harbor and principal wharf with U.S. transports at Ponce Porto Rico, 1898. (*Library of Congress*)

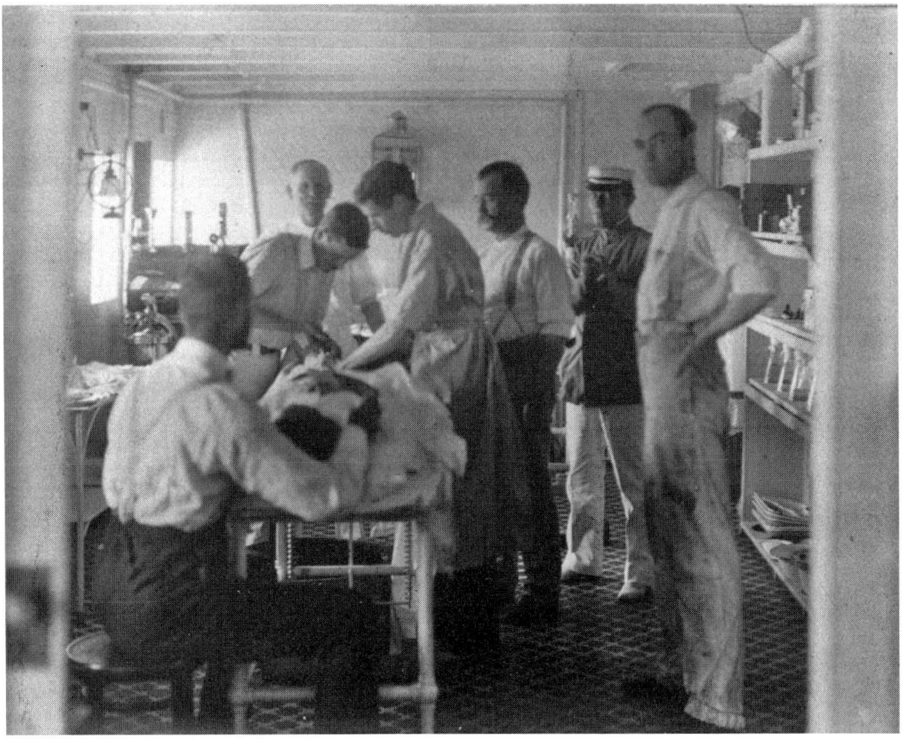

An operation by Dr. George Torney, Jr., directed by Colonel Nicholas Senn on hospital ship *Relief*, 1898. (*Library of Congress*)

He further stated: "Ninety-one percent of the U.S. Army casualties during the Spanish-American War occurred in Cuba, where major land battles of the war took place. In contrast, the short-lived campaigns in Puerto Rico and the Philippines were relatively bloodless."[15]

With so many troops succumbing to disease, the provision of medical care became a growing issue. In a communication to Secretary of War Alger in Washington, D.C., sent from Ponce on 11 August 1898, General Miles reported: "Following is result of conference and recommendation by Surgeons Greenleaf, Torney, Daly, regarding case [*sic.*] sick of army in Porto Rico: 'General Miles: Hospital of lumber can be built, but one of tents preferable. We, however, urgently recommend speedy return of sick to the United States on properly equipped transports or hospital ships. Fifty doctors and 150 trained male nurses required at once.'"[16] Miles' earlier warnings to the War Department about the likelihood of disease having a negative impact on the war were proving true. Yellow fever, typhoid, and dysentery spread like wildfire and quickly debilitated entire units. He found he could not wait for Washington to respond.

Miles took quick action in response to the suggestions of his surgeons. Shortly after he sent his report to Secretary Alger, Daly was assigned a role in evacuating many of the sick. At 4 p.m. on 04 September, the transport steamer *Panama* set sail with Daly in command with the support of three assistants. That afternoon, 246 convalescent soldiers were on their way home.[17] By 13 September, all of the sick had been transported to medical facilities in the States. A news article in the *New York Sun* on 18 September 1898 reported:

> The surgeon in charge of the transport *Panama*, which brought convalescents from Porto Rico back to this country, was Major W. H. Daly, Chief Surgeon U.S. Volunteers. Major Daly gives this account of the measures taken for the health and comfort of the men: "As a member of his personal staff, Gen. Miles had selected me for this duty, and enjoined me by both special written and verbal orders to bring these sick men to their homes in such a manner as to prove to be above reproach. Before his departure Gen. Miles sent for me to come to his ship, and, expressing his confidence in my judgment, again enjoined me to leave nothing undone for the care and comfort of his sick soldiers on their way home, expressing to me what he always feels, and which is a leading trait of his life and character, viz.: solicitude for the life and health of his soldiers, such as the tenderest solicitude of a father could not exceed. For all my labor and anxiety I had my reward in seeing the sad, wan and wasted faces of the men grow happier day by day, and their tottering, staggering footsteps growing firmer, and, in their daily warm personal thanks and words of appreciation, and I take this opportunity of acknowledging my indebtedness to all the help I had from my executive officers and surgeons alike on board, and also Capt. Prout, master of the *Panama*.
>
> It ought to be understood that the *Panama* was not a hospital ship, but only a transport that was turned over to me in a filthy condition. I first had it thoroughly sprinkled with chloride of lime and swept out, then several times thoroughly scrubbed out and flushed with sea water, and when dried out I fumigated the whole ship with the fumes of burning sulphur (nascent sulphurous acid gas) for eighteen hours, personally all through the night seeing that the sulphur was kept burning; then a heavy coat of the following wash was applied: Fresh-burned lie, sulphate of iron (copperas) and carbolic acid. After this, the ship was not only surgically and antiseptically clean, but it looked and smelled clean. I then hung hammocks and put up cots for the men.[18]

There is no doubt that Daly's ship contained a significant number of ill and wounded troops. In a report sent to Surgeon General George Miller Sternberg from Lexington, Kentucky, on 11 October 1898, Daly wrote:

> I have the honor to report myself on duty as follows. 1st to 13th September 1898, on duty under Special Field Orders, No. 37, Commanding General of the Army in charge of preparing S.S. *Panama* and bringing 255 convalescents from Arroyo and Ponce, Porto Rico to the United States. 13th to 30th on duty under Special

Orders, No. 218, Headquarters of the Army pertaining to inspection of Medical Department of the several regiments of U.S. Vol. Infantry, stationed at Jacksonville, Chickamauga, and Lexington, Kentucky.[19]

Written with the best interests of the sick and wounded soldiers in mind, Daly transmitted another communication on 21 September 1898 (Daly later testified the date should have been 21 October) to the Headquarters of the Army that would bedevil him for months. With the strike of a telegraph key, he ignited a national debate over the quality of beef being fed to the military—and the public by implication—and unintentionally became immersed in a political battle that would soon play out in Washington, D.C., and major newspapers across the country. In his report to the Assistant Adjutant-General of the Army, Daly wrote:

I have the honor to report, in the interest of the service, that in the several inspections I made in the various camps and troopships at Tampa, Jacksonville, Chickamauga, and Porto Rico, that I found the fresh beef to be apparently preserved with secret chemicals, which destroys its natural flavor, and which I also believe to be detrimental to the health of the troops.

While on duty at headquarters of the army at Tampa at the time of the embarkation of the "Shafter expedition," Colonel Weston, the efficient chief commissary, showed me a quarter of beef that had already, as a test, been sixty hours in the sun without being perceptibly tainted, so far as the sense of smell could detect.

It is impossible to keep fresh beef so long untainted in the sun in that climate without the use of deleterious preservatives, such as boric acid, salicylic acid, or nitrate potash, injected into it in quantities liable to be hurtful to the health of the consumer.

At Ponce, Porto Rico, much of the beef I examined arriving on the transports from the United States was also of the same character, being apparently preserved by injecting chemicals to aid deficient cold storage.

Where efficient cold storage is impossible transporting beef alive is the method that should receive the fullest consideration by the Government as being safest for the health of the consumer. When detailed to take charge of the transport *Panama*, for conveying convalescents to the United States, I obtained 2,000 pounds of fresh beef from the commissary at Ponce. It looked well, but had an odor similar to that of a dead human body after being injected with preservatives, and it tasted when first cooked like decomposed boric acid, while after standing a day for further inspection it became so bitter, nauseous, and unpalatable as to be quite impossible for use. I was therefore obliged, owing to its condition, and the just complaints of the sick about it, and the disgustingly sickening odor it emitted when being cooked, and its mawkish, flat taste when served, and the safety of my patients—255 convalescent soldiers on board—to organize a board of survey, condemn and throw 1,500 pounds, all we had, overboard; consequently the convalescents were entirely without much-needed

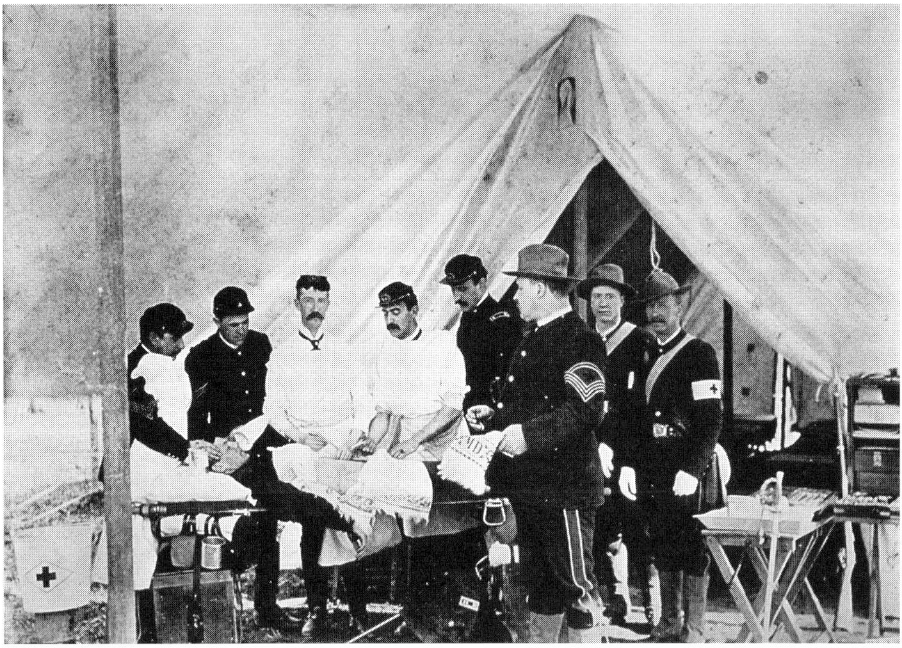

Tent operation during the Spanish-American War, 1898. (*National Library of Medicine*)

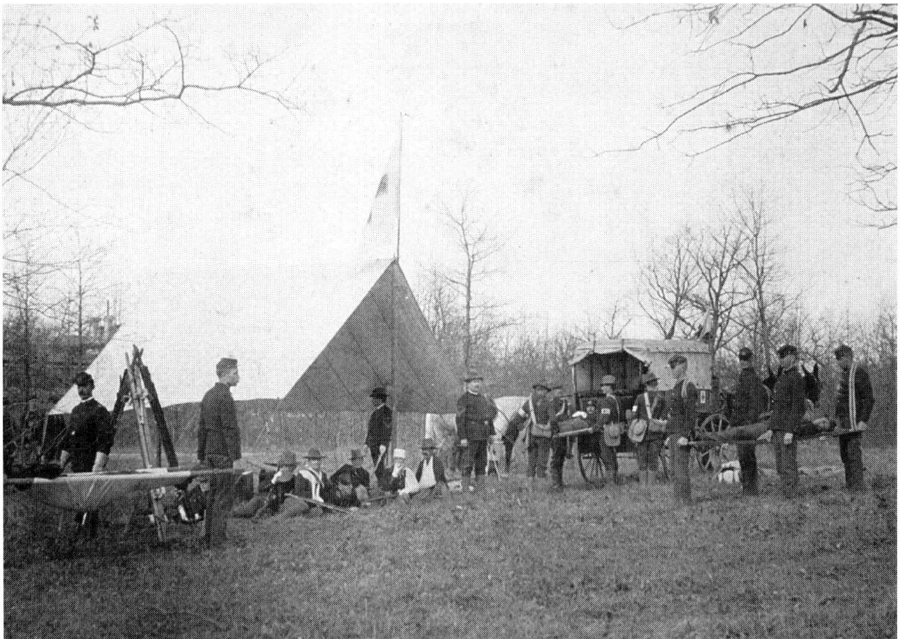

Horse drawn ambulances transporting wounded during the Spanish-American War, 1898. (*National Library of Medicine*)

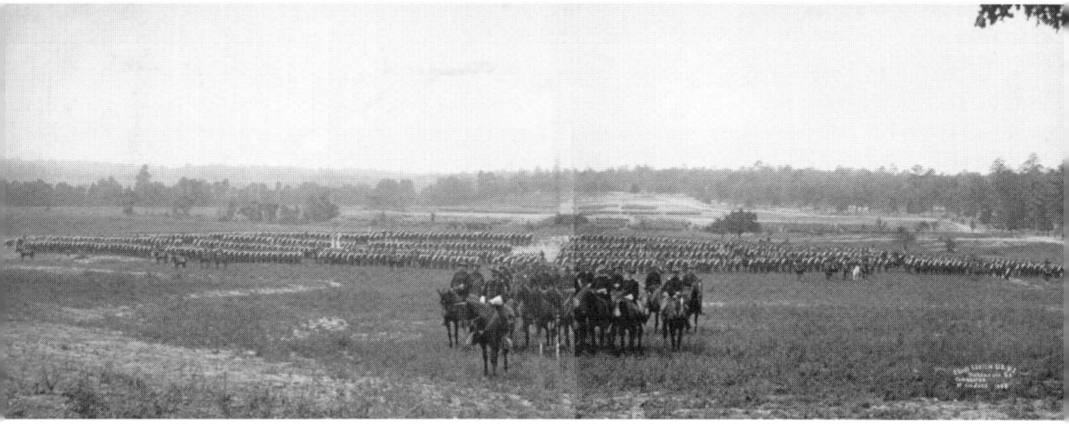

Grand Review U.S. Volunteer Infantry, Chickamauga Georgia, 1898. (*Library of Congress*)

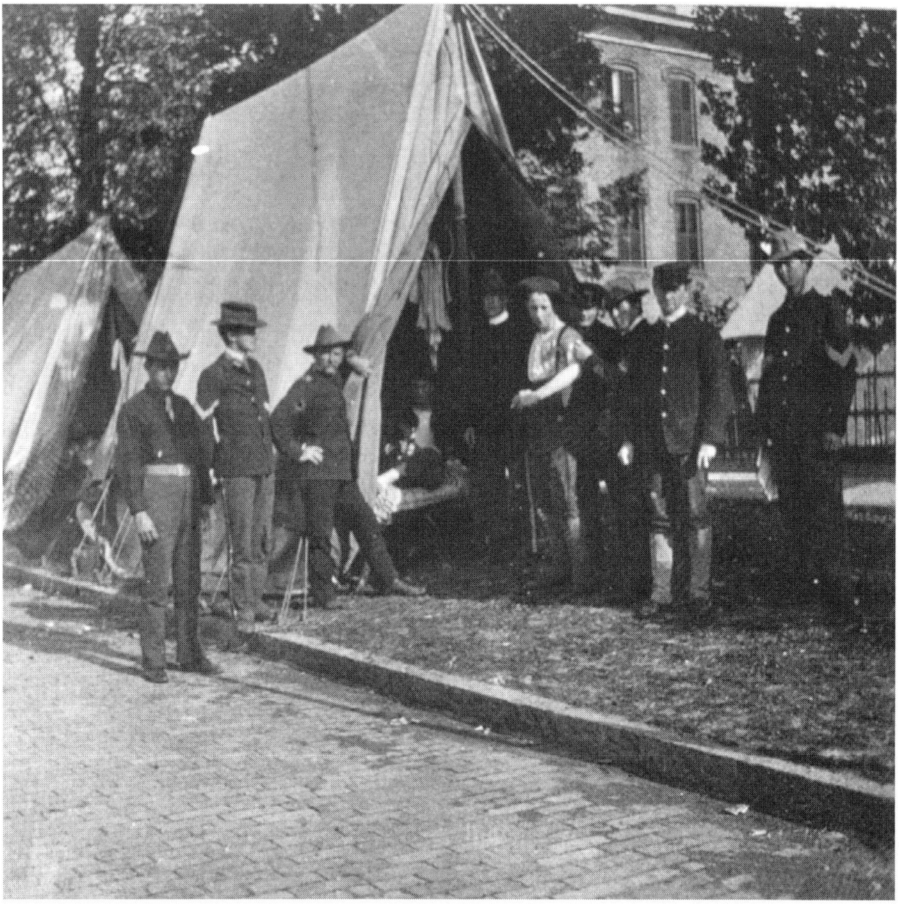

Exterior view showing group of officers and enlisted men standing around a tent at the Jacksonville Emergency Hospital, 1898. (*National Library of Medicine*)

> fresh beef, making the duty of bringing the men to the United States in an improved condition a very difficult matter.
>
> In my inspection of the Fourth United States Volunteer Infantry at Jacksonville recently I observed the same odor and taste upon the fresh beef, but not so marked, and at camp of Sixth United States Volunteer Infantry at Chickamauga I also, at severally inspections, observed it markedly. I there inspected a lot of beef just issued to that regiment, and, while it looked well, was of a sickening odor, like a human body dead of disease and injected with preservatives, and when cooked was quite unpalatable, consequently likely to prove an efficient cause of ill health. The men complained of its insipid and mawkish flavor that high seasoning could not conceal.
>
> Believing that the Commissary Department has been imposed upon by the misdirected commercial spirit of persons furnishing beef, I respectfully recommend that the matter be investigated by experts making a quantitative and qualitative chemical analysis of the several preservatives suspected to be used by getting samples of beef furnished for export to Cuba and Porto Rico.
>
> If the question arises that a report should have been made by me earlier, I beg to say that I have endeavored, with all my opportunities, to first inform myself, by observation, of the conditions above noted sufficiently to warrant my drawing the attention of the Adjutant-General at Headquarters of the Army to the matter.[20]

The previous concerns Miles conveyed about sickness, and more recent suspicions Daly expressed about the quality of beef supplied to troops and its impact on the general health of the Army, were not the only ones heard. Theodore Roosevelt, commander of the First Volunteer U.S. Cavalry Rough Riders, was part of the Army's Fifth Corps that was being decimated by disease and imposed upon by the poor quality of food during late summer after the fall of Santiago. More than 5,000 soldiers in the corps were ill at the time. In concert with several commanding officers, Roosevelt composed and delivered the following letter to Major General Shafter:

> In a meeting of the general and medical officers called by you at the Palace this morning, we were all, as you know, unanimous as to what should be done with the army. To keep us here, in the opinion of every officer commanding a division or brigade, will simply involve the destruction of thousands. There is no possible reason for not shipping practically the entire command North at once. Yellow fever cases are very few in the cavalry division where I command one of the two brigades, and not one true case of yellow fever has occurred in this division, except among the men sent to the hospital at Siboney, where they have, I believe, contracted it. But in this division, there have been fifteen hundred cases of malarial fever. Not a man has died from it, but the whole command has been so weakened and shattered as to be ripe for dying like rotten sheep, when a real yellow fever epidemic, instead of a fake epidemic like the present, strikes us, as it is bound to if we stay here at the height

> of the sickness season, August, and the beginning of September. Quarantine against malarial fever is like quarantine against the toothache. All of us are certain, as soon as the authorities fully appreciate the conditions of the army, they will order us to be sent home.
>
> If we are kept here, it will in all human possibility mean an appalling disaster, for the surgeons here estimate that over half the army, if kept here during the sickly season, will die. This is not only terrible from the standpoint of the individual lives lost, but it means ruin from the standpoint of the military efficiency of the flower of the American Army, for the great bulk of the regulars are here with you. The sick list, large although it is, exceeding four thousand, affords but a faint index of the debilities of the army. Not ten percent are fit for active work.
>
> Six weeks on the North Maine coast, for instance, or elsewhere, where the yellow fever germ can not possibly propagate, would make us all as fit as fighting cocks, able as we are, and eager to take a leading part in the great campaign against Havana in the Fall, even if we are not allowed to try Puerto Rico.
>
> We can be moved North, if moved at once, with absolute safety to the country, although, of course, it would have been infinitely better if we had been moved North or to Puerto Rico two weeks ago. If there were any object in keeping us here, we would face yellow fever with as much indifference as we face bullets. But there is no object in it. The fever immune regiments ordered here are sufficient to garrison the city and surrounding towns, and there is absolutely nothing for us to do here, and there has not been since the city surrendered. It is impossible to move into the interior. Every shifting of camp doubles the sick rate in our present weakened condition, and, anyhow, the interior is rather worse than the coast, as I have found by actual reconnaissance. Our present camps are as healthy as any camps at this end of the island can be.
>
> I write only because I can not see our men, who have fought so bravely and who have endured extreme hardship and danger so uncomplainingly, go to destruction without striving, so far as lies in me, to avert a doom as fearful as it is unnecessary and undeserved.[21]

Among the group of officers that took part in preparing the letter, Roosevelt was the only volunteer, so he was most at ease in its delivery since he had little to lose relative to his military status. The rest were regular Army officers who initially feared reprisal. Once the letter was delivered, however, the others in the cabal reconsidered their position and signed their names to a follow-up letter to Shafter. For the most part, its contents reiterated the first. They ended the second letter, however, by emphatically stating: "This army must be moved at once or perish. As the army can be safely moved now, the persons responsible for preventing such a move will be responsible for the unnecessary loss of many thousands of lives."[22]

Following protocol, General Shafter transmitted the contents of the documents to Secretary of War Alger. Immediately after Shafter referred the matter to Alger, but before the Secretary could react, the letters were leaked to the press. Much to the chagrin of Secretary Alger, and with the second communication now being referred to as the "round robin" letter, the issues of illness and poor food would soon be tried in the court of public opinion.

While ill feelings over the "round robin" letter festered in Washington and the press, there were no immediate consequences other than the prompt removal of many troops from Cuba, just as the letters suggested. Alger fought back with a range of recriminations against Shafter for allowing the letter to go public and denials that the letters had motivated the evacuation. Shafter responded by disavowing any involvement with the leak; but complied with orders to withdraw much of the Army from the island.

Daly's written communication to the Assistant Adjutant-General of the Army and verbal reports to General Miles in the fall of 1898, however, seemingly became the straw that broke the camel's back. Since the invasion of Cuba in July 1898, and the "round robin" letter at the end of August, official military reports and subsequent newspaper articles had started to bring attention to the high rates of illness affecting the troops in training camps and on the front. By the time Daly's message was sent, it was already clear that Miles' forewarnings to President McKinley and the War Department in May and June were justified relative to the negative impact of disease on troops and the logistical challenges of supplying food and materials to forces spread across the Caribbean islands. While sensational at the time, the "round robin" letter was one log on a fire that Miles and Daly were now stoking.

Despite Miles' earlier admonitions, little was done by the War Department initially to respond. At the onset, national fervor for war was high and the need for quick action imperative. There were political considerations that required expediency; midterm elections were only a few months away.

Whether it was General Miles' soldier-first mentality, his growing animosity toward Secretary of War Alger caused by perceived slights in assigning military leadership to the war effort, or political aspirations as others would later suggest, the situation soon took on a life of its own in the public arena. While actual military battles were few and the war short, reports on the alarming numbers of soldier deaths from disease increased during the summer of 1898. As the mortality reports reaching the homes of parents and spouses grew, the public and the press soon began asking how such a thing could happen in a country so rich and powerful. Soon, the public outcry—amplified a hundredfold by the press—for assigning culpability was too loud to ignore and the din forced President McKinley to take action. Miles grabbed the reins and made his case to the public by way of a series of newspaper interviews that appeared across the country. He let the public know he had warned those responsible, but his warnings had gone unheeded. J. D. Whelpley, a journalist for the *Kansas City Star* supposedly first reported the general's apprehensions in July 1898.[23] However,

Miles later disavowed granting such an interview from Porto Rico. Whether the interview was real or fabricated, it nevertheless caused great excitement. In later denying that he gave the interview, Miles' rebuttal contained many of the same recriminations of the War Department. Either way, the damage was done.

The 20 August 1898 edition of *The Literary Digest* contained an article that summed up the situation playing out in the halls of government and newspapers across the country. The article stated:

> A terrific storm of newspaper criticism pertaining to the conduct of army affairs prevails in all parts of the United States. The demand that responsibility for the conditions revealed must be located has led to the publication of a mass of statements, personal and official, by way of explanation. In substance, these statements consist of defenses made by the several branches of the army organization, each of its own conduct, and attempts to shift the responsibility upon another branch.[24]

Things quickly got out of hand for all involved. Political mischief was afoot, and Secretary of War Alger and Commissary General Charles P. Eagan soon bore the brunt of national disenchantment. Feeling the heat but remaining self-righteous, Alger requested President McKinley open an investigation into the conduct of the War Department during the war. He was certain his actions would be vindicated. McKinley, seeking political cover, responded promptly by appointing a special commission to investigate the matter. On 24 September 1898, little more than a month after the war's end, the President's Commission to Investigate the Conduct of the War Department in the War with Spain began deliberation.

Within a few months, William H. Daly would get caught in the crosshairs between the politicians, General Miles, and the public.

9

One Swallow Doesn't Make a Summer

There was little room for President McKinley to maneuver in the public arena once the alleged interview with General Miles was published in the *Kansas City Star* in late August 1898. Much to the chagrin of McKinley and Alger, the general's many grievances over the handling of the war were set in print. The article created a maelstrom of public discontent over the administration's handling of the war with Spain.

Miles arrived in New York on 07 September. The following morning the *New York Journal* provided insight into the tumult Miles was causing Washington, D.C., when it reported:

> He salutes the official authority of the Secretary of War, but he can hardly be suspected of entertaining either respect or affection for Mr. Alger. Nor is General Miles the man to quail even at the august frown of Mr. McKinley himself. "I shall neither oppose nor court an official inquiry," he said to the *Journal* yesterday, "but I stand ready to answer for my part in the conduct of the war." That is a glove thrown at the feet of Mr. Alger.
>
> "I have been willing to give General Shafter all the credit due him, but I do not believe in being robbed." That is another glove, cavalry size. The interview with Mr. Whelpley, of the *Kansas City Star*, which took Washington aback and stirred the country, General Miles stamps as substantially correct. That interview charges the War Department with duplicity, with conspiring to undermine the authority of the General of the Army, with failure to keep secret the plans for the invasion of Porto Rico, with neglect to furnish promised landing apparatus, and with rejection of precautions proposed by General Miles that would have saved the army in Cuba from being assailed by preventable diseases. That interview is a glove of steel, the clang of which lands before Secretary Alger, Corbin [Adjutant General] and McKinley, wakes echoes which travel to every corner of the United States. It is a

> notification to all concerned that Nelson A. Miles, soldier and gentleman, comes ashore with lance in rest and visor down, resolved to hold the pass of his rights and to charge for his honor and the truth's sake should the challenge be accepted.[1]

The article appeared on the front page of the paper adding yet another voice to the growing number of publications across the country coaxing the President to action. McKinley would now be forced to deal with the matter whether he wished to or not.

Secretary of War Alger was not at all happy about the prospects of an investigation of the War Department, but political realities were now creating too much pressure to be ignored. In reality, McKinley had already determined the necessity of an official investigation after the Miles article appeared; but he needed Alger's consent to provide political cover to make it appear to the public his administration had nothing to hide.

Evidence suggests Alger finally agreed to an investigation after receiving promises the matter would be dealt with in quick order and his integrity, and that of the War Department, would be preserved. Ostensibly in a display of political showmanship Secretary Alger wrote to the President on 08 September 1898 officially requesting the investigation. In his letter, Alger wrote:

> I have the honor to ask that a board, consisting of from five to seven members, of the most distinguished soldiers and civilians that can be selected, be appointed by you, with full power to investigate thoroughly every bureau of the War Department in connection with the mustering, clothing, supplying, and arming of troops, transportation, the letting of contracts, and chartering vessels, and all expenditures of every kind, as well as of orders issued by this Department—indeed, that everything connected with the Army be thoroughly investigated for your information.[2]

McKinley reacted immediately through presidential decree and established the Commission to Investigate the Conduct of the War Department in the War with Spain. Alger would later come to regret his acquiescence.

The commission met for the first time in the Lemon Building in Washington, D.C., on Monday, 26 September 1898. While the full name of the commission was used for official purposes, the press and public very quickly began referring to it simply as the "Dodge Commission," in recognition of its president, General Grenville M. Dodge.

Members of the commission included General Grenville M. Dodge, Iowa, (president); Colonel James A. Sexton, Illinois; Colonel Charles Denby, Indiana; Captain Evan P. Howell, Georgia; ex-Governor Urban A. Woodbury, Vermont; Brigadier General John M. Wilson, Chief of Engineers, U.S.A.; General James A. Beaver, Pennsylvania; Major General Alexander McD. McCook, U.S.A.; and Dr. Phineas S. Conner, Ohio. Others who were subsequently added for administrative

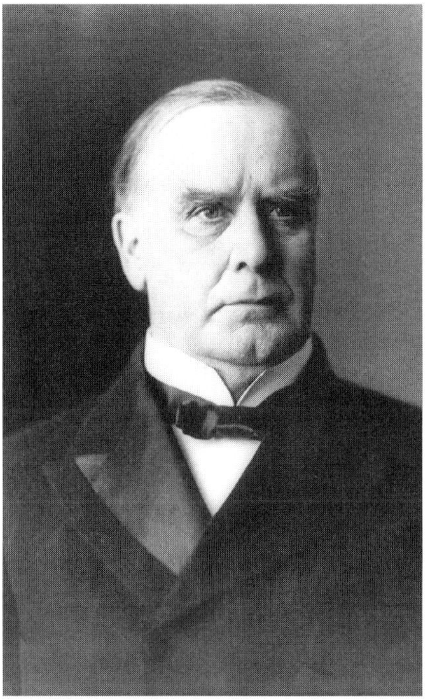

President William McKinley, 1900. (*Library of Congress*)

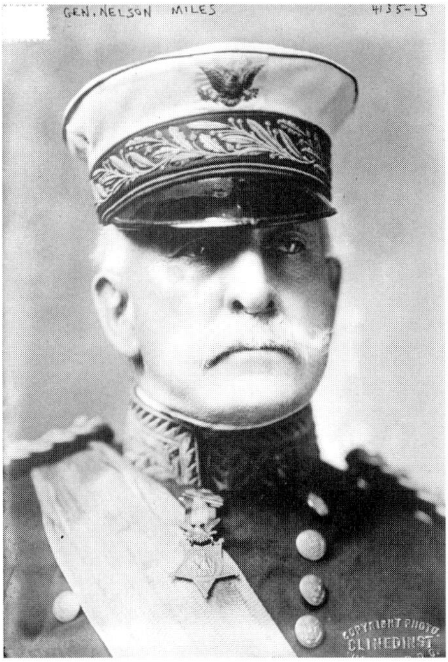

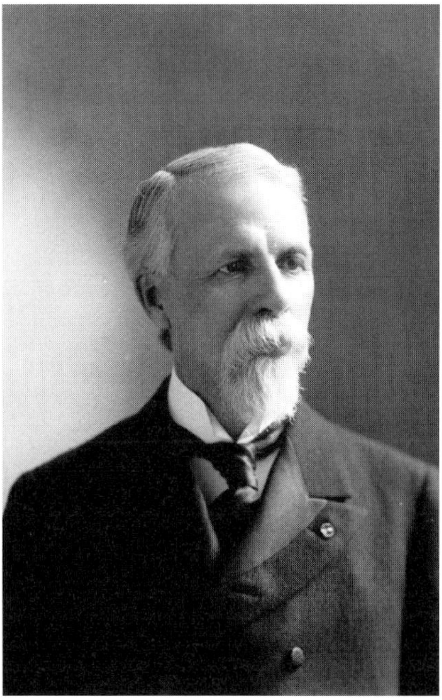

Above left: Gen. Nelson A. Miles. (*Library of Congress*)

Above right: U.S. Secretary of War Russell A. Alger. (*Library of Congress*) purposes included Richard Weightman, (secretary); Lieutenant Colonel F. B. Jones, Chief Quartermaster of Volunteers, (disbursing officer); and Major Stephen C. Mills, (recorder).[3] The group consisted of previous cabinet members, elected officials, active duty and retired military officers, a physician, and business leaders.[4]

Upon engaging the commission, the president wrote a letter to its members, stating:

> Before suggesting the matters which shall come before you for investigation, I desire to express my appreciation to each of you for your willingness to accept the patriotic service to which you have been invited. You are to perform one of the highest public duties that can fall to a citizen, and your unselfishness in undertaking it makes me profoundly grateful.
>
> There has been in many quarters severe criticism of the conduct of the war with Spain. Charges of criminal neglect of the soldiers in camp and field and hospital, and in transports, have been so persistent that, whether true or false, they have made a deep impression upon the country. It is my earnest desire that you shall thoroughly investigate these charges and make the fullest examination of the administration of the War Department in all of its branches, with the view to establishing the

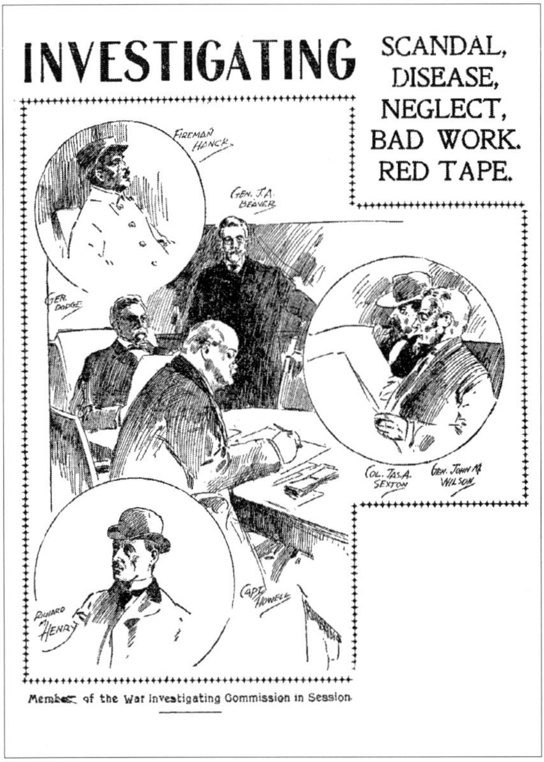

War Investigating Committee. (*New York Journal*, *19 November 1898*)

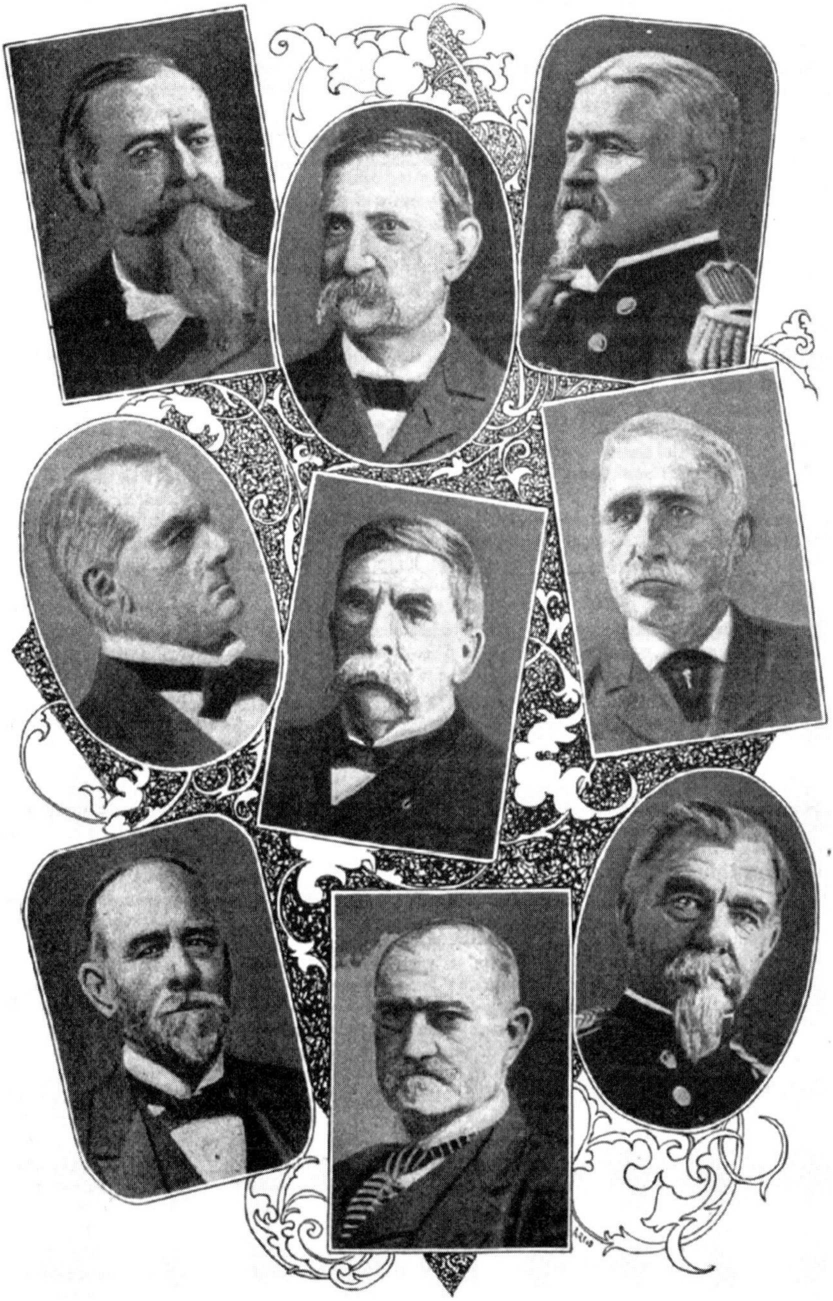

Col. James A. Sexton.
Col. Charles Denby.
Gen. James A. Beaver.

Dr. Phineas D. Conner.
Gen. Grenville M. Dodge (Chn.)
Capt. Evan P. Howell.

Maj.-Gen. Alex. McD. McCook.
Hon. Urban A. Woodbury.
Brig.-Gen. John M. Wilson.

THE WAR INQUIRY COMMISSION.

The War Inquiry Commission. (*The Literary Digest, Volume 17, 05 Nov 1898*)

> truth or falsity of these accusations. I put upon you no limit to the scope of your investigation. Of all Departments connected with the Army, I invite the closest scrutiny and examination and shall afford every facility for the most searching inquiry. The records of the War Department and the assistance of its officers shall be subject to your call.
>
> I can not impress upon you too strongly my wish that your investigation shall be so thorough and complete that your report, when made, will fix the responsibility for any failure or fault by reason of neglect, incompetency, or maladministration upon the officers and bureaus responsible therefore, if it be found that the evils complained of have existed.
>
> The people of the country are entitled to know whether or not the citizens who so promptly responded to the call of duty have been neglected or misused or maltreated by the Government to which they so willingly gave their services. If there have been wrongs committed, the wrongdoers must not escape conviction and punishment.[5]

The letter was immediately released to the press in an effort to engender favorable public response. The public was not entirely impressed.

With the exceptions of General Dodge and Colonel Sexton, all of the other members of the commission attending the first meeting were not President McKinley's original choices. The replacements were nonetheless considered solid choices by the administration; their prestigious backgrounds deemed sufficient to eschew public censure. Regardless of their first-rate credentials and the president's best efforts to gain public support, newspaper editors immediately began speculating McKinley had handpicked commission members as politically expedient appointments to help "whitewash" the entire matter.[6]

Between 26 September 1898 and 09 February 1899, the president's commission held 109 meetings and interviewed 495 people. The roster of those interviewed was not only extensive; it was also by outward appearance, well rounded. Government officials, military officers, enlisted personnel, civilians, and representatives of the meatpacking and railroad industries were included.

While the McKinley–Alger–Miles drama played out in the press during late summer and early fall 1898, William H. Daly was busy fulfilling his responsibilities as an army medical officer. In late August, he received orders from General Miles to take charge of a medical transport, the S.S. *Panama*, and outfit the vessel for evacuation of sick and wounded soldiers from Porto Rico. At that point, Daly had no idea he would soon become personally involved in the political kabuki playing out in the States, or of later becoming a star witness in the Dodge Commission hearings.

Events leading to Daly's entanglement were innocuous and more in line with the routine responsibilities of a physician and military officer than otherwise might be construed from subsequent newspaper headlines. No signs of him having an interest in political intrigue have ever come to light. He was by all accounts a good soldier; he followed orders and made decisions reflecting both his medical expertise and good judgment. He always upheld General Miles' mantra for doing everything possible to assure the safety and wellbeing of his soldiers.

While Daly was never simply a bystander, he nonetheless became a target for those wishing to aim at Miles. The general, however, always proved an elusive target. His military acumen was second to none; his ability to wage "political" war, however, was largely underestimated. Miles' enemies, unable to strike their main objective with blows of sufficient force to have him court-martialed or censured in a manner that would harm his career and high public standing, were easily deflected. The ricochet, however, hit Daly head-on after General Miles gave testimony to the commission in late 1898. Daly did not emerge unscathed.

The story of how Daly's name and routine military medical activities became so well recognized throughout the country during the fall of 1898 is interesting. It all began shortly after his arrival with General Miles in Tampa on 01 June 1898.

By the time they arrived, troops from across the country were being assembled for the planned expedition to Cuba. As General Miles later noted in his testimony to the Dodge Commission:

> The troops were assembled first at New Orleans, Mobile, and Tampa. Then other troops were mobilized at Chickamauga—some at the same time—cavalry and artillery. The cavalry and artillery were afterward moved to Tampa. There were three expeditions practically ordered—first, the movement of the troops to those points which I have mentioned; then the concentration of almost the entire regular cavalry and infantry and light artillery at Tampa; and then, later, about the 8th or 9th of May, an army of 70,000 men was ordered to Cuba, and supplies for 70,000 men for ninety days were ordered sent to Tampa, and thirty days' supplies for the animals.[7]

He went on to note that the arrival of so many troops "... occasioned much confusion on the railroads. At one time there were nearly 1,000 cars loaded with munitions of war of various kinds. Of course, it was impossible to unload them, because there were no government storehouses at Tampa at the time, and they were side-tracked, at one time as far back as Columbia, S.C."[8] The chaos that ensued was not limited just to troop movements, arms, and munitions, but also to medical and food supplies. As confusion reigned, orders for an additional 10,000 troops from Chickamauga were issued further complicating the situation.

The War Department thought it necessary to muster a force of more than 25,000 troops for deployment in a matter of several days. Upon receiving telegrams from Washington urging haste in outfitting the invasion force, Miles found "it was impossible to put more than 15,877 officers and men on transports ... equipped as well as possible under the circumstances."[9] Despite Miles' misgivings, the Santiago expedition commanded by General Shafter was launched from Tampa on 12 June with as many troops and as much equipment as could be carried.

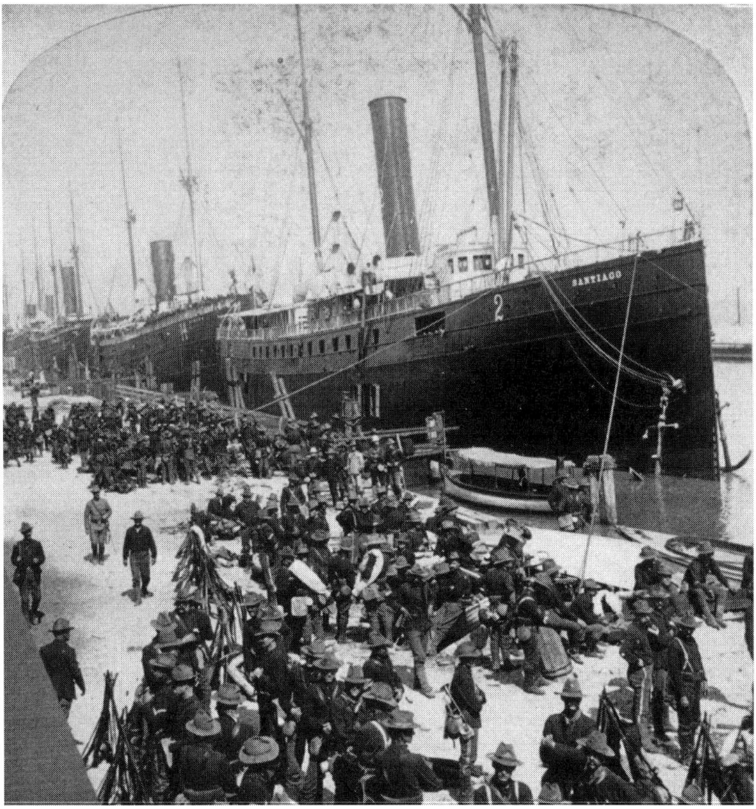

Above: Stereograph view showing dock at Tampa on the day of sailing for Santiago de Cuba, 1898. (*Library of Congress*)

Below: Maj. Gen. Miles and army transports on sailing day at Tampa, 1898. (*Library of Congress*)

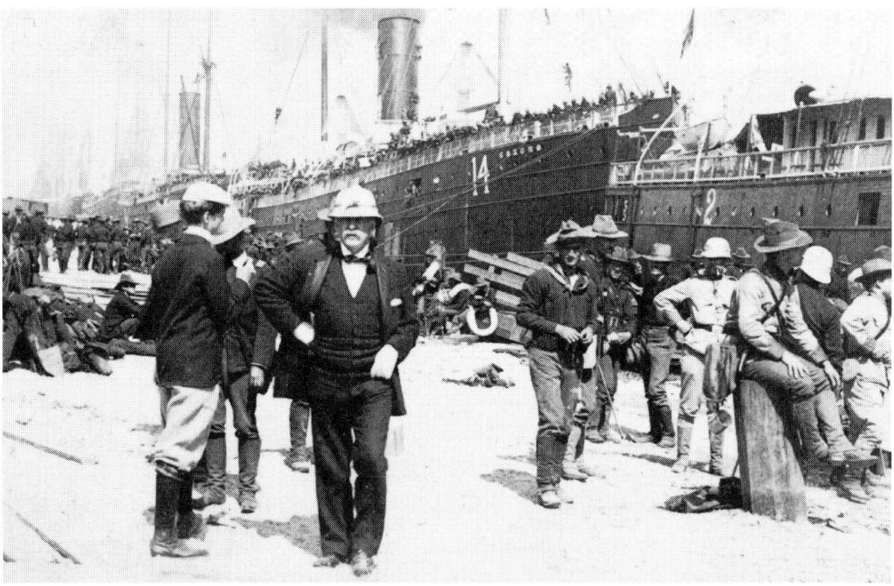

During the Dodge Commission hearings in late December 1898, Miles was questioned: "To what extent was this expedition supplied, as far as your observation enabled you to judge of it, with commissary and quartermaster stores, with ammunition and medical supplies?" He responded:

> As regards quartermaster stores—of course, the troops took with them the clothing which they were accustomed to wear. Some of the troops, a few, came from the Southern States. Most of the regular regiments came from the Middle States, from the lakes, and from the Northwest, where they were accustomed to wear woolen underclothing. There had not been time to obtain suitable clothing for the Tropics. As far as the camp equipage and arms are concerned, the regular troops were fairly well equipped. They had the modern rifle. The volunteer troops were not so well equipped. They had the Springfield rifle and black powder, and they had no opportunity for target practice. I think in the Seventy-first New York Regiment it was reported to me there were 800 men who had never fired a shot before going to Tampa. As far as the commissary stores were concerned, I think there was a sufficient amount of the kind furnished; that is, of the kind that was furnished. The medical supplies were not sufficient.[10]

Daly was among those who reported the medical supply deficiencies. While the supply reports were routine in nature, they were not the only thing Daly made a note of during his inspections.

As stated previously, Daly was very busy inspecting troops, health services, and the above-mentioned medical supplies during preparation for the expedition's launch. While on a routine inspection of one of the transport ships, the S.S. *Comal*, Daly encountered something he had not seen before: a quarter side of beef was hanging exposed on the deck. It was the beef he later spoke about with General Miles and subsequently communicated to the assistant adjutant-general in his report on 21 October. As Daly later noted:

> Colonel Weston, the efficient chief commissary, showed me a quarter of beef that had already, as a test, been sixty hours in the sun without being perceptibly tainted, so far as the sense of smell could detect. It is impossible to keep fresh beef so long untainted in the sun in that climate without the use of deleterious preservatives, such as boric acid, salicylic acid, or nitrate potash, injected into it in quantities liable to be hurtful to the health of the consumer.[11]

At the time of the inspection, the ship was being prepared to carry officers and enlisted men of the 5th Artillery, 7th U.S. Infantry Company "I," 1st U.S. Artillery, Light Battery "E," 1st U.S. Artillery, Light Battery "K," as well as gear and provisions for the 10th U.S. Cavalry for the planned invasion of Cuba. Daly was uncertain as to whether or not the side of beef had any relationship to the health of the troops, but it nevertheless piqued his interest.

Daly later reported he was so curious about the meat he went back several times throughout the day to inspect it. On one of his visits, he carved off a small piece of meat and stuck it in his pocket. A day later, while on special assignment to assist the town of Tampa in cleaning up its poor sanitary condition causing problems for the troops, he had an opportunity to cook the beef over an open fire while waiting for a horse at the nearby corral. He noted:

> It did not smell natural when I was cooking it, but it did not arouse any suspicion that anything was wrong. It did not taste good when I ate it. I was very busy after eating it, and afterwards went over into the corral, selected a big strong horse, and helped the men lasso him out of the four or five hundred there, put a saddle and bridle on him, and started over toward Tampa Heights, some 5 or more miles. The horse proved to be wild and unruly and threw himself once or twice. In the heat of the day and struggle with the horse I got ill with a burning in my stomach, nausea, and vomiting, which I first attributed to my exertion and activity in the sun; but when I vomited there was a taste in my mouth that recalled an experience of some years before which I had long forgotten. It was an experience with some chemically prepared antelope and elk meat.[12]

Despite his illness, and the unpleasant reminder of previous bad experiences with preserved meat it elicited, he was still not convinced there was anything wrong with the beef. His feelings about the matter would soon change.

His uncertainties about the potential harmfulness of the beef intensified once he discovered issues with the supply of beef on the *Panama* while transporting sick troops in early September 1898. As previously mentioned, Daly was assigned to take charge of the ship on 23 August. During the next week, he spent time inspecting the vessel, directing its cleaning, and organizing it in a manner that would allow the transport of sick and wounded troops. He assumed official command of the ship on 01 September and began issuing orders for medical and food supplies. After appointing Captain R. J. C. Irvine of the 11th Infantry as ship commissary, he directed him, among other things, to obtain a sufficient supply of beef to feed the troops and staff on their voyage from Porto Rico to Fortress Monroe on the Virginia Peninsula. Irvine initially had difficulties locating both a sufficient supply of beef and an adequate amount of ice necessary to refrigerate the beef once it was obtained. Before the ship left Ponce, Porto Rico, on 04 September to pick up troops in Arroyo, a small amount of beef was acquired, but only enough to cover the short trip to Arroyo and back. When the ship arrived back at Ponce, they were able to obtain another 2,000 pounds of beef and 1½ tons of ice. On 05 September, they set sail for Mayaguez to pick up additional troops. While there, they were able to pick up another 10 tons of ice. At that point, they had 11½ tons of ice, which they considered sufficient to preserve 1 ton of beef—or so they thought. There was a problem with the beef obtained from the commissary at Ponce that went unnoticed except for a "peculiar odor" while it was being transported to the ship in the open air. Once the beef and ice were stored in the ice room for a short period, however, "it was soon discovered that the beef was very offensive."[13]

The problem was first noticed by the 150 convalescent troops billeted nearest the ice room. As Daly later reported: "When the butchers opened the ice room there would be a great outcry on the part of the patients about the horrible stench, and it was horrible, and there was a good deal of discussion about it at officers' call in the morning." Daly unsuccessfully attempted to quell their disdain by telling them there was nothing wrong with the beef. He quickly found he was unable to mitigate the situation and decided another action was necessary. Recalling his orders from General Miles "to leave nothing undone for the care and comfort of his sick soldiers on their way home," he felt compelled to take action. Besides the general's directive, he later recalled: "… my conscience and judgment told me there was much wrong."[14]

On 06 September, Daly called together his officers for a board of survey (an inspection and assessment group) to consider what might be done about the beef problem. Their decision was made promptly: the meat was to be discarded and thrown overboard immediately. Before throwing 1,500 pounds of beef overboard, however, Daly took time to collect "a quart measure of the beef tea, before any seasoning was put in, from one of the large caldrons on the deck of the vessel that the soup or stews were made in, and after filtering it once or twice through absorbent cotton, so as to free it from fat, put it in a couple of empty aerated water bottles that had nothing but aerated water in them, and put the bottles in my portmanteau and kept it under lock and key."[15]

His suspicions were raised, but he knew he could not just make an informed guess about the matter. He needed to apply scientific rigor that would separate fact from intuition. While he had sufficient foresight to collect and preserve samples of the beef, he now needed time and a laboratory to test his hypothesis that the meat had been chemically treated with unknown preservatives. For the time being, however, he was busily engaged with official duties, and his tests would have to wait.

Most of the convalescent troops on board the *Panama* were dropped at Camp Josiah Simpson Army General Hospital at Fortress Monroe on 10 September. The remaining fifty were left at hospitals in Washington, D.C., on 12 September.

On his trip to Washington, Daly came down with malarial fever, just like many of the troops he had recently transported. His case was severe enough to force him to request sick leave. It also caused him to ask General Miles to delay orders he had just received to inspect some military camps where the so-called immune troops were based.[16] Temporary leave was granted, and he went to his home in Pittsburgh to recover. During his recovery, he used the time to analyze some of the beef he had collected on board the *Panama*.

Sufficiently recovered from his illness to resume the inspections General Miles had requested before sick leave, Daly arrived in Jacksonville on 23 September 1898. While there, he inspected the 4th Volunteer Infantry Regiment. Three days later, on 26 September, he inspected troops of the 6th Volunteer Infantry Regiment at Chickamauga, Georgia. He then went to Lexington, Kentucky, to inspect the 7th and 10th Volunteers Infantry Regiments and then back to Chickamauga to examine the 8th Volunteer Infantry, which had only returned to camp after his initial visit a few weeks earlier. All of these inspections involved examinations of "immune regiments." On 11 October, while at Lexington, Daly sent his monthly report to the U.S.A. Surgeon General Sternberg, stating:

> I have the honor to report myself on duty as follows. Station Headquarters of the Army by Special Orders, No. 125, War Department, Adjutant General's Office, dated May 28, 1898. 1st to 13th September, 1898, on duty under Special Field Orders, No. 37, Commanding General of the Army in charge of preparing S.S. *Panama* and bringing 255 convalescents from Arroyo and Ponce, Porto Rico to the United States. 13th to 30th on duty under Special Orders, No. 218, Headquarters of the Army pertaining to inspection of Medical Departments of several regiments of the U.S. Infantry, stationed at Jacksonville, Chickamauga, and Lexington, Kentucky.[17]

Daly's inspections of the military bases would be his last official military duties. In his communications to the surgeon general in early November 1898, December 1898, and January 1899, he reported from Pittsburgh that he was on approved sick leave due to "malarial fever contracted in Porto Rico."[18]

During his 28 September inspection of the troops at Chickamauga, he encountered another problem with beef, which he generalized in his previously mentioned 21 October report to the assistant adjutant-general. During his commission testimony in January 1899, he later recounted: "I inspected a lot of beef that had just been brought from the post commissary to the regiment, and there were a lot of soldiers working with it, cutting it up. I examined it, smelled it, and it had a very strong odor ... not so very pronounced, but so much so that to one who had smelled it before it was plainly discernible."[19] When asked if others were present and whether they had the same impression, he said: "I do not know who was present, but after examining and smelling it they said it looked all right but it did not smell right."[20] He added: "This beef looked all right and looked very nice, except it had the peculiar odor. I tasted some cooked the next day and it had this same unnatural, disagreeable, and unpalatable taste."[21]

When questioned later about why he was not more forceful in expressing his opinion that the beef was tainted by the use of chemical preservatives, and why he waited until 21 October 1898 to file his report with the assistant adjutant-general, Daly responded:

> "One swallow doesn't make a summer," and one observation doesn't give conclusive proof. I have lived fifty-seven years in this world, and I have grown a little cautious. I do not feel like jumping at conclusions, even with a chemical analysis. I think I used the ordinary discretion—waiting for my own observations to be confirmed—and I have no excuses to offer. If I withheld any private experiments, that was my own private affair, because I had recommended the Government to make investigations for itself [referring to his 21 October report to the assistant adjutant-general]. Although a student of chemistry for thirty years, and although I graduated very high in chemistry, I did not suppose the Government would care to take my analysis as conclusive, notwithstanding I believe it was carefully made.[22]

Daly's observations and reports on the beef might have gone unnoticed by anyone except General Miles and the assistant adjutant-general if not for the Miles' testimony in front of the Dodge Commission in December 1898. Miles was not a willing witness; he had no interest in becoming involved in what he considered little more than a case of political intrigue and War Department cover-up. Miles, like many others around the country, had read reports suggesting there was something remiss about the hearings. Just a few weeks earlier, an article in the *American Monthly Review of Reviews* reported:

> The manifest intention of the commission is to be entirely fair and just. Its methods thus far, however, would indicate that its attitude is lenient and that it proposes to throw the burden of proof very strictly upon any one who may have an accusation to make. The witnesses it called at the outset were mostly men who had received high honors at the hands of the War Department, and who showed a loyal disposition to approve of almost everything, and to brush aside complaints and criticisms.[23]

Miles knew there would be little to gain by his participation. However, after receiving a personal entreaty from General Dodge, he acquiesced and agreed to testify.

On 21 December 1898, exactly eighty-six days after the hearings began, the commission raised the lid on Pandora's Box. Initially, Miles' testimony was little more than a restating of the remarks he had purportedly made to the *Kansas City Star* newspaper reporter in August and those mentioned earlier in this chapter about the logistical and supply issues in Tampa. He did take the opportunity to offer his opinion on the less than optimal conditions he found on several military bases, offering a particularly derogatory emphasis on the general unsuitability of Camp Alger, which was located near Falls Church, Virginia.[24]

Approximately three-fourths the way through his testimony, Miles introduced allegations about the unsatisfactory quality of the refrigerated beef supplied to the troops. With no forewarning, Miles offered a statement: "There was sent to Porto Rico 337 tons of what is known as so-called refrigerated beef, which you

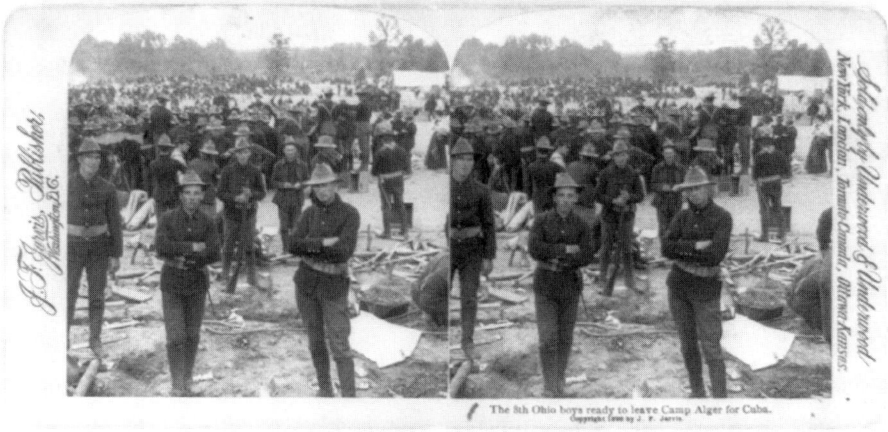

Stereograph view of the 8th Ohio Infantry ready to leave Camp Alger for Cuba, 1898. (*Library of Congress*)

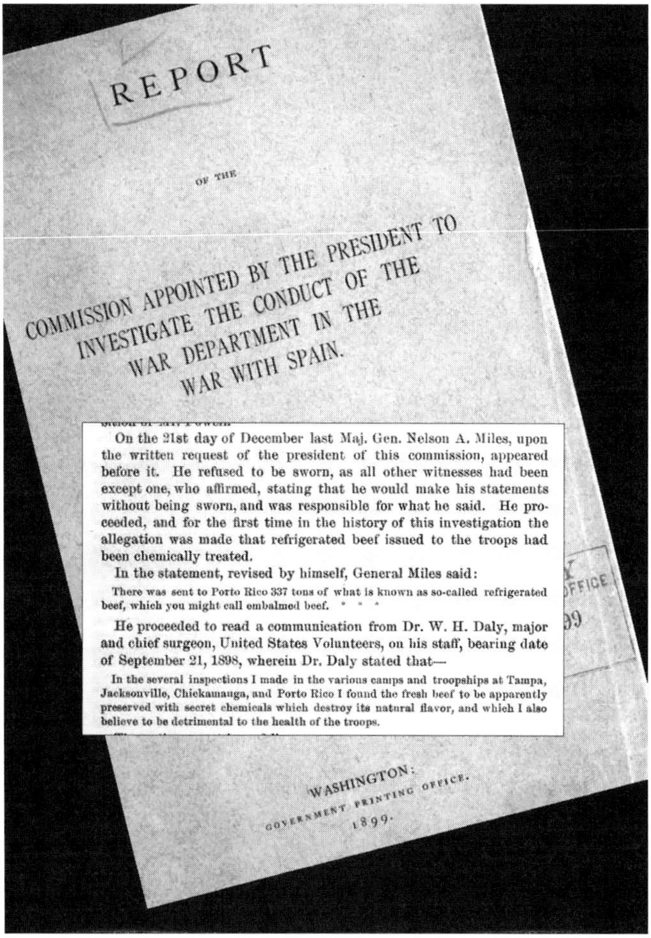

REPORT

OF THE

COMMISSION APPOINTED BY THE PRESIDENT TO INVESTIGATE THE CONDUCT OF THE WAR DEPARTMENT IN THE WAR WITH SPAIN.

On the 21st day of December last Maj. Gen. Nelson A. Miles, upon the written request of the president of this commission, appeared before it. He refused to be sworn, as all other witnesses had been except one, who affirmed, stating that he would make his statements without being sworn, and was responsible for what he said. He proceeded, and for the first time in the history of this investigation the allegation was made that refrigerated beef issued to the troops had been chemically treated.

In the statement, revised by himself, General Miles said:

There was sent to Porto Rico 337 tons of what is known as so-called refrigerated beef, which you might call embalmed beef. * * *

He proceeded to read a communication from Dr. W. H. Daly, major and chief surgeon, United States Volunteers, on his staff, bearing date of September 21, 1898, wherein Dr. Daly stated that—

In the several inspections I made in the various camps and troopships at Tampa, Jacksonville, Chickamauga, and Porto Rico I found the fresh beef to be apparently preserved with secret chemicals which destroy its natural flavor, and which I also believe to be detrimental to the health of the troops.

WASHINGTON:
GOVERNMENT PRINTING OFFICE.
1899.

"Embalmed Beef" investigation report and testimony, 1899. (*National Library of Medicine*) might call embalmed beef, and there was also sent 198,508 pounds of what is known as canned fresh beef, which was condemned, as far as I know, by nearly every officer whose command used it."[25] He then offered into evidence Major Daly's critical report to the assistant adjutant-general of 21 October about the issues encountered with "refrigerated beef" on the S.S. *Panama*, and the suspected chemical treatment of beef ("embalmed beef") on the S.S. *Comal*.

Miles' invention of the phrase "embalmed beef" to refer to the meat Daly described in his report as having "a sickening odor, like a human body dead of disease and injected with preservatives" was provocative. Commission members considered it outrageous; the public found it disconcerting, but highly amusing. In a matter of minutes, the general had turned the hearings upside down. The proceedings would not recover and the matter of "embalmed beef" would soon take on a life of its own.[26]

Aside from describing issues with the "embalmed beef," Miles widened the discussion to include problems with canned beef rations as well. Surprising commission members even further, he advised them that, after receiving Major Daly's reports, he had requested written statements from his officers about the beef he wished to submit into evidence. A few examples of the initial group of remarks offered by regimental commanders include:

> Brigadier-General Viele—First Cavalry
> The meat was a miserable apology for food in a hot climate, a slimy-looking mass of beef scraps, unpalatable to the taste, and repulsive to the sight.
>
> Lieutenant-Colonel Miner—Sixth Infantry
> The meat was utterly unfit as an article of diet for either sick or well. It had no nutriment in it and turned the stomachs of men who tried to eat it.
>
> Major Humphreys—Twelfth Infantry
> The meat issued presented such a repulsive appearance that men turned from it in disgust. "Nasty" is the only term that will fitly describe its appearance.[27]

In many minds, Miles' statements confirmed the public's worst suspicions about maltreatment of Army troops. In one fell swoop, his testimony changed the trajectory of the hearings and brought Daly directly into the fray. Once the general testified about how he was instigated to action upon receiving Major Daly's report and gave the bad beef its new name, Daly joined the general in the administration's bull's-eye. The fact Miles used Daly's report to set in motion the canvassing of regimental officers asking their opinions on the quality of beef opened a wound that would not soon heal. In addition to the above declarations, the general would later submit into evidence many other testimonials as to the unfitness of the beef ration, including one from Theodore Roosevelt:

> The so-called canned roast beef that was issued to us for travel rations, both on the transport and on the train, and which we occasionally got even at the front, was practically worthless. Unless very hungry, the men would not touch it, and even when suffering from lack of food, they never ate a fifth of it. At the best it was tasteless; at the worst it was nauseating. There was also a supply of beef (in the shape of quarters), which was put aboard our transport at Tampa. It was supposed to be fitted by some process to withstand tropical heat. It at once became putrid and smelt so that we had to dispose of it for fear of its creating disease. I think we threw it overboard. At any rate, it was condemned. The beef we got in Santiago, after about the 24th or 25th of July—that is, after the siege had ended, and when my brigade had been without fresh meat or vegetables for a month, was generally good. By that time the cavalry division was in a sickly condition. The fact that the meat ration was so bad as generally to be inedible caused very great hardships to my men, and reduced the supply of food below what was necessary to keep them in proper condition.[28]

It is interesting to note Roosevelt's report indicated, like Daly's report on the quarter of beef he encountered on the *Comal*, another of the beef quarters "supposed to be fitted by some process to withstand tropical heat."[29]

Miles' testimony and his submission of many additional testimonials from regimental officers greatly annoyed Secretary of War Alger and incited open hostility from Commissary General Charles P. Eagan. The Spanish-American War was by no means over as far as its organization, management, and food procurement efforts were concerned. At this point, it had simply moved from the islands in the Caribbean to the Lemon Building in Washington, D.C.

Commissary General Eagan had already testified before the commission on 12 and 13 December 1898, but his testimony dealt with routine matters in a rather innocuous manner that ruffled few feathers. Miles' testimony several days later on 21 December caused Eagan to erupt in a fit of rage. Eagan reacted indignantly to Miles' charges and immediately requested the commission grant him an opportunity to respond. On 22 December 1899, Eagan wrote to the president of the investigating committee, General Dodge:

> General: I have the honor to inclose [*sic.*] herewith newspaper clippings from last evening's *Star* and this morning's *Post*, purporting to be the statements made before your committee by Gen. Nelson A. Miles in regard to the beef furnished by this Department for the use of the Army in Porto Rico and elsewhere. The astounding nature of some of the statements requires, in justice to the Government and myself and for the proper information of your committee, the truth and the facts in regard to the matters stated by General Miles, and which statements, the papers state, were not made under oath, as mine and all others were. I respectfully ask that the committee furnish me with a copy of General Miles's statements and any reports he may have submitted in so far as they refer to this department or myself, and that I be

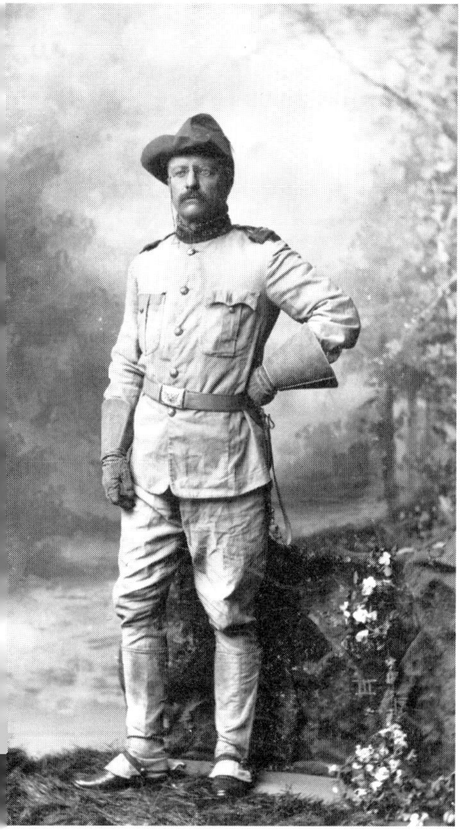

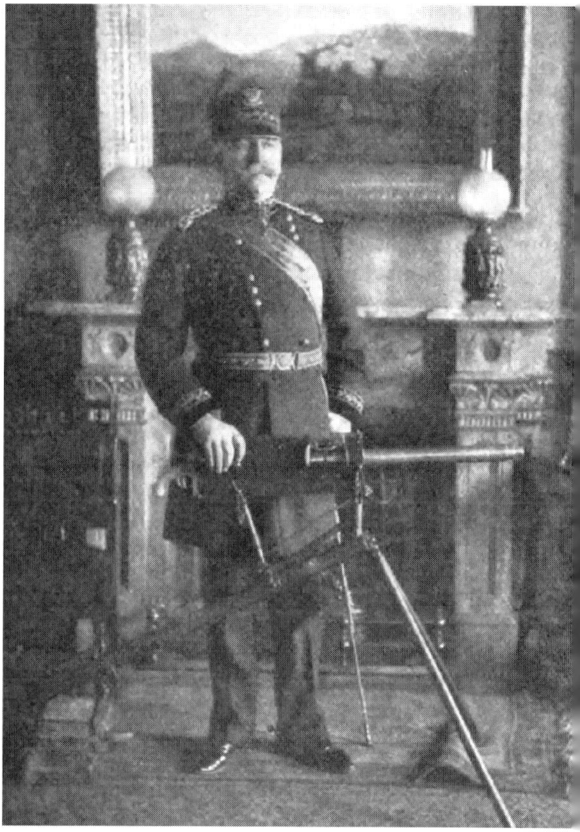

Above left: Col. Theodore Roosevelt, in uniform, 1898. (*Library of Congress*)

Above right: Gen. Nelson A. Miles, 1899. (*Literary Times, Volume 18, Number 4, 28 January 1899*)

summoned before your committee to give my sworn evidence on all the facts in my possession in rebuttal of the statements alleged to have been made by General Miles. This course is all the more imperative because among other statements that I am prepared to rebut is the following, which I quote: "General Miles suggested that the food was sent to his large army under pretense of an experiment." I contend that the only proper interpretation to be placed upon this statement, and the interpretation that will be placed upon it by the public at large, is that if this food was sent under the "pretense of an experiment" it must have been because there existed corruption or some other equally improper motive. I refrain from characterizing here this statement in terms. A court of justice can do that.

While it is very far from my intention to involve the committee in controversy of any kind, I respectfully submit that it is not just that the statements alleged to have been made by General Miles should go unchallenged or unrefuted, and claim

> the right to be heard in rebuttal; and to enable me to do this it seems but fair and necessary that I should be furnished with a correct report of his statements to your committee in regard to the Subsistence Department and myself. I desire to appear before the committee and under oath meet the statements herein referred to.[30]

General Dodge agreed to the request. On 12 January 1899, General Eagan reappeared in front of the commission. He was eager to respond to General Miles' charges and his hostility toward both Miles and Daly was quickly expressed. His rebuttal, read from a prepared statement, was long and exhausting. It started with Eagan stating: "Gentlemen: I hold in my hands the official copy of the statements made to your commission by the senior major-general of the United States Army, Nelson A. Miles."[31]

He began by noting his irritation over Miles' selection of commissary officers of his choosing instead of those Eagan thought more appropriately suited to the role. From there he went on to discuss his issue with the general's involvement in beef procurement discussions (Miles had suggested the use of live cattle stock instead of refrigerated or canned beef). Eagan then noted his annoyance over the general's negative comments about problems with foodstuffs on transports—canned beef, refrigerated beef, and purported "embalmed beef," during the Cuba and Porto Rico campaigns.

Surprisingly, at an early point in his statement, the commissary general thought it necessary to attest to the integrity of the beef contractors. He stated, "I take this occasion to say, [they] have lived up to the letter of their contracts faithfully, honorably, honestly, and caring apparently for no expense that might be entailed in the proper execution of their contract; honorable men in every way, so far as I know, and these are the men whose merchandise was permitted to spoil, entailing serious loss upon them, because due and proper effort seems not to have been made, as we have seen, to issue this beef to the troops."[32]

It was not long before Eagan targeted Major Daly. He stated: "General Miles was asked by you [the Commission] if he based his cablegrams [soliciting testimonials from regimental commanders] upon the opinion given by Dr. Daly. He replies: 'I did not know so much about the character of beef at that time as I know now, because, as I say, I have been investigating the subject, and the matter will be still further investigated.'"[33]

With Daly now in his crosshairs, he referred to Miles' comments about Daly's report and went on to state:

> He [meaning Dr. Daly] made an expert examination of it (refrigerated beef) as a medical officer who was accustomed to the use of chemicals of the description that are used for embalming bodies. "Did he make any chemical analysis of it General?" was asked by your commission, to which he replies: "The understanding is that this is a secret process of preserving beef;" and, further, General Miles states: "It has a

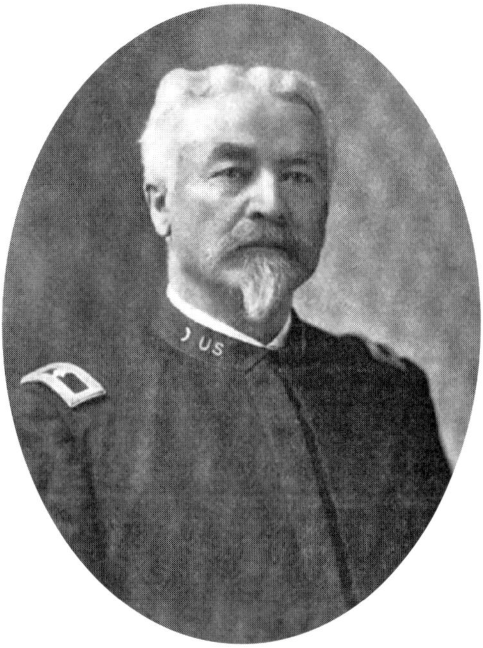

Commissary Gen. Charles P. Eagan, 1899. (*Literary Times, Volume 18, Number 4, 28 January 1899*)

> Keeley-motor effect on the health of the men." What General Miles means by Keeley-motor effect on the men can only be understood by connecting the remark with the others that he has made. The implication, of course, is that it had an improper effect upon the men, probably upon their health. Assuming this to be the intent of his statement, I desire to say that it had no such effect, and I do not believe that Dr. Daly ever made an expert examination of it.[34]

Eagan next went into a lengthy dialog countering Daly's comments about the beef at Ponce, on board the *Panama*, and at Tampa. In special reference to the beef that Daly encountered in Tampa aboard the *Comal*, Eagan stated: "... it was not meat intended for the soldiers nor beef the Subsistence Department had anything whatsoever to do with. On the contrary, Colonel Osgood [referring to H. B. Osgood, Acting Commissary-General of Subsistence who testified earlier] tells you that it was processed beef, being experimented upon by a man named Powell."[35]

With Osgood's testimony, the mystery of the beef Daly found on the *Comal* was solved. Alexander B. Powell was a principal of Powell Brothers Company, a New York City meat vending company. The firm specialized in using a proprietary preservative process to prepare meats for shipment to southern locations. In a letter to President McKinley in early May 1898, Powell offered his firm's services to the government in support of the war effort. In his communication to McKinley, he described the preservation process: "It so purifies the meats that they will stand any climate for from four to ten days after leaving the ice house. I simply so purify the germs of the meats that they will stand the destroying elements of any climate."[36]

The company never received a government contract for beef; however, as Eagan noted, the commissary general's office had allowed Powell to prepare and hang six beef quarters on ships to demonstrate his preservation process. Major Daly and Colonel Roosevelt had each documented their observations of two of the six quarters.

Eagan then questioned why Daly waited until 21 September (not 21 October as Daly testified) to report the beef issue to General Miles and had not reported the matter sooner to authorities Eagan considered more appropriate. Regarding Daly's report, he added: "If it seemed to him that soldiers were being diseased and made sick by bad beef, embalmed beef, chemically processed beef, why did he not make a chemical analysis of the alleged chemicals or preservatives or embalming fluid?[37] At this point in the commission's hearings, Daly had not yet testified he had tested the beef while on sick leave in Pittsburgh in late September.

Eagan further expressed his irritation with Major Daly by stating:

> As we see, he kept this report to himself, as we know he never furnished it to the War Department, but first introduced it to this commission, thus proclaiming to the world that the beef fed to the soldiers was chemically treated, caused sickness, and, by clear inference, that each and every one of the large packing houses who were contractors for furnishing this beef were cheating the Government, violating their contracts, imposing on the Subsistence Department, and that the Commissary-General himself, by insisting upon its use, was a party to this fraud upon the troops.[38]

He then turned again to his discomfort with General Miles for implying the commissary had sent the beef to the Army as an experiment:

> ... which implies corruption, which ninety-nine out of every one hundred people will understand to mean corruption, because it was "a pretense of experiment," he says, not even giving credit to me for furnishing it as an experiment, but that I furnished it under the "pretense of an experiment." This is a serious charge; should not be made by any man lightly nor without ample evidence to support it.[39]

Charles Eagan's testimony on 12 January 1899 covered more than thirty-five pages of responses to Miles and Daly's assertions and included numerous exhibits he thought important in making a case he had been wronged. His longwinded retort might well have been successful in turning public opinion if it had not been for an acrimonious outburst he made as part of the aforementioned "pretense of experiment" remarks. As soon as his offensive words were uttered, they were deemed inappropriate for an Army officer and government official. It was quickly decided they should be struck from the official hearing records.

Despite the commission's action to strike them from official documents and preference they be omitted from reports of the hearing, Eagan had already distributed copies to the press. He was later allowed to edit the most egregious parts of his statement for inclusion in the final report. However, there was no way to put the genie back in the bottle as far as the press was concerned. Accounts of his testimony began appearing quickly. The next morning, for example, a *New York Sun* headline read "Gen. Eagan hotly denies the story about Army beef. Calls Gen. Miles a Liar."[40] Less than two days after Eagan's testimony was given, a detailed report of the officially omitted language was printed in *The Army and Navy Journal.* After providing background on Eagan's "pretence for experiment implying corruption" testimony, they reported his pejorative statements:

> This is a serious charge, should not be made by any man lightly or without ample evidence to support it. Taking the statement in the sense that was probably intended, the sense that will be accepted by the country at large, the sense that already the press almost wholly of the United States has accepted it—indeed, some of that press because of it called for my dismissal from the Army and my court martial—I answer that it was not furnished under the pretence of experiment, nor even as an experiment, and when Gen. Miles charges that it was furnished as "a pretence of an experiment," *he lies in his throat, he lies in his heart, he lies in every hair of his head and every pore of his body; he lies willfully, deliberately, intentionally and maliciously.*
>
> If this statement is true that this was furnished under "pretense of an experiment," then I should be drummed out of the Army and incarcerated in State prison. If this statement is false, as I have asserted it to be, then he should be drummed out of the service and incarcerated in prison with other libellers. His statement is scandalous libel, reflecting upon the honor of every officer in the Department who has contracted for or purchased this meat, and especially and particularly on the Commissary General—myself. In denouncing Gen. Miles as a liar when he makes this statement itself, I wish to make it as emphatic and as coarse as the statement itself. I wish to force the lie back into his throat, covered with the contents of a camp latrine. I wish it branded as a falsehood of whole cloth, without a particle of truth to sustain it, and unless he can prove his statement he should be denounced by every honest man, barred the clubs, barred from the society of decent people, and so ostracized that the street bootblacks would not condescend to speak to him, for he fouled his own nest, he has aspersed the honor of a brother officer without a particle of evidence or fact to sustain in any degree his scandalous, libelous, malicious falsehood, *viz.*, that this beef or anything whatever was furnished the Army under pretense of an experiment.
>
> If I have used harsh language before the Commission in dealing with the subject I ask the Commission to bear in mind that the grouping together of the statements made by Gen. Miles means that I have furnished or allowed to be furnished to the Army embalmed beef which has diseased soldiers, and that a great deal of sickness

> arose from its use; that I have furnished meats to the Army under the "pretence of experiment," meats that made the soldiers sick, and this under the pretence of experiment; this because of corruption. Also, that these statements of Gen. Miles were held back by him, not furnished to the Government for its appropriate action and use, but sprung upon you and the country at a time when the country, from falsehoods that have been told in regards to the starvation and supplies for the Army. The subject I have treated here is a filthy subject, and you cannot touch pitch without being defiled; you cannot touch base, malicious, libelous falsehoods, misrepresentations, without calling a spade a spade, and telling the whole truth and characterizing things as they are. The damage that has been done by these statements is believed to be very great, but I indulge the hope and belief that my statement, when published to the country, when read by the representatives of foreign countries, will offset the statements made by Gen. Miles, and will, in some measure at least, do justice to others that have been wronged, maligned and libeled. For myself, I content myself with expressing my profound belief that either Gen Miles or I should be put out of the service; either he is right or I am right, either he dishonors his uniform with his false statements and libels, or I dishonor mine in feeding soldiers with poisonous beef, causing their sickness and doing so under "pretence of experiment."[41]

Talk of possible censure began among commission members even before Eagan left the hearing room. Things moved fast, and it was almost as if a tornado had just struck. In the same issue of the *Army and Navy Journal* in which Eagan's statements were reported, editors wrote: "Brig. Gen. Charles P. Eagan, Commissary General of Subsistence, is an Irishman by birth and we should be at liberty to suppose that his fighting Irish blood had got the better of his judgment in his attack upon the Major General Commanding the Army."[42] The editors further commented:

> It can hardly be that General Eagan wishes to provoke a court martial in which he will have the manifest advantage of defence. His proper course would be to demand a court of inquiry. He has put the matter now in such a position that if a court martial is ordered the charges brought would naturally be "conduct unbecoming an officer and a gentleman," or "conduct subversive of good order and military discipline." It is difficult to see how General Eagan could escape conviction of both of these offences, if his testimony, which we quote elsewhere from the daily papers, is correctly reported.[43]

On 18 January 1899, less than a week after reading his statement before the commission, Brigadier General Charles P. Eagan, Commissary General of Subsistence, U.S. Army, was court-martialed. Two charges were entered: Charge I—"Conduct unbecoming an officer and gentleman," for use of "grossly insulting" and "ungentlemanly" language in denouncing General Miles as a liar; Charge

II—"Conduct to the prejudice of good order and military discipline," for use of "grossly abusive and unmilitary language with reference to the Major General Commanding the Army."[44] Adjutant General's Charge II included much of Eagan's language as was quoted in the 14 January edition of the *Army and Navy Journal.*

Eagan pled not guilty to the charges, but he did acknowledge his use of the language. On 17 February, the court-martial board's decisions were reported. He was found guilty on the specifications and charges for both counts and sentenced "To be dismissed the service."[45] The findings and sentence were transmitted to the president for action.

McKinley approved the action of the board but commuted Eagan's sentence. In his response, he wrote:

> In view, however, of his [Eagan's] gallant conduct in battle, upon more than one occasion, which merited and has received the warm commendation of his superiors, and of his long and honorable record of service, extending over a period surpassing in duration that usually allotted to a generation; having regard, also, to the mitigating circumstances which were developed during the trial of the case, and in deference to the recommendation to clemency submitted in his behalf, the sentence imposed by the court is commuted to suspension from rank and duty for six years.[46]

In commuting Eagan's sentence and suspending him with pay for six years, McKinley also effectively allowed Eagan to retire with full military benefits.

On 18 January, on the same day as Eagan's court-martial began, Major William Hudson Daly resigned his military commission. Four days later, on 22 January, he was scheduled to testify before the commission at 10 a.m. in the Lemon Building in Washington, D.C. He was witness number 442.

There seems little doubt Daly communicated with General Miles over the previous few weeks, and the general had forewarned him about what might be asked—or suggested—during his questioning. Daly timed his resignation to occur after the general's appearance before the commission but before his own. He also took time in Pittsburgh to confer with an attorney. A copy of a recently discovered invoice read: "To professional services, advice, direction, preparation of papers, examination, instruction in regard to the law in the matter of Embalmed Meat Investigation, and advice for himself and others, and advice for himself as to their obligation to obey subpoena to go to Washington, D.C."[47]

The main facts of Daly's testimony before the commission have already been noted. During his questioning, members of the commission took turns probing him on what he saw, what he knew, and what he had reported. Many of the questions were asked multiple times in different ways in an obvious attempt to trip him up and catch him in a lie. Daly did not fall for the gambit.

Much of the questioning was rather antagonistic, with many questions insinuating Daly had failed to make reports to the commissary general or surgeon general's office. Daly repeatedly replied he reported directly to General Miles, and by rendering reports to him and the adjutant-general, he had fulfilled his responsibilities as an officer. He expressed his opinion that it was entirely up to the general or adjutant-general whether or not they wished to pursue the matter further. Other questions were asked in such a manner as to suggest Daly was not a scientist, and in as much as he was not an expert in chemical analysis, his judgment was somehow lacking. When questioned again about why it took him so long to write his report of 21 October, and implying he was on trial, Daly claimed the high ground and responded:

> I had no explanation to make except so far as my report there goes, with the supplemental information that I have tried patiently to give you today. I don't propose to be put on trial by this commission or anybody else, with all due respect to you. I do not believe this country will put me on trial. I am not afraid for one moment that my fellow-countrymen will ever put me on trial for having simply done my duty and reporting with due deliberation and without unnecessary delay.[48]

The commission's proceedings certainly must have made it feel like a trial to Daly. Before entering the hearing chamber that morning, he was undoubtedly aware of the fact dozens of witnesses had already been questioned about him, his actions, his reports, and just about everything he did during the war. Throughout the proceedings and even under the most intense questioning, however, Daly remained calm and collected. Much to the chagrin of his interrogators, he handled even the most hostile questions in a polite and professional manner. To Daly's relief and delight, Professor Frank W. Clarke, Chief Chemist of the Department of the Interior, United States Geological Survey, issued a report on what he had found in the samples of the beef extract powder Daly had tested in Pittsburgh. Clarke wrote to the commission:

> In accordance with your request we have examined the powder submitted by Dr. W. H. Daly for boric and salicylic acids. Both the flame test and the turmeric paper test give distinct evidences of the presence of boric acid. We submit herewith the slips of turmeric paper showing the red coloration given by the sample examined, and also a slip showing the reaction obtained by boric acid alone. We also obtained good reactions with ferric chloride, showing the presence of salicylic acid in the powder.[49]

Daly held his ground that day, but the beef matter was not about to go away any time soon.

The Commission Appointed by the President to Investigate the Conduct of the War Department in the War with Spain ended its deliberations on 09 February 1899. At the end of the day, on the 109th day of their investigation, they delivered a final report to President McKinley at the Executive Mansion. The report filled eight volumes with thousands of pages of testimony and exhibits. William H. Daly's name was cited hundreds of times.

When hearings began back in September 1898, nobody anticipated beef would end up usurping so much of the commission's attention. By the time the final report was issued, the matter of refrigerated and canned beef had been so thoroughly examined it ended up consuming a significant part of the official record. For the press and public, it was also one of the most eagerly anticipated parts of the report.

The commission, in its report, did its best to end the beef matter once and for all. In regard to the refrigerated beef, it wrote: "In view of the facts above set forth, the commission is of the opinion that no refrigerated beef furnished by contractors and issued to the troops during the war with Spain was subjected to or treated with any chemicals by the contractors or those in their employ."[50] Relative to the canned beef, the commission noted:

> After careful consideration, we find that canned meat, as issued to the troops, was generally of good quality, was properly prepared, and contained no deleterious substance. At times probably material of poor quality is issued; in one of the cans sent to us and examined by the chemist large amount of gristle was found. That was not issued "under pretense of an experiment" is indicated by the fact that has been in use in the Army for more than twenty years.[51]

The general public was very interested in the beef matter but paid little attention to the commission's many other findings and recommendations about the operation of the Army's departments and bureaus, or its intended rebukes of Miles and Daly. Despite the commandeering of the commission's work to investigate beef, and its suggestion no further action need be taken, many of its recommendations subsequently proved useful in reorganizing the Army. However, much to the annoyance of President McKinley, the beef trusts and the money the industry represented, the beef problem would simply not go away.

Politically, the "embalmed beef" scandal, as it was now billed in the press across the country, upended the president's best-laid plans for delivering political cover. It humiliated Secretary of War Alger and caused him to offer his resignation to President McKinley in September 1898 (which was not accepted until August 1899), cost Commissary General Eagan his position in February 1899, and, perhaps most importantly, had the potential to damage McKinley's chances of winning reelection in 1900.

While it was suggested the president had no advance knowledge of the commission's findings, evidence suggests otherwise. Shrewdly, McKinley once again took control of the situation by forming another investigating commission to deal specifically with the "beef problem." On 03 February 1899, McKinley initiated a court of inquiry and directed it "to investigate certain allegations

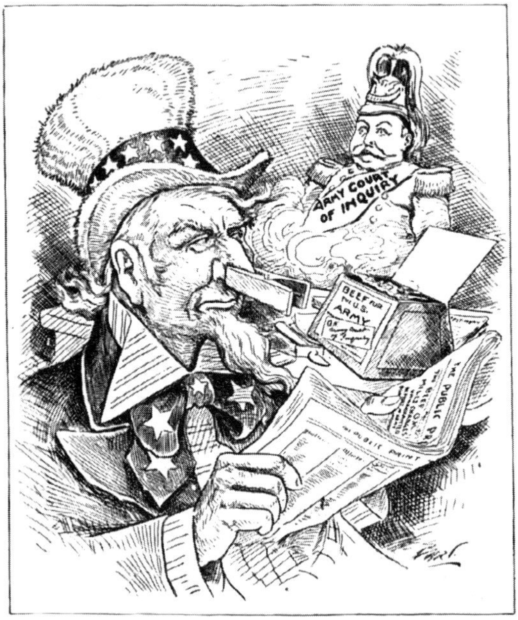

UNCLE SAM'S VERDICT.

UNCLE SAM: "Well, close the thing and take it away. It may be O. K., but the whiffs I have had have been very unsavory."

—*The Journal* (*Rep.*), *Minneapolis.*

Uncle Sam's verdict, 1899. (*The Literary Digest, Volume 18, Number 19, 13 May 1899*)

of the Major-General Commanding the Army [Nelson A. Miles] in respect to the unfitness for issue of certain articles of food furnished by the Subsistence Department to the troops in the field during the recent operations in Cuba and Porto Rico. In addition to its findings of fact, the court will submit an opinion upon the merits of the case, together with such recommendations as to further proceedings as may seem to be warranted by the facts developed in the course of the inquiry."[52]

On 09 February 1899, the exact day the Dodge Commission ended its work and delivered its findings, the Food Furnished by Subsistence Department to Troops in the Field Court of Inquiry began its deliberations. William H. Daly would once again play an integral part in the new proceedings.

10

No Trifling Matter

William H. Daly soon found he was deceiving himself to have considered his involvement in the beef matter ended with his testimony in front of the Dodge Commission. It had been a grueling experience, almost as nerve-racking as his time at the front during the Civil War. Instead of dodging bullets while a young man in the woods of Virginia, at the age of fifty-seven, he had just survived a series of attacks on his professional qualifications and his service as an Army officer in Washington, D.C. He was not happy about the outcome of the commission's work, but he was confident he had done his best to make his case about the potential harmfulness of the preserved beef. Even more importantly, in his mind, he had supported his friend General Miles in a manner like no one else could under the changed circumstances that now prevailed with Miles openly engaged in political battle against Secretary Alger and the War Department.

President McKinley's move to form the Food Furnished by Subsistence Department to Troops in the Field Court of Inquiry was breathtakingly quick and caught many outside the president's administration by surprise. General Miles seemingly took the matter in stride. William H. Daly, on the other hand, was not at all thrilled about the prospects of being called back to Washington, D.C. Even if it was his verbal and written reports that had roused the general's interest in the poor quality of beef, he thought his entanglement in the matter was over once the Dodge Commission issued its final report.

Much like what occurred with the name of the Commission to Investigate the Conduct of the War Department in the War with Spain becoming known as the "Dodge Commission," the same occurred with the Court of Inquiry. The "Wade Beef Board," as it was later known, was composed of Major General James F. Wade, U.S. Volunteers (chairman); Brigadier General George W. Davis, U.S. Volunteers; Colonel George L. Gillespie, Corps of Engineers; and Lieutenant Colonel George B. Davis, Deputy Judge Advocate General, U.S. Army (recorder). In addition to the regular members, John W. Hulse of Washington, D.C., was

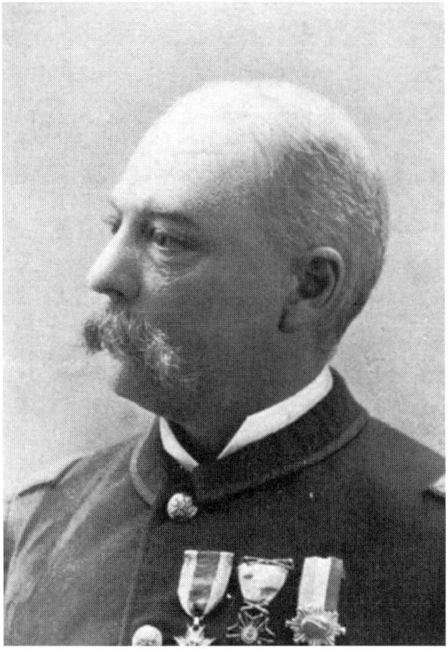

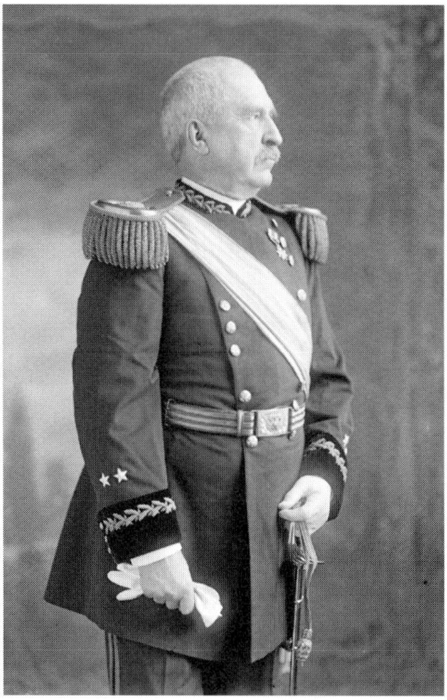

Above left: Brig. Gen. James F. Wade, 1899. (*Wikimedia Commons*)

Above right: Gen. George W. Davis, 1905. (*Library of Congress*)

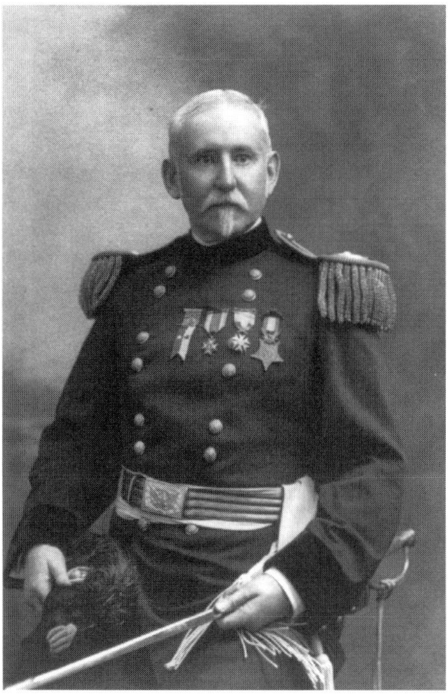

Brig. Gen. George Lewis Gillespie, Jr., 1898. (*Wikimedia Commons*)

employed as reporter. Like its predecessor, the Court of Inquiry used the Lemon Building in Washington, D.C., for its deliberations.

In creating the Court of Inquiry, President McKinley described the subjects of inquiry:

> 1. To investigate certain allegations of the Major-General Commanding the Army [Miles] in respect to the unfitness for issue of certain articles of food furnished by the Subsistence Department to the troops in the field during the recent operations in Cuba and Porto Rico.
> 2. To determine if the beef furnished the army was wholesome and of good quality and sufficient in quantity, and to inquire with care into the allegation that it was treated with acids or chemicals by the contractors or others, or in any way made deleterious to the health of the consumers.[1]

In addition to its findings, McKinley also requested "the court will submit an opinion upon the merits of the case, together with such recommendations as to further proceedings as may seem to be warranted by the facts developed in the course of the inquiry."[2]

While the "Wade Beef Board" officially began its work on 09 February 1899, the first several days were filled with routine preparatory tasks. On Monday 20 February 1899, immediately before the court's first hearing, President McKinley presented the following list of questions he wished members to address:

> 1. The character and quality of the meat, refrigerated and canned, furnished to the Army; how purchased; how shipped to the soldiers; if good when shipped; what was the cause of its deterioration, if there was any?
> 2. If the meat was doctored, did the Commissary-General or any of his officers have any knowledge of it or means of knowledge?
> 3. Was it the meat of commerce?
> 4. Was it inspected by the Government inspectors as provided by law?
> 5. Was it an authorized ration in the Army?
> 6. If good when purchased, what made it bad?
> 7. Was it anybody's neglect or fault; and if so, whose?
> 8. When unfit for use, if you should so find, was the fact made known to the War Department? When, and by whom?
> 9. If, after leaving the depot commissary, it was not cared for and properly preserved, whose fault?
> 10. Was it a suitable ration for the campaigns in Cuba and Porto Rico?
> 11. Was there anything better that was practicable?
> 12. Would it have been prudent for our troops to have made the expeditions to Santiago and Porto Rico without the preserved meats, either refrigerated or canned, with which they were supplied?

13. Could the Army, with any certainty, rely upon the cattle on the hoof on these islands?
14. Did the commanding officers in Santiago or Porto Rico or the Major-General Commanding report during the war that either the refrigerated or canned beef was an unfit ration?
15. When were these reports first made, and by whom?
16. If the allegations of the Major-General Commanding are established, I want the court to find the cause and fix the responsibility for the fact, that the guilty may be properly punished.
17. Did the cattle in Porto Rico make a wholesome beef ration?
18. If the packers of the country are guilty, it must be known.
19. If officers of the Commissary Department are guilty, it must be known.
20. If any officer of the Army is guilty, it must be known.[3]

As a civilian, Daly could have easily ignored the inquiry's invitation to testify as some other witnesses did. His friendship with General Miles, however, suggested he abandon the thought. Daly knew Miles was in a pitched battle with the War Department over the beef and Miles had a festering political confrontation brewing with the White House over real and perceived slights during the war. As such, his testimony could prove critical to the general's case, so he knew he had to submit to another round of hearings. Whether or not Daly was aware of Miles' political aspirations remains unknown, but it is likely he did since they continued to correspond and hunt together throughout the period.

General Miles was called as the inquiry's first witness at noon on 20 February 1899. Covering twenty-two pages of testimony, Miles did little more than rehash the statements he had made before the Dodge Commission in late December the previous year. What was new in this investigation was the submission of a voluminous list of witnesses General Miles recommended for interview. Relative to the general's list, the inquiry later noted that he had submitted names of 441 potential witnesses, out of which 104 were called to testify. Not to be outdone by the general, the inquiry called 163 of its own witnesses, including twenty from the Subsistence Department, thirteen from the Agricultural Department, fifty-one representatives of the meat industry, and seventy-nine others, including military officers, enlisted soldiers, medical officers, ex-officers, and soldiers of the volunteers. William Hudson Daly was one of the 267 witnesses. During the proceedings, General Miles also offered 340 official written reports into evidence.[4]

Notably, meat industry witnesses represented almost 20 percent of those called to testify. Members of the inquiry either ignored or were oblivious to the public sentiment expressed in countless news articles over the previous several months since the Dodge Commission began its work the previous fall. By the time the Wade Beef Board held its first session in February 1899, suspicions of a government cover-up were rampant, secondary only to a total mistrust of the meatpacking industry. Headlines and articles suggesting the McKinley administration of a whitewash were evident throughout the country. One example of the public view of the Dodge Commission proceedings appeared in *Harper's Weekly* in November 1898, when its editors wrote:

> The investigation of the army administration is going on, the commissioners traveling the circuit. They are conducting the examination of officers who have received favors from the administration, and they are neglecting a good many opportunities, apparently, to learn the truth. Their report is likely to find that affairs were conducted about as well as could be expected from the nature or the demand made upon the staff corps; but whatever the report may be, it will be of no importance. We refused to attack the commission in advance, but now we are forced to the conclusion that it is not diligently seeking the truth. The facts are, not only that we began the war before we were prepared for it, but that we went into Cuba like a mob, at a time when Northern soldiers should not have been sent there, and that the men were badly clothed and badly fed, owing to the incompetency of the staff officers, most of whom were civilians appointed for political reasons.[5]

There were many other instances of articles and editorials written in a similar vein before the Wade Beef Board's first meeting. Most relied on facts and testimony to present their case throughout the Dodge Commission's tenure; others took the route of humor and sarcasm as the *New York Journal* did in its editorial pages in mid-October 1898:

> When the Dodge Commission went into executive session yesterday after members had removed their disguises, which they were forced to wear to avoid recognition and unpleasant questioning on their way to daily work, there was an air of happy expectancy on each face. Nobody mentioned Credit Mobilier behind the Chairman's back and the subject of Alger's son having real estate in camp land in Florida was not hinted at. "It seems evident," remarked Colonel Denby, "that we will be enabled now to prolong our sessions until after the election. I have prepared an entirely new set of questions which, for general irrelevancy and pure inapplicability to the subject, can scarcely be excelled."[6]

Following the same pattern, the *Evening Times* of Washington, D.C., came to a similar conclusion several weeks after Miles' testimony on 20 February, when it reported:

> It is announced that the Court of Enquiry will be able to complete its work in Chicago in time to leave for Washington tomorrow evening. This is not because there are no more witnesses, but because it is not considered necessary to take any more evidence in defense of General Miles' charges. A correspondent quotes Colonel Davis as saying that it has been abundantly proved that bad meat was sold to the Government and issued to the soldiers.

It should be noted that this does not mean the experimental beef referred to by the Alger Relief Commission in its whitewashing report, but that twenty-five percent of all the refrigerated beef had to be buried and twenty-five percent of the rest had to be cut off and thrown away. How large a proportion of the canned beef was unfit or dangerous has not been estimated. It has been established, too, on the testimony of many surgeons and regimental officers, that the beef caused a large amount of sickness; that the enormous increase of the sick list corresponded with the issue of bad beef. There is evidence that the refrigerated beef was, in fact, chemically treated, at least by the Armours and Swifts, and that the chemicals were injurious to health.

These are findings that would be surprising if the report of the recent Commission had been received with anything but contempt. The explanation made by that body, though without reason, was that an irresponsible person had, on his own account, transported beef to Florida to prove that by a patent process he could preserve it; and that it was this meat that Major Daly saw and examined. Perhaps some persons who did not follow the proceedings closely accepted this explanation and thought the packers had been slandered by General Miles and Major Daly. To help along this opinion, one of the Commissioners said, in a public address, that if the Court of Enquiry had the same experience the Commission did, General Miles would be dismissed from the army. Fortunately for the cause of truth, the Court has not limited its enquiry to persons in the commissary service. It has even placed Mr. Marshall, who was refused a hearing by the Commission, on the stand.

The object of the Alger Relief Commission, even the avowed object, was to give a certificate of honesty to the packers. The members seemed to think it was more important that the reputation of American meat should be protected than that justice should be done, and the soldiers saved from the fraud and danger of diseased beef. The facts brought out in the present investigation make it impossible for the Court to give a certificate to save the meat business from injury. Unless a refutation of the testimony of any number of apparently honest and disinterested witnesses is effected—and that seems wholly impossible—nothing can save the packers from prosecution.[7]

Amid the background of public distrust of the Dodge Commission's findings and the Wade Beef Board's initial hearings over the previous several weeks, William H. Daly was summoned as a witness. He appeared before the Court of Inquiry on 22 February 1899. An article in the *New York Times* the following day documented Daly's testimony:

When the Court of Inquiry met this morning Col. Davis, the Recorder, announced the examination of witnesses so far summoned and reported was about concluded. They should consider now, he thought, the questions of further summons and procedure, and at his suggestion the court went into secret session.

When the executive session was concluded Dr. William H. Daly of Pittsburg, who was Major and Chief Surgeon of Volunteers during the war, who testified before the

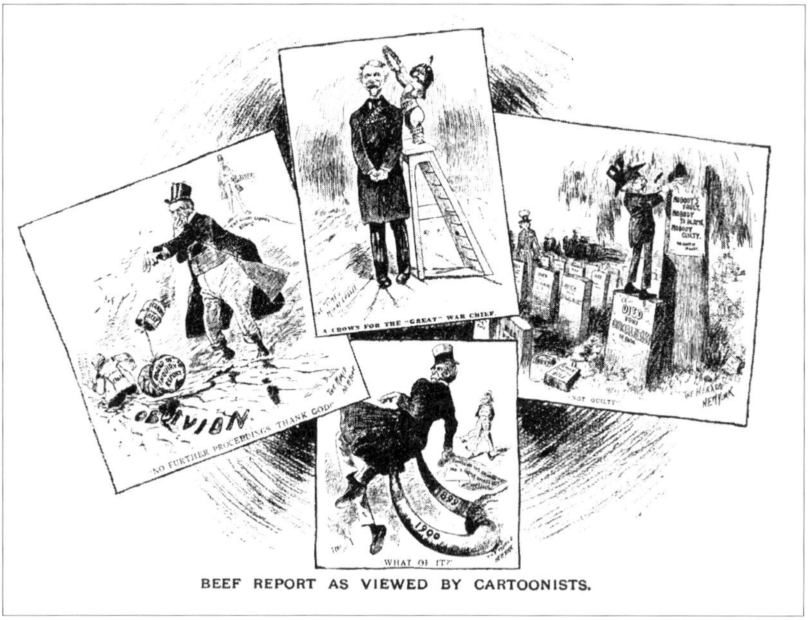
OBLIVION
NO FURTHER PROCEEDINGS THANK GOD
A CROWN FOR THE "GREAT" WAR CHIEF.
"NOT GUILTY"
1899
1900
WHAT OF IT?
BEEF REPORT AS VIEWED BY CARTOONISTS.

Above: Beef report as viewed by cartoonists, 1899. (*The Literary Digest, Volume 18, Number 20, 20 May 1899*)

Below left: Secretary of War Russell A. Alger, "Suppose a little of the beef was spoiled—what of that" cartoon. (*Life Magazine, Volume 33, Number 860, 18 May 1899*)

Below right: "The Country Will Not Swallow That Beef" cartoon 1899. (*New York Journal and Advertiser, 03 February 1899*)

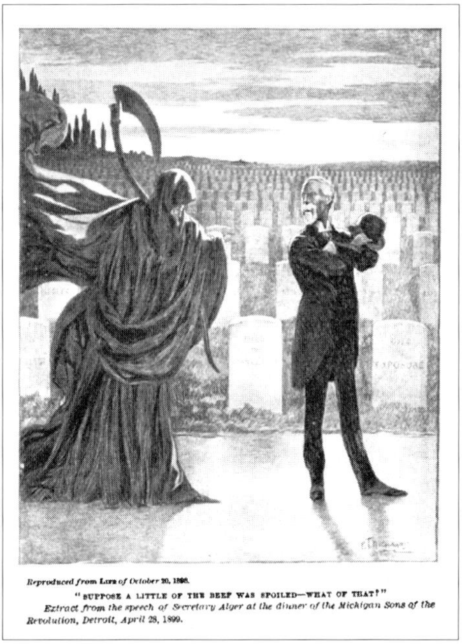
Reproduced from Life of October 20, 1898.
"SUPPOSE A LITTLE OF THE BEEF WAS SPOILED—WHAT OF THAT?"
Extract from the speech of Secretary Alger at the dinner of the Michigan Sons of the Revolution, Detroit, April 28, 1899.

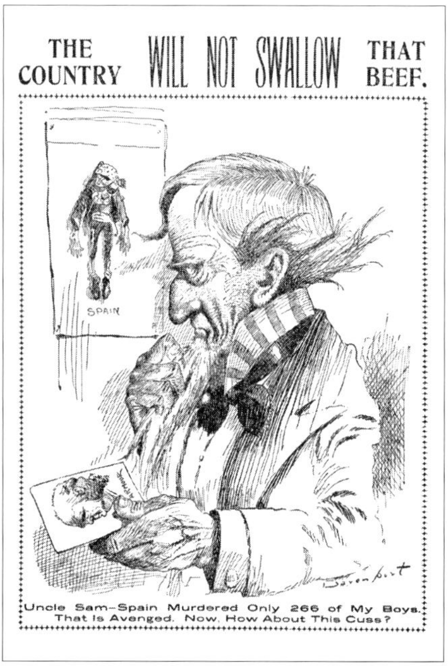
THE COUNTRY WILL NOT SWALLOW THAT BEEF.
SPAIN
Uncle Sam—Spain Murdered Only 266 of My Boys. That Is Avenged. Now, How About This Cuss?

War Commission that he had discovered by chemical analysis boracic and salicylic acid in refrigerated beef furnished the army, was introduced. His examination by the Recorder was conducted slowly and with great care, developing with minuteness all of Dr. Daly's duties while attached to Gen. Miles's staff. These, besides those of an army Surgeon, consisted of making special reports to Gen. Miles on camp sites, water supply, and the like.

The Recorder very carefully developed the fact that most of these reports were verbal or telegraphic, therein differing from the now famous meat report which was the cause of Dr. Daly's being summoned as a witness. Therein the examination differed considerably from the previous witnesses.

Dr. Daly testified that he was assigned to duty on the staff of Gen. Miles and remained at Tampa until a few days after the Shafter expedition sailed, his duties being miscellaneous under direction of the army Medical Department. Thence he went to Key West, Miami, and other points to study proposed camp sites, Later he came North, and finally joined Gen. Miles at Guánica, Puerto Rico, sailing from Charleston subsequent to the latter's departure.

In all of this very detailed recital the question of beef was not once broached by the court, but when Dr. Daly had been chronologically carried through his term of service and out of the army, the Recorder handed him the famous "embalmed beef" report, and asked him if he recognized it. Dr. Daly said he did, and to the best of his recollection the exact date was Oct. 14. The date, however, he said, was not essential, the report being genuine, and in the opinion of Dr. Daly perfectly accurate.

Col. Davis then addressed the court briefly, saying that it was only within twenty-four hours that he had been able to study this report of Dr. Daly, and he found therein certain allegations against certain persons who had made contracts for supplying food material to the Government. To continue the examination of the witness on this subject in the absence of those persons against whom his charges were directed would be to deprive them of rights accorded them by law. He therefore suggested that the other parties interested (the meat contractors) should be given reasonable notice of proceedings, and that the witness be excused subject to recall when examination could be continued with the other interested parties present.

Prior to leaving the stand, Dr. Daly was examined in regard to the Powell experiment with beef preservatives at Tampa, Col. Davis pointing out that it was merely experimental and no contractor was involved. Dr. Daly and Col. J. F. Weston called his attention to a quarter of beef, which was hanging on a transport, and which, Col. Weston said, had been for sixty hours in the open, and he was waiting to see what would happen.

Dr. Daly did not recall anything of Col. Weston's statement indicating the beef was other than a part of the general supply or that it had been treated with a chemical as an experiment. He noticed that flies would not remain on the beef, and that no larvae were deposited. He thought that strange, and that beef would not putrefy in the Tampa air after sixty hours' exposure.

> Witness finally cut a piece from the beef and later cooked and ate it. After riding on horseback he became nauseated. He did not suspect preservatives on the beef, although his taste suggested an experience he had with preservatives on antelope some years before while hunting. Nevertheless, Dr. Daly said, he remarked to no one about the matter. Witness wanted it made plain that Col. Weston had said nothing about the quarter of beef being experimental, and he had no reason to suspect the Government was conducting an experiment as to the efficacy of any chemical preservative.
>
> Replying to Col. Davis, witness said he supposed the beef was a part of a consignment from the contractors, supposed to keep for seventy-two hours in the sun, and perhaps Col. Weston was merely curious to see if the beef would stand the test. Recurring to the taste of the beef as suggesting an experience with preserved antelope meat, witness said some years ago, while en route to hunting grounds in the West, he secured in Chicago what was recommended as a preservative—a white powder. It was used in camp and preserved the meat; but the latter, when eaten, nauseated him. An analysis disclosed the presence of boric and salicylic acids.
>
> In regard to the Tampa experience, Dr. Daly said it did not arouse any suspicion; he did not look upon the incident as a Government experiment, and did not feel called upon to report or take any official action about it. He gave it little thought then, and replying to Col. Gillespie, said he first considered his Tampa experience sufficiently serious to present to the department when he had experience with contract beef on the *Panama*. Dr. Daly was then excused.[8]

Daly was recalled as a witness on 04 April. This round of interrogation covered little more than what had already been accomplished during his testimony before the Dodge Commission. The difference this time, however, was his examination was even more contentious. Examiners did their best to test his memory, medical background, and scientific acumen. As in previous testimony, Daly held his ground. Despite protests, he even managed to introduce the 21 January 1899 report of Dr. P. S. Connor of the Department of the Interior, United States Geological Survey, that confirmed the presence of both boric and salicylic acids in the beef broth specimen (residuum) that Daly had previously and correctly asserted. Since Connor was a government expert witness, Daly effectively made his case. The only other differences between the previous Dodge Commission questioning were additional questions about Daly's knowledge of the Powell beef experiment on the *Comal* and an attempt to get him to weigh in on the canned beef issue. Daly adroitly responded he did not know about the Powell experiment before reading about it during the Dodge Commission hearings. Regarding the canned beef, he offered no professional opinion other than to respond: "Do not understand me to be discourteous, sir. I wish to answer any question that the court desires me to answer. I must say that my observations were such that they would lead me to give an opinion that the so-called canned roast beef was not a proper thing for soldiers."[9]

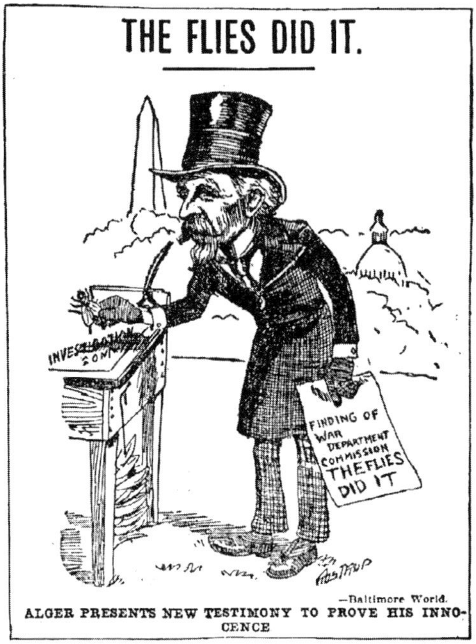
THE FLIES DID IT.
FINDING OF WAR DEPARTMENT COMMISSION THE FLIES DID IT
—Baltimore World.
ALGER PRESENTS NEW TESTIMONY TO PROVE HIS INNOCENCE

Secretary of War Russell A. Alger "The Flies Did It" cartoon. (*The Literary Digest, Volume 17, Number 19, 05 November 1898*)

Before ending his testimony, the Wade Beef Board questioned whether he had any other relevant information to share. With the opening, Daly shocked the Court of Inquiry by indicating he had a list of thirty to forty names of individuals who could attest to the chemical treatment of beef. When requested to turn the list over, Daly demurred. The corroborative evidence he had collected was offered only on condition that names of those offering the information remain confidential. Daly presented one example by stating:

> Well, one instance occurred like this, sir. I was riding in the streetcar with an old acquaintance, and he said, "Doctor, you do not know all about the chemical treatment of beef yet." "Well," I said, "I don't suppose I do. I am under the impression that there are others that can tell me a good deal if they will." He said, "Surely; but we don't like to have our business destroyed." "Well," I said, "it seems a queer thing that patriotism comes in last after business and money and everything else; that the lives and health of our soldiers should be considered as a trifling matter compared to a few dollars."[10]

Colonel Gillespie, who was questioning Daly at the time, was not amused. Gillespie responded to the Court of Inquiry: "I do not know whether this should continue. He has not given names."[11] The line of questioning abruptly ended.

Daly's second round of testimony before the Wade Beef Board would cover twenty-four pages. Probably the best that could be said about this last round of testimony was the Court of Inquiry checked all the boxes it felt necessary to profess thoroughness. Daly had certainly been abused, but in his mind, his professional stature remained unsullied. His feelings would change, however, once the Court of Inquiry issued its final report.

Daly was among the last witnesses called before the Court of Inquiry. Over the following few weeks, additional written testimony was accepted, closing arguments were made, and a final report drafted. Among the most interesting statements made during closing arguments were those offered by Major Jesse M. Lee on behalf of General Miles on 24 April 1899. In his summation, he reiterated the general's rationale for calling attention to the beef problem. Regarding Dr. Daly, he stated:

> Among these witnesses is Dr. W. H. Daly, who, we claim, has not been successfully contradicted by any reputable witness. He testifies in substance that "on the *Panama*, he observed that the beef had an odor similar to a dead body injected with preservatives. He later made a chemical analysis of the soup from this beef with due care and precaution and, in conjunction with a well-known chemist, found boric and salicylic acids." Dr. Daly's inspections and reports, read in evidence before this court and sworn to by him, appear to fully corroborate his evidence in the first instance as to chemicalized beef. There has been conclusive evidence that the beef examined by Dr. Daly was refrigerated beef which came from the *Manitoba*.[12]

Lee's comments about canned beef were equally absorbing. He stated for the record:

> We venture the assertion that there are enough abandoned cans around Santiago, left there by the heroes who charged San Juan Hill and El Caney, to erect a monument sacred to the memory of every packing house in Chicago, Omaha, and Kansas City; and in years to come the line of march and of battle can easily be traced by the discarded "Helmet Brand," which did not protect, and by the "Prize Winner," which won nothing in the fight for humanity, and Armour's "Prime roast beef," which was in fact a "roast" on the soldier who tried to eat it.[13]

Lee went on to take both the government and meatpacking industry to task by stating:

> The day has not yet come in this land, we hope, when great establishments shall be exempt from the rules, regulations, and laws requiring careful inspection of their products when purchased for the American soldier. If, like the king, they can do no wrong, then let the Agricultural Department withdraw its hundreds of inspectors from the packing houses and give them free scope for reputation's sake, and save the people the expense of looking after those whose infallible honesty would be as well assured without it.[14]

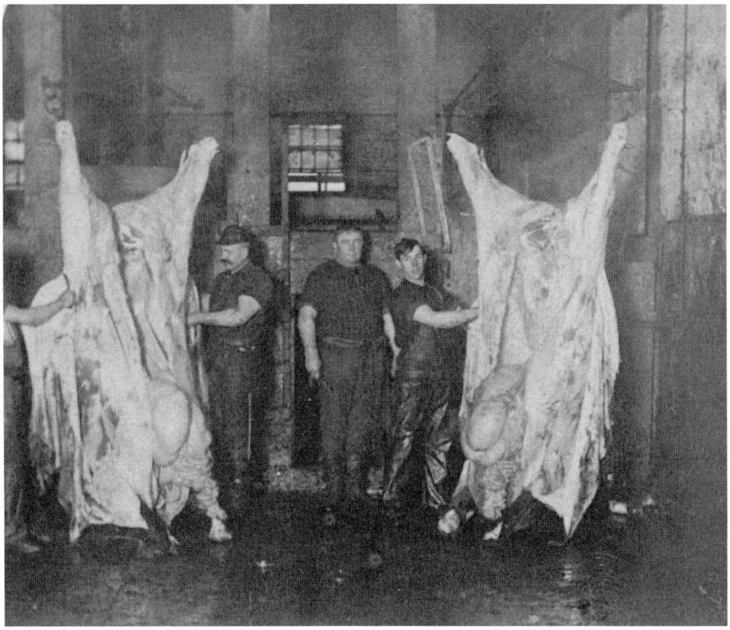

Above: Workers dressing the beeves in Armour's great meat packing house, Chicago, 1892. (*Library of Congress*)

Below: Cutting up the hogs in Armour's great packing house Chicago, 1893. (*Library of Congress*)

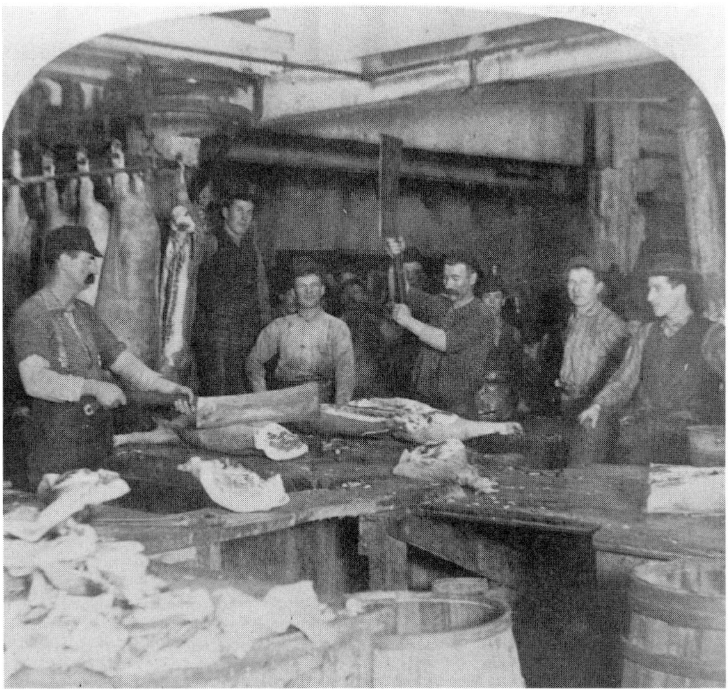

President McKinley approved the Court of Inquiry's findings on 06 May 1899, after which they were released to the public. In concluding its work, the Court of Inquiry offered this assessment:

> The court, with a deep sense of the responsibilities devolving upon it, has labored zealously to bring out the truth and believes that it has fully covered all the matters referred to it for investigation. The calling of more witnesses from the large number suggested by the Major-General Commanding, including all those who had taken part in the operations of the war, would only have resulted in additional testimony on the same lines as those pursued, without throwing further light upon the questions involved. Several witnesses who were duly subpoenaed to appear before the court did not obey the summons. Some of these were called at the instance of the Major-General Commanding, others at the instance of the court. Having knowledge of the fact that the statutes do not make it possible to punish witnesses who refuse to testify before a court-martial or court of inquiry, the court took no steps to compel their attendance.
>
> It has been developed in the course of the inquiry, as recited in this report, that in some instances certain individuals failed to perform the full measure of duty or to observe the proprieties which dignify high military command, but the court is of the opinion that the mere statement in the official report of the facts developed meets the ends of discipline, and that the interests of the service will be best subserved if further proceedings be not taken.[15]

In the main body of its final report, the Court of Inquiry responded to each of the twenty questions originally posed by President McKinley. In total, more than 4,700 pages of testimony were collected along with a large number of exhibits. In summarizing the findings, the *Literary Digest* reported:

> The findings of the military court appointed to investigate the charges made by Major-General Miles, commanding the army, to the effect that the beef supplied to the troops during the recent war was unfit for use, was made public Sunday, May 7, by order of the President, who approved the report. The court finds that the refrigerated beef were not treated with chemicals, or "embalmed," as General Miles charged; but finds that the "canned roast beef" was not suitable for a continuous ration, ought not to be used oftener than one day in five, and should be cooked before using; that very little beef was spoiled, and that the spoiling of that was due to the tropical climate more than to any other cause; and that the illness of the troops was due to the climate, exposure, malarial influences, bad water, and similar causes, but not to the beef. The court finds that the beef was not thoroughly inspected, but also that there was no law compelling a thorough inspection.
>
> The court criticizes General Miles, finding that he had no sufficient justification for alleging that the refrigerated beef was embalmed or was unfit for issue to the troops. It also finds that he erred in that, having belief or knowledge, as claimed, that the food

> was unfit, that it caused sickness and distress, that some of it was supplied under the pretense of experiment, and that other beef was embalmed, he did not immediately report such knowledge or belief to the Secretary of War, to the end that a proper remedy might be promptly applied. The court finds that he made no official complaint until December 21, when he appeared before the War Investigating Commission. The court criticizes General Shafter for not responding to the appeal of the Swift Company's agent at Santiago to have a shore refrigerator landed July 27. The refrigerator was not landed until September 21. Commissary-General Eagan is severely criticized for buying the enormous amount of 7,000,000 pounds of canned roast beef, which had not been sanctioned as a field ration, and whose value was untried and unknown. The court characterizes his action as "a colossal error, for which there is no palliation." Failure to provide cooking facilities on the transports; failure to transport the refrigerated beef properly, and to provide wagons, clean and protected from the sun; and failure of the general officers to report promptly on the unfitness of the food during the field operations in Cuba and Puerto Rico, are also criticized. It could not possibly have been foreseen, the court finds, that native beef would have been available in Puerto Rico, for if the American landing had been opposed, as was expected, the Spanish would have driven the cattle inland or destroyed them.
>
> The report concludes with the opinion that its criticisms meet the requirements of discipline, and recommends that no further proceedings against the officers criticized be taken.[16]

In offering its overview of the Court of Inquiry's findings, editors of *Literary Digest* felt compelled to also offer quotations from newspaper articles around the country. Several positive and negative examples were offered. Perhaps the most poignant was the one highlighted from the *Philadelphia Public Ledger*:

> The Public the Final Court—"Whether this criticism or censure of General Miles be just under the circumstances, or whether any of the findings of the court be sustained by the published testimony, the case must now be remanded to the great jury of the public, who penetrate the motives and acts of public men ofttimes with inerrant sagacity, and assign praise and censure with the good judgment which is vindicated by time and more light. There were suffering and 'neglect' in the American army during the operations in the Spanish islands. It is surprising and regrettable that one of the generals, who took the unpleasant initiative and concealed nothing in calling the country's attention to the conditions complained of, should receive the crown of censure, while those really responsible for a lamentable situation are unnamed. The mind of the country is quite capable of arriving at a correct judgment in these matters, and to that tribunal, the issues before the board will now be appealed. Without imputing infallibility to General Miles, it is firmly believed that his only motive in his frank statement of his belief as to the army rations was a humane and patriotic motive, and was intended solely for the good of the service which he

> has helped to make illustrious. The findings will not displace him in the popular affection and respect. If it have any effect at all in this respect, it will be that of enhancing his popularity as a soldier and a friend of the rank and file of the army."[17]

The *New York Journal and Advertiser* put it more succinctly when they wrote under the headline "Whitewash for Beef and Boodle." The paper's sub headlines read: "Court of Inquiry's Report scores Miles as much as it dares, hits Eagan with a padded club, feebly reprimands Shafter and ends with the happy suggestion that the whole matter be quietly buried. Sweeping condemnation of the beef by Miles, Roosevelt, Dr. Daly and scores of officers ignored. Eagan only blamed for buying too much."[18]

Once the Court of Inquiry's work was completed and the report issued, Daly thought the ordeal was over. He was now ready to resume a normal life, or so he presumed. What he did not yet realize was he had unknowingly accomplished something others had long believed impossible; he opened the door to government malfeasance and critical assessment of meatpacking industry practices. His official reports and testimony about the use of chemical preservatives on meat being fed to the Army unleashed a tsunami of negative public sentiment about the beef industry that would not go away. Misgivings that he expressed about the tainted meat would reverberate among the public in a powerful and ultimately productive way, and repercussions would play out over the next several years.

The *Philadelphia Public Ledger*'s editorial comment about Miles proved prescient when it suggested "The findings will not displace him in the popular affection and respect." Their assessment was dead-on as the public view was entirely supportive of the general and Dr. Daly, with many feeling the pair had been maligned to the benefit of the government and beef industry. Furthermore, the *Ledger*'s idea that the outcome of the Court of Inquiry would enhance the general's popularity as a soldier and a friend of the rank and file of the Army was equally accurate. What went unstated in the editorial, however, was that the same would hold for Daly. He was now a person of great interest across the country.

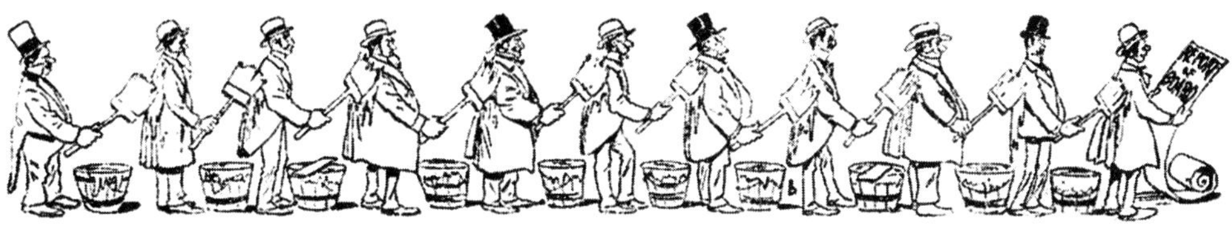

Washington whitewash cartoon, 1898. (*New York Journal and Advertiser, 14 October 1898*)

11

A Grievous Surprise

Following his last round of testimony in front of the Court of Inquiry on 04 April 1899, Daly returned to Pittsburgh. He went about things that made it appear he was comfortable resuming his normal day-to-day activities, much like those he left behind in May 1898 when he departed Pittsburgh for service during the Spanish-American War. He resumed his medical practice and social activities, and once again began thinking about hunting. However, his new normal was different than his previous. His mood had changed, and he was conspicuously less gregarious and increasingly more circumspect. Daly was less inclined to seek new patients to enlarge his practice, and he exhibited little interest in doing any further writing. He also struggled with lingering health issues resulting from his recent bout of malaria and his long-term back injuries from the Big Horn elk that attacked him many years earlier.

Daly's relationship with Miles was now even better than before the war. They were certainly proud of their accomplishments during the war, but this was different. Now, they had walked the halls of power in Washington, D.C., and taken on the meatpacking industry and the War Department's vast bureaucracy. It felt like they were an army of two. While they did not emerge unscathed, their friendship grew stronger.

In early spring 1899, Pittsburgh labor leaders invited General Miles to visit the city. Many things were happening in Pittsburgh at the time, including initial planning for the merger of Andrew Carnegie's steel interests with those of Elbert Gary's Federal Steel Company and William Henry Moore's National Steel Company, which when combined in early 1901 would become known as U.S. Steel Corporation. Miles was to be the guest of "organized labor." The labor group initially appointed 100 people to a planning committee but quickly realized it was too large a group to function well. A revised scheme called for Pittsburgh Mayor William J. Diehl to appoint a smaller executive committee to organize Miles' visit. Diehl would serve as chairman and its other members limited to three

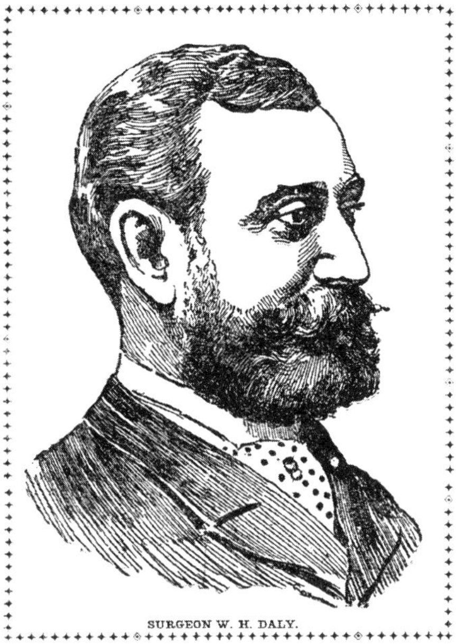

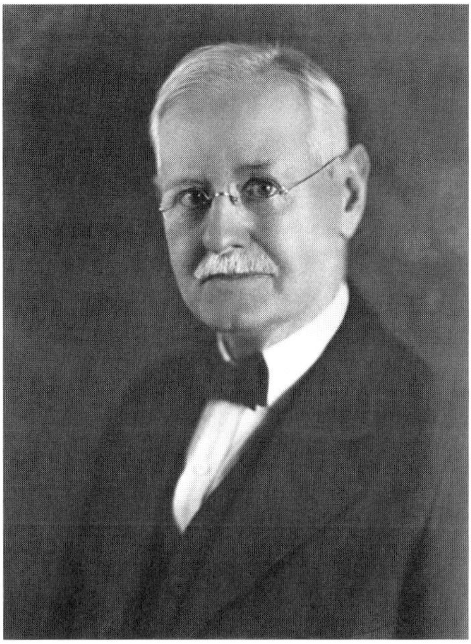

Above left: Surgeon William H. Daly, 1899. (*Salt Lake Herald, 05 April 1899*)

Above right: William Diehl, Mayor of Pittsburgh, 1899–1901. (*Historic Pittsburgh, University of Pittsburgh*)

of the region's leading citizens: Allegheny City Mayor, James G. Wyman; Major William H. Daly; and Major Albert J. Logan.[1]

As a long-term friend of the general, William H. Daly was an easy, logical choice. Logan, like Daly, was another favorite son of Pittsburgh. He had a long involvement in the military, starting in 1875 when he joined the area's famous Duquesne Greys infantry regiment. He subsequently became involved in the Homestead Steel Strike of 1892, the Pittsburgh Railroad Riots in 1877, and Luzerne County Coal Riots the same year. During the Spanish-American War, he served as an officer in the Pennsylvania National Guard and was largely responsible for organizing and transporting the state's troops during the war. Daly and Logan also shared another common bond: they were both affiliated with the Western Pennsylvania Hospital. Daly was a member of the hospital's senior medical staff, and Logan would soon serve as a board member appointed by the State of Pennsylvania.

The general's visit was scheduled for 30 June 1899. Up until late June, it was uncertain whether Mrs. Miles would participate. Upon confirmation of Mrs. Miles' planned attendance several days before the scheduled visit, quick plans were drawn up to host her at venues different than her husband's. William's wife, Athalia, became the chief architect of plans for hosting Mrs. Miles. On 01 July, a newspaper account offered insight into the previous day's activities:

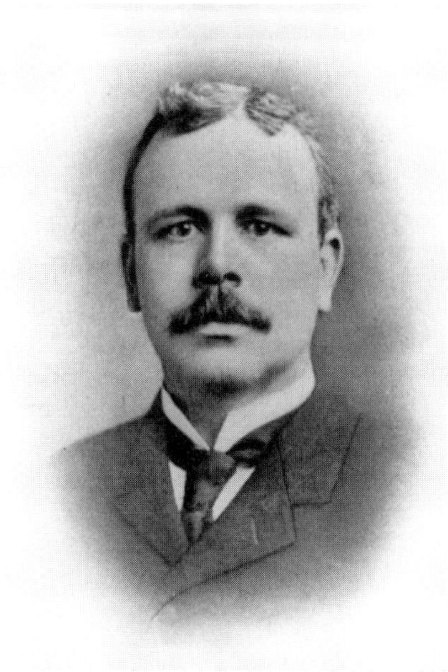

Col. Albert J. Logan, *c.* 1905. (*Carnegie Library of Pittsburgh*)

The coming of Major General Nelson A. Miles, who is in this city as a guest of "all organized labor," has been the crowning event of the week. The enthusiasm with which Governor Roosevelt was received upon his tour through the west to join his comrades of the rough riding fame was scarcely more intense than that which was manifested in this city on the appearance of the commander in chief of the United States army, whose unsullied record as a fighter and a general having the welfare of his troops at heart has won for him a place in the bosoms of the masses that can never be usurped by another.

The representatives of organized labor and the citizens of Pittsburg generally vied with each other in paying homage to the commander whose keen foresight enabled him to protect his men from the dangers of impure food from unscrupulous purveyors in the rear, which threatened to work more mischief than the bullets of the enemy at the front. Everywhere the brave warrior who has been the idol of his troops through many a dreary campaign on the western planes [*sic.*] was given ovations that demonstrated the whole-souled patriotism of Pittsburg.

General Miles had a busy time all day, sightseeing, holding receptions and addressing meetings. In the morning the general was taken through the Homestead armor plate works and other mills, in the afternoon he held a public reception, and in the evening he addressed two large audiences in the Grand Opera house and avenue theater. Preceding the evening entertainment General Miles was escorted through the principal streets by several of the local military organizations. The route of the parade was lined with thousands of people anxious to see and cheer the distinguished guest.

> Mrs. Miles was entertained today by Mrs. Dr. Daly and other prominent ladies by a drive over the boulevard and through the parks, after which she was warmly greeted by many visitors at the Schenley.[2]

Predictably, William H. Daly accompanied the general throughout his visit. While there is no evidence to confirm the full range of their discussions, it is likely they used the opportunity to refine plans for their next hunting trip to Montana and Wyoming, scheduled for October and November 1899. As previously noted, it was on 22 November 1899, just a few weeks after the hunting trip, that William's wife, Athalia, died at her brother's home in Garner, Iowa.

Daly was still intermittently struggling with his illness from malaria at the time of Athalia's death. With her passing, he became despondent and suffered from depression for the remainder of his life. Ill and without his wife, and with decreasing interest in his practice, he struggled to go through the motions of everyday life. The enjoyment he previously had in living was all but gone.

Perhaps sensing his mortality, in the early weeks of 1900, he responded to a solicitation from the *National Cyclopedia of American Biography*. He had never before shown traits of vanity, but he nevertheless agreed to purchase a subscription to the publication under the condition that a future volume contain a sketch of his life, along with a "marginal vignette."

Whether or not he saw this as an opportunity to document what he thought the public should know about his life is uncertain. What is undeniable, however, is he subsequently regretted purchasing the subscription after he started receiving dunning notices for payment of $10 each for the first nine volumes of the *Cyclopedia*. Daly argued to no avail that his understanding was payment would not be expected until after his biography appeared in print. The publisher disagreed. Numerous pieces of correspondence between the two parties attest to the frustration felt by both Daly and the publisher. The matter was finally settled after Daly received a letter from Pittsburgh attorney Harry L. Christy dated 06 April 1900 threatening suit if payment was not immediately forthcoming. On 28 May, Daly paid the $93 due for the first nine volumes. On 12 January 1901, he paid an additional $10 for the tenth volume. It was in this volume his biography and vignette appeared.[3]

The biographical information Daly provided was substantial and covered much of his life and military career. The section written about his involvement in the Spanish-American War was perhaps the most interesting. It read:

> At the outbreak of the Spanish war he was appointed major and chief surgeon U.S. volunteers, was assigned to duty on the staff of Gen. Nelson A. Miles, and participated in the active campaign of the war and performed services of a varied character. It was upon the report of his observations made to the commanding general of the armies that the "embalmed beef" supplied to the army was made a

> subject of investigation. In this, Dr. Daly's reputation for accuracy was sustained by the testimony of the army and supported by the confidence of the medical profession; the result being the improvement of the army commissariat.[4]

By his statement, it is obvious he was still struggling with frustration over the beef controversy. Even though many dozens of newspapers across the country supported his views for many months, and the general public believed his testimony, the ordeal of the Dodge Commission and Wade Beef Board still troubled him. His comment about the "confidence of the medical profession" is interesting. It likely refers to the endorsements he received from the Allegheny County Medical Society and the American Medical Association in February 1899 during the period when the Dodge Commission was ending its deliberations and the Wade Beef Board was beginning its hearing. The *Journal of the American Medical Association* included the endorsements in its 18 February 1899 issue:

> Allegheny County Medical Society—At the fifth annual reception banquet of this Society, held at Pittsburgh, Pa., Dr. James T. Whittaker of Cincinnati, Ohio, was the guest of honor and presented the principal paper of the evening, on "Arterial Sclerosis." One of the features of the evening was the adoption of the resolution endorsing the position taken by Dr. W. H. Daly, a member of the Society, who was on the staff of General Miles, and was Surgeon-in-Chief, United States Volunteers, regarding his recent testimony as to the "embalmed" beef furnished the soldiers.[5]

In early 1900, Daly was dealing with some real estate issues. For several months, he had been involved in a legal case attempting to force the purchase of property in the city. The owners supposedly signed papers of intent to sell and subsequently changed their minds. Daly was not happy and sued to force the sale. Available evidence suggests he lost the case. In the spring, he had another real estate problem. This time it was for failure to pay taxes on a property he owned. Why he chose not to pay the taxes is unknown, but authorities did not wait long before executing a sheriff's sale on the property. On Monday 04 June, the real estate he owned on Pittsburgh's Hazelwood Avenue was sold at a sheriff's sale.

By early summer, Daly appears to have regained an interest in traveling, and he began making plans for a trip to Europe. It is not known when or how Daly connected with Miles during this period, but it appears that General Miles may have instigated the trip. Correspondence Daly received from Miles and Surgeon General (Army) George Miller Sternberg suggests Daly's plans to visit European military installations, watching troops maneuvers, and inspecting sanitary and food supply conditions were not impulsive or for recreational purposes. A clue to Daly's ulterior motives may be found in a piece of correspondence he received from Miles dated 09 July 1900. The communication indicated the general had just sent Daly "a letter of introduction to U.S. Military Attaches in care of London

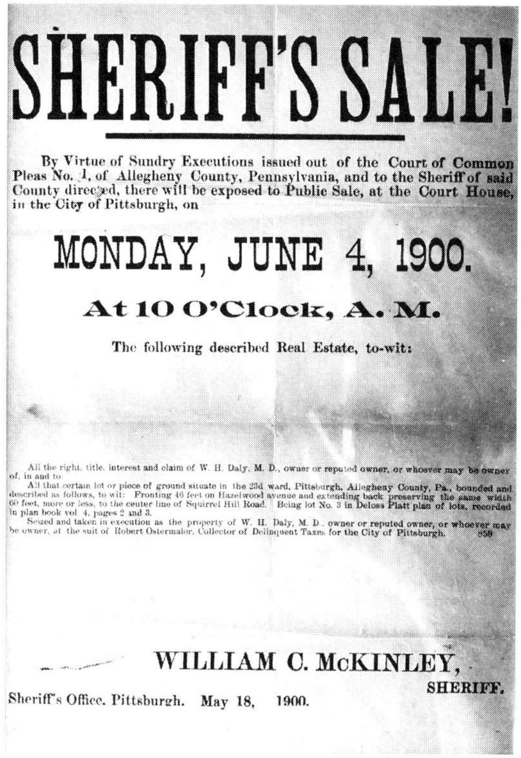

SHERIFF'S SALE!

By Virtue of Sundry Executions issued out of the Court of Common Pleas No. 1, of Allegheny County, Pennsylvania, and to the Sheriff of said County directed, there will be exposed to Public Sale, at the Court House, in the City of Pittsburgh, on

MONDAY, JUNE 4, 1900.

At 10 O'Clock, A. M.

The following described Real Estate, to-wit:

All the right, title, interest and claim of W. H. Daly, M. D., owner or reputed owner, or whoever may be owner of, in and to:

All that certain lot or piece of ground situate in the 23d ward, Pittsburgh, Allegheny County, Pa., bounded and described as follows, to wit: Fronting 46 feet on Hazelwood avenue and extending back preserving the same width 60 feet, more or less, to the center line of Squirrel Hill Road. Being lot No. 3 in Deloss Platt plan of lots, recorded in plan book vol. 4, pages 2 and 3.

Seized and taken in execution as the property of W. H. Daly, M. D., owner or reputed owner, or whoever may be owner, at the suit of Robert Ostermaier, Collector of Delinquent Taxes for the City of Pittsburgh. 858

WILLIAM C. McKINLEY,
SHERIFF.

Sheriff's Office, Pittsburgh. May 18, 1900.

William H. Daly sheriff's sale poster, 04 June 1900.

Bankers, Brown, Shipley & Company." In his closing remarks, the general wrote: "I will hold your application, and in case there is any prospect of going to China for war purposes, I will put it in."[6]

Considering the general's words and the timing of the Boxer Rebellion then taking place in China, it is obvious Miles and Daly had discussed the possibility of Daly rejoining the Army. In July 1900, the situation in China was uncertain, as was how much U.S. military involvement would be required to handle the situation. The fact that Daly once again volunteered his service was telling. Despite the uncertainty over China, however, Daly continued planning for his trip to Europe. On 03 July, he applied for his passport, indicating that he planned to return "within two years."[7] On 05 July, he received his passport. Little else is known about his trip to Europe or whether it was ever actually taken. Evidence suggests he elected to delay the trip until the summer of 1901 when his brother, Thomas, could accompany him.

In late fall 1900, Daly was once again thinking about hunting. It was his favorite time of year for such things. He joined Miles and family members for a short hunting trip. This time it was to the duck swamps of North Carolina. The area's wood ducks were a favorite target. In one of the last known photographs of Daly, he is seen relaxing at a campsite with a rather large group of friends and relatives that included his brother, Thomas Lafayette Daly; General Miles; and a small

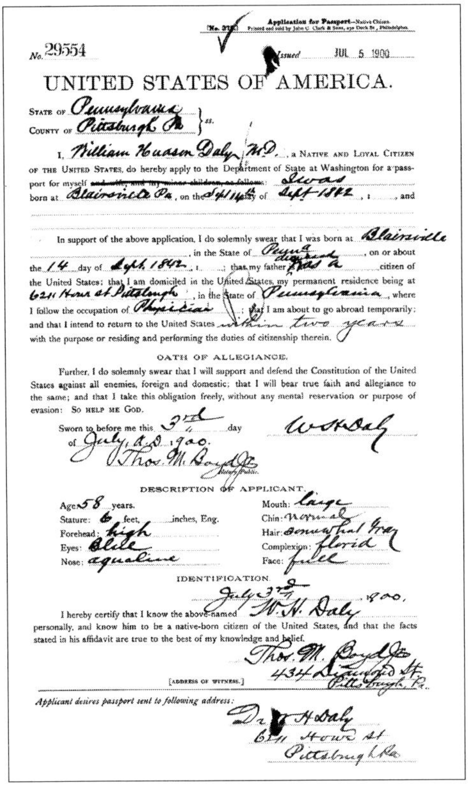

Application for Passport—Native Citizen.

No. 29554 Issued JUL 5 1900

UNITED STATES OF AMERICA.

State of Pennsylvania
County of Pittsburgh Pa } ss.

I, William Huasin Daly M.D., a Native and Loyal Citizen of the United States, do hereby apply to the Department of State at Washington for a passport for myself alone, born at Blairsville Pa, on the 14th of Sept 1842, and

In support of the above application, I do solemnly swear that I was born at Blairsville in the State of Penna, on or about the 14 day of Sept 1842; that my father was a citizen of the United States; that I am domiciled in the United States, my permanent residence being at 6211 Howe St Pittsburgh, in the State of Pennsylvania, where I follow the occupation of Physician; that I am about to go abroad temporarily; and that I intend to return to the United States within two years with the purpose of residing and performing the duties of citizenship therein.

OATH OF ALLEGIANCE.

Further, I do solemnly swear that I will support and defend the Constitution of the United States against all enemies, foreign and domestic; that I will bear true faith and allegiance to the same; and that I take this obligation freely, without any mental reservation or purpose of evasion: So help me God.

Sworn to before me this 3rd day of July, A.D. 1900. W. H. Daly
Thos. M. Boyd Jr. Notary Public.

DESCRIPTION OF APPLICANT.

Age: 58 years. Mouth: large
Stature: 6 feet, inches, Eng. Chin: normal
Forehead: high Hair: somewhat gray
Eyes: blue Complexion: florid
Nose: aqualine Face: full

IDENTIFICATION.

July 3rd, 1900.

I hereby certify that I know the above-named W. H. Daly personally, and know him to be a native-born citizen of the United States, and that the facts stated in his affidavit are true to the best of my knowledge and belief.

Thos. M. Boyd Jr.
434 Diamond St. Pittsburgh, Pa.
[Address of Witness.]

Applicant desires passport sent to following address:
Dr. W. H. Daly
6211 Howe St
Pittsburgh Pa

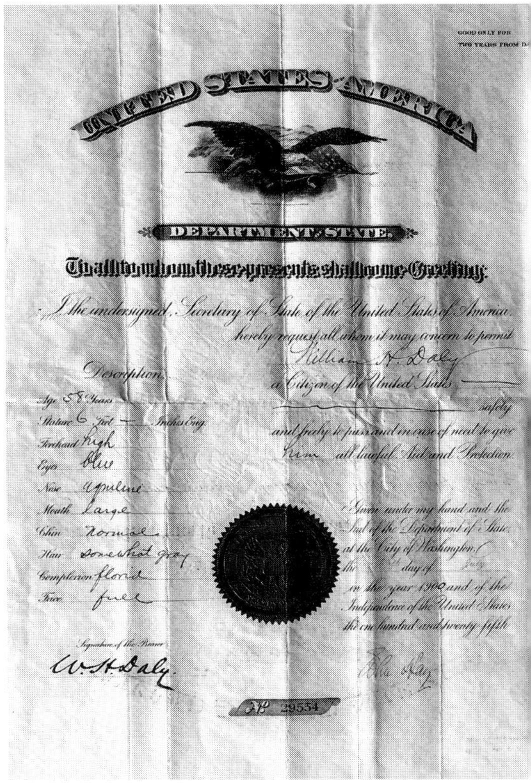

GOOD ONLY FOR TWO YEARS FROM DA

UNITED STATES OF AMERICA

DEPARTMENT OF STATE.

To all to whom these presents shall come, Greeting:

I the undersigned, Secretary of State of the United States of America, hereby request all whom it may concern to permit William H. Daly a Citizen of the United States safely and freely to pass and in case of need to give him all lawful Aid and Protection.

Description.
Age 58 Years
Stature 6 Feet Inches Eng.
Forehead high
Eyes blue
Nose aquiline
Mouth large
Chin normal
Hair somewhat gray
Complexion florid
Face full

Given under my hand and the Seal of the Department of State, at the City of Washington the day of July in the year 1900 and of the Independence of the United States the one hundred and twenty fifth

Signature of the Bearer
W. H. Daly

John Hay

No. 29554

Above left: William H. Daly passport application, 1900.

Above right: William H. Daly passport, 05 July 1901.

contingent of military aides. It appears he was once again in his element and at ease with the world around him. The effects of his lingering illness and his struggle with depression were not evident. It was a respite that would not last long.

For General Miles, it was a time to relax and regroup. His battles with the War Department and confrontations with President McKinley had tested his perseverance, but he was used to the pressure. With the presidential election concluding and McKinley winning reelection, it was time to regroup. Military life was his lifeblood, but political ambition was now a more pressing imperative and one that would play out in a more visible fashion over the next few years.

Not long after his hunting trip, Daly again traveled to Washington, D.C. This time, however, it was not to testify, but rather a trip to witness the second inauguration of William McKinley on 04 March 1901. While the "embalmed beef" matter was still evident but appearing less frequently in the press, the beef scandal continued to haunt Daly personally. His remarkable military career and widely acknowledged medical prowess had all of a sudden become less important

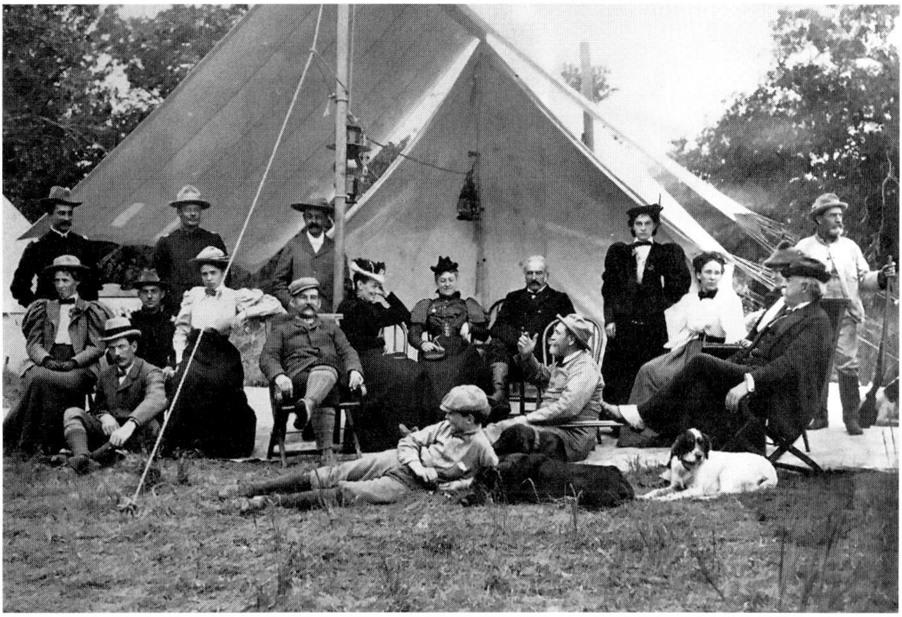

Daly family hunting encampment photograph. Probably taken in North Carolina during fall 1900. The individual sitting on the right front ground with the dogs is believed to be William H. Daly. General Nelson A. Miles is thought to be the person immediately behind Daly to the right. The individual standing with a rifle on the far right is probably William's brother, Thomas. The presence of the three military figures on the left support the premise that Miles participated in the hunt. The dogs also support the hypothesis that Miles is sitting in the chair as Thomas Daly had given him a prize English setter a few years earlier. The dogs on the ground next to William appear to be Retrievers, which he preferred as best suited for waterfowl hunting. (*Photo courtesy of Bruce B. Wilson, St. Davids, PA*)

than his involvement in the beef matter. His role in the government debacle was now more widely recognized than all of the other important things he had accomplished. It followed him wherever he went and played heavily on his mind.

For a few months in late 1900, he again mistakenly thought the beef matter might be coming to a close, and he could get back to the routine of a normal life. He was mistaken. Upon his return from the hunting trip in North Carolina, Daly found the matter again making the news. This time it was ex-Secretary of War Alger bringing the beef debacle back into public view. Upon his resignation from office on 01 August 1899, Alger went about writing his memoirs of the Spanish-American War. He saw it as his opportunity to set the record straight by offering the public a polished, positive view on his accomplishments as Secretary of War, and explanations of why so many things went wrong, including the "embalmed beef" and canned beef scandals. Naturally, he took little blame for the problems encountered and laid it squarely on the shoulders of inept military officers and insufferable government bureaucracy.[8]

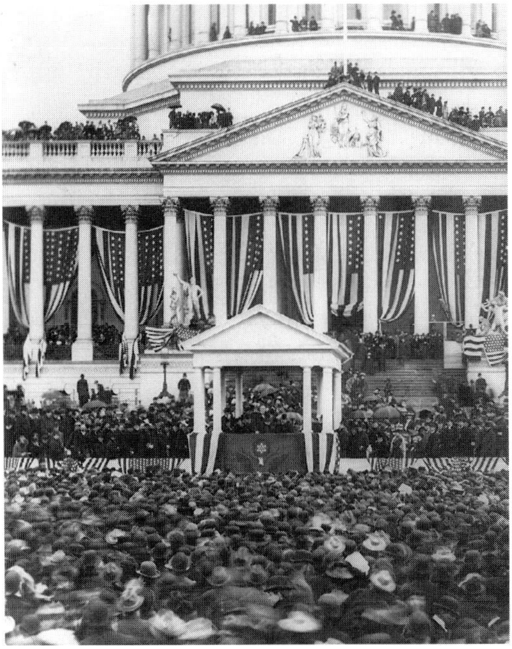

President McKinley's second inauguration, Washington, D.C., 04 March 1901. (*Library of Congress*)

Before completion and publication of Alger's book, *The Spanish-American War*, in October 1901, a serialized version appeared in the literary review magazine, *The North American Review*.[9] On 09 January 1901, the *Daily Inter Mountain* newspaper in Butte, Montana, took notice of the most recent chapter published in the magazine and reported on an interview with Daly in Pittsburgh:

> Major W. H. Daly, chief surgeon on General Miles' staff during the Spanish American war, has just returned to his home in this city from a hunting trip with General Miles. Concerning ex-Secretary Alger's recently published magazine article, Dr. Daly said: "It seems to be a hodge-podge of inaccuracies as to the facts and the testimony I gave. What Mr. Alger calls my 'verbal statements' and a 'single letter' was in fact just one typewritten official report to the commanding general of the army, and it seems to me to have been a rather efficient report in fulfilling its objects made manifest by the prompt abatement of the issue of improper foods to our army. I made the chemical analysis after my return to my laboratory in Pittsburg, because there was no opportunity for the accurate examination in a military campaign in a foreign country, and I wanted to see whether or not I was correct. The government chemical experts sustained my analysis in every detail, in fact, 'the Alger relief commission' suppressed this report of their own chemist and merely said in their report to the public, that 'inasmuch as Mr. Daly's analysis was not sustained by the government's own expert chemist, he was not worthy of credence.' The report written by Chief Chemist Clarke and his assistants ought to refute any impeachment of my credibility. Fortunately, I have a copy of the report of the government

> chemists in my possession else it would have been a question of veracity as between Alger, his commission and me. That Mr. Alger re-opened the matter at this late day when everyone but himself seems to have considered it a closed incident is unfortunate. To me, it seems another case of a man sitting down without a chair behind him."[10]

Daly was annoyed over Alger's article. His statement to the press confirmed his wish—and preference—that the matter would go away. That was not to be the case.

Over the next few months, Daly went about managing his dwindling medical practice, his substantial real estate holdings throughout the City of Pittsburgh, and other business investments. During this period, he also continued to fill notebooks with copious medical notes, seemingly to keep abreast of the latest diagnostic procedures and treatments.

The income he derived from real estate provided the financial resources he needed to continue enjoying a comfortable existence. In total, he owned twenty-seven properties, a majority of which were rental properties, that included twenty-three homes in the city; three properties (including a "mansion," farmhouse, and a home) in Baden, Pennsylvania (located in Beaver County along the Ohio River approximately 20 miles north of Pittsburgh); and a rental property in Etna, Pennsylvania (a Allegheny County borough located just outside of Pittsburgh along the Allegheny River).[11] At the time, it was estimated he derived an annual income of approximately $15,000 from the rentals.

It was during this period that Daly decided to make a significant investment in the Gottlieb-Bauernschmidt-Straus Brewing Company, a new business venture forming in Baltimore, Maryland. The company had recently emerged as a consortium of businessmen intent on consolidating Baltimore's brewing industry. With funds from investors like Daly, the new company acquired seventeen brewing companies, including the Globe and National Breweries.[12] William's decision to invest in the company was likely based on advice he received from his brother, Thomas, who was still an executive at Gibsonton Mills distillery in Westmoreland County, Pennsylvania.

Sunday 09 June 1901 was eventful. It was the day that Daly's pain and anguish stopped. Early that morning, Mary Short, Daly's live-in housekeeper, arose to make breakfast, much like so many previous mornings while in the doctor's employ. At first, nothing seemed unusual. She heard what she thought were normal noises coming from the second floor above where Daly's bedroom, office, sitting room, gunroom, and bathroom were located. She was accustomed to Daly's typical Sunday morning routines and behavior, so nothing seemed amiss. It was a fine morning she thought.

Mid-morning, around 9:45 a.m., she thought it wise to roust Daly from his second-floor redoubt for breakfast. It was getting late, past the usual time the doctor normally ate, and she thought he might have just lost track of time. As she ascended the stairs and landed on the second floor, she found all the doors to Daly's living quarters locked, which was rather odd she thought. After trying a few

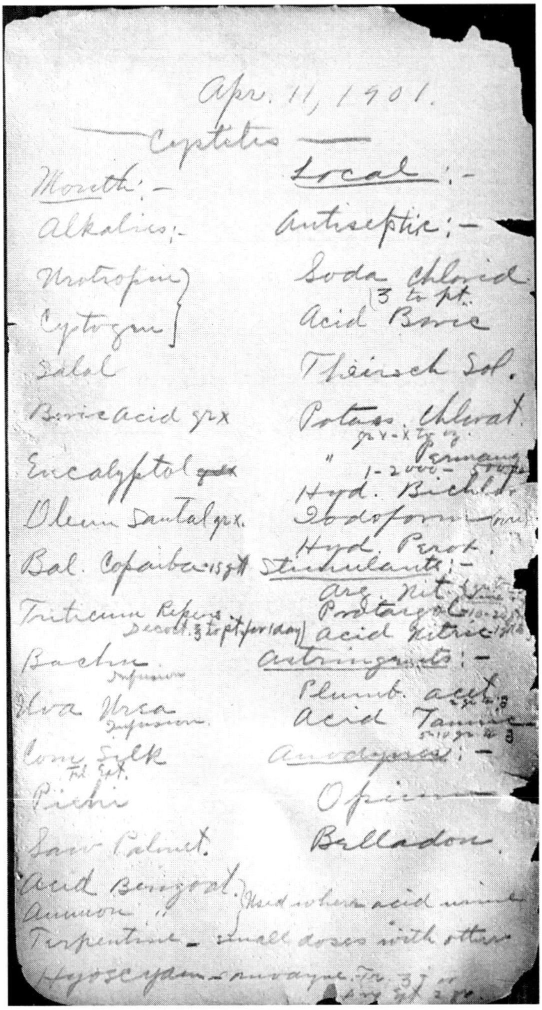

Left: William H. Daly's handwritten notes on cystitis, 11 April 1901.

Below: William H. Daly's personal bank check payable to Gottlieb-Bauernschmidt-Straus Brewing Company dated 10 June 1901, the day after his suicide. Daly committed suicide on Sunday 09 June 1901. This check was written before his death.

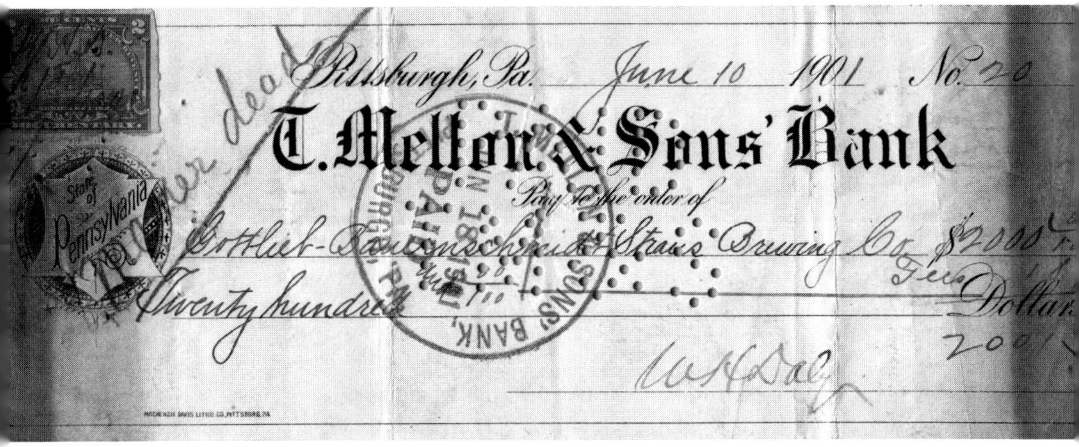
Pittsburgh, Pa. June 10 1901 No. 20
T. Mellon & Sons' Bank
Pay to the order of
Gottlieb-Bauernschmidt-Straus Brewing Co. $2000
Twenty hundred Dollars
W H Daly
State of Pennsylvania

doors, she moved on to the bathroom and found that door unlocked. With the door slightly ajar, she called out for the doctor but received no response. As she opened the door further, she saw the doctor's body lying on the floor in a pool of blood with his favorite Merwin and Hulbert 38-calibre revolver on the floor next to him.

Mary Short later stated that she screamed and quickly notified his family. From what she saw, she thought he was dead. She was not certain, however, if there was anything that could be done to revive him, so she recomposed herself and immediately went about contacting two of the doctor's friends who lived nearby. Allegheny County Court Judge John M. Kennedy and Dr. W. S. Foster arrived promptly but quickly assessed there was nothing that could be done.

Just three months shy of the age of fifty-nine, Daly was dead from a self-inflicted gunshot wound to the head. His anguish ended in a pool of blood.

Dr. Foster then summoned the Pittsburgh city coroner. While awaiting the coroner's arrival, Kennedy, Foster, and Short removed Daly's body from the bathroom floor and placed him on his bed. At a coroner's inquest the following day, Daly's death was ruled a "suicide of shooting while temporarily insane."[13] During the inquest, Foster testified the doctor had shot himself "under temporary derangement and mental aberration," stemming from his medical problems.[14]

On the same day as the coroner's hearing, local newspapers reported on Daly's death. The report carried in the *Pittsburg Dispatch* contained a wonderful tribute to the doctor. Under the headlines "Revolver Shot Ends The Life Of Dr. W. H. Daly; Famous Physician And Army Surgeon Found Dead By His Own Hand In His Home; Act Undoubtedly Done During Deep Dejection. Death A Grievous Surprise And Shock To Social And Professional Friends; His Career One Of Honor," it read:

> The many professional and social friends of Dr. William Hudson Daly were painfully shocked yesterday by the announcement that he had taken his own life. While suffering from severe dejection and mental aberration he shot himself at his home, 6211 Howe Street. His body was found in the bathroom by his housekeeper a few hours later. Dr. Daly enjoyed a confidence and respect from the City that were, perhaps, unsurpassed by any other member of his profession, and in his widespread acquaintance, there was scarcely a man who would be less expected to commit such an action. He was naturally of a buoyant disposition, fond of outdoor life and athletics and a passionate devotee of hunting. His sunny disposition naturally won him a legion of friends and the earnest love and admiration of them all.
>
> While never aspiring to leadership in society he was nevertheless a social favorite, and during the life of his wife was a notable figure in social functions. Since her death, which occurred November 22, 1899, he had greedily changed his everyday life, and many of his most intimate friends had remarked about the apparent difference. Unquestionably he missed her society greatly and secretly grieved at her loss. They had been markedly affectionate and companionable, and her death came as a blow from which he never recovered.

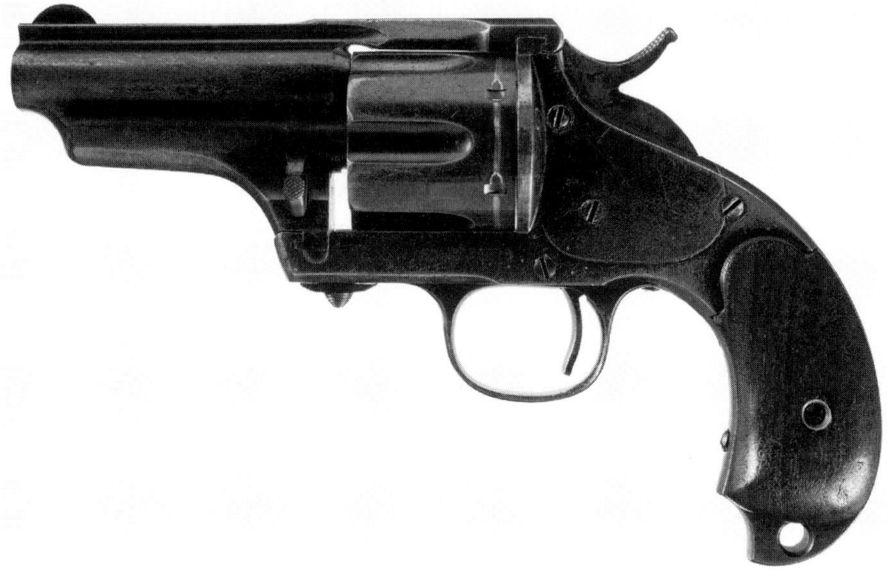

Merwin and Hulbert 38-caliber revolver like Daly used to commit suicide.

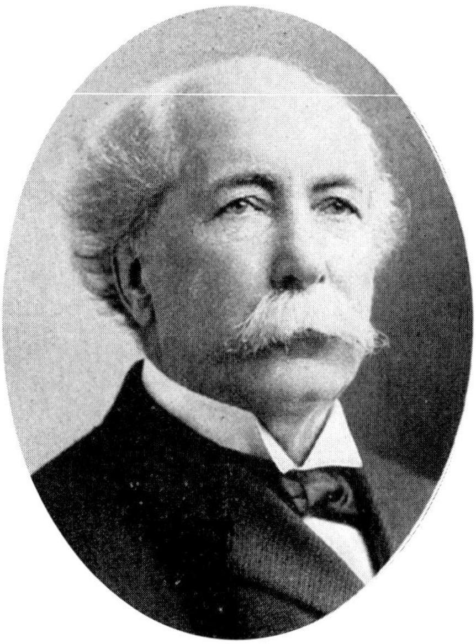

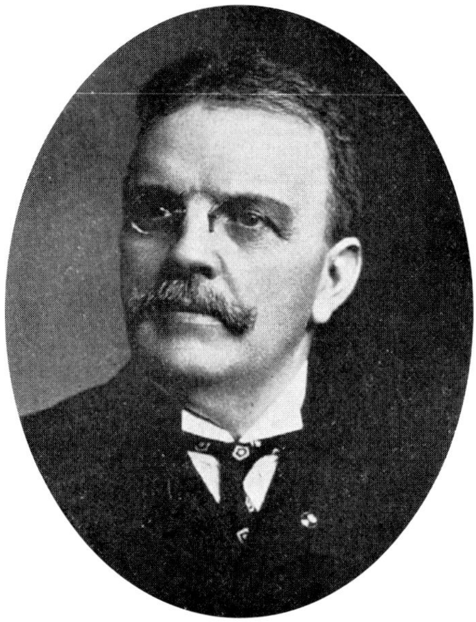

Above left: Allegheny County Court Judge John M. Kennedy. (*Carnegie Library of Pittsburgh*)

Above right: William S. Foster, M.D., professional friend of William H. Daly. (*Carnegie Library of Pittsburgh*)

Lately, it had been noticed that he was aging rapidly, his former good spirits were deserting him, and his fits of melancholy to which he had been ever subject became more and more frequent. His interest in social matters waned, and he was seldom seen at the club, where he had been an erstwhile ever jovial companion. In brief, the death of his wife changed the whole tenor of his life, and in the minds of his friends, there is a general admission that indirectly the cause of his action yesterday was the irreparable injury suffered when he lost his companion of a lifetime.

He was eminently successful in his chosen profession; wealthy to a degree that permitted him to spend life as he pleased; enjoyed the luxuries of a fine home, rich in mementos of many trip through the west and Europe; was recognized as an authority in several lines of specialists treatment and wore his deserved honors with a modesty which eminently became him.[15]

The article went on to discuss what was understood about Daly's health status:

The deceased had been in ill health for some months, his ailment taking the form of insomnia with attendant attacks of indigestion. Nearly two months ago he went to Atlantic City, remaining there until three weeks ago. Since his return, he has been troubled more than ever with sleeplessness. His melancholia had also been more pronounced, but at no time had it been sufficient to occasion alarm with either his friends or members of his household. He has been attending regularly to his practice and only last Saturday prescribed for patients who visited his office, among them being two sons of a relative, William Gass of this city.

So far as could be learned, he was in his usual frame of mind Saturday and remained nearly all the day at home, taking a short walk in the evening. He dined at home at the usual hour and retired rather earlier than usual. At no time Saturday had he given expression to any depressing sentiments, but had seemed entirely his usual self. The suicidal dementia appears to have come upon him suddenly. There were no letters, no notes upon any of his recently attempted manuscripts, that would indicate the tendency of his mind and nothing in his recently laid aside books that dealt with the subject.[16]

Also found in the obituary are several testimonials made by friends and professional associates:

Dr. Jacob Wolf—
… the deceased physician called on him several days ago and seemed to be mentally depressed and imbued with the idea that he was ill. At his request, Dr. Wolf examined him thoroughly. Beyond a general nervous depression, he found him in perfect health, though a trifling inclination to indigestion was apparent. But there was no promise of serious complications, and when so advised the doctor was naturally much encouraged. He came a second time, however, and was again advised that he

needed rest and a change of scene. He explained that he had taken a shooting trip through the South, but, instead of improving his condition appeared to grow worse. He contemplated a Western trip, and possibly one to Europe. Dr. Wolf declared last night that from his knowledge of the condition and temperament of the dead man he would say that the case was one of emotional suicide. There was evidence of nervous exhaustion at the time of the examination, but he had not for an instant considered it likely to develop into dementia.

Dr. R. S. Sutton of Allegheny—
Dr. Daly's rank in the medical profession was good. He was an accomplished doctor. He was formerly a general practitioner and senior physician on the staff at West Penn Hospital. In 1880 he went to London and devoted himself to the study of throat diseases under Dr. Sir Morrell Mackenzie, now dead, who attended the crown prince of Germany and was knighted. Dr. Daly had a flourishing practice here from the time he returned from London in 1882 until 1893. After the latter date, the country filled up with throat specialists. For the last three years, Dr. Daly had not devoted much time to his profession. Besides contributing articles to home and foreign medical journals, he wrote on sporting, hygiene, and climate. If not the discoverer of the fact that asthma was a reflex from a disease of the nose he was the first to call attention to it.

Dr. C. B. King of Allegheny City—
Dr. Daly stood very well in the medical profession. Besides, he was a fine man and well respected among his professional brethren. Not long ago I talked with General McCook of the United States Army, and Dr. Daly came up in the conversation. I learned then that he was not popular with the regular army men, but that was attributed to the fact that he had been drawn into the beef controversy through his close friendship for an association with General Miles. I know that Dr. Daly was greatly worried over the beef matter and I believe that it was one of the things that led to his death.

Dr. J .C. Lange—
Dr. Daly was a very excellent man and stood high in the profession. I think his position in the Army Beef scandal was generally supported by the local medical fraternity.

Dr. W. D. Huselton—
Dr. Daly stood well in the profession here. He was formerly a general practitioner, but some time ago became a specialist in throat diseases. He was perhaps the pioneer in that field in this city. I believe that in practice and in public opinion he was rather endorsed in the stand that he took in the Army Beef matter.

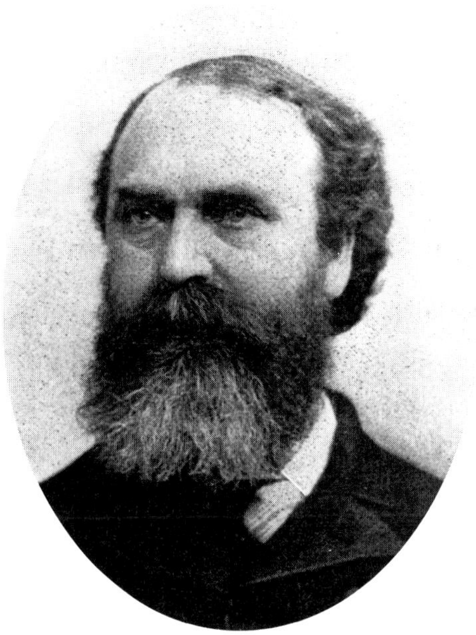

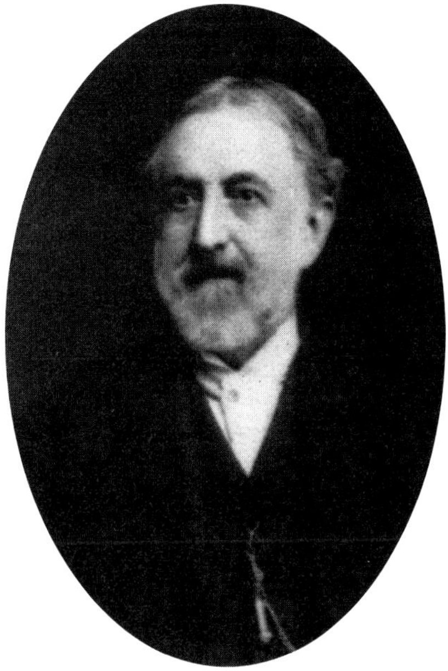

Above left: Rhodes S. Sutton, M.D., professional associate of William H. Daly. (*Carnegie Library of Pittsburgh*)

Above right: C. B. King, M.D., professional associate of William H. Daly. (*Carnegie Library of Pittsburgh*)

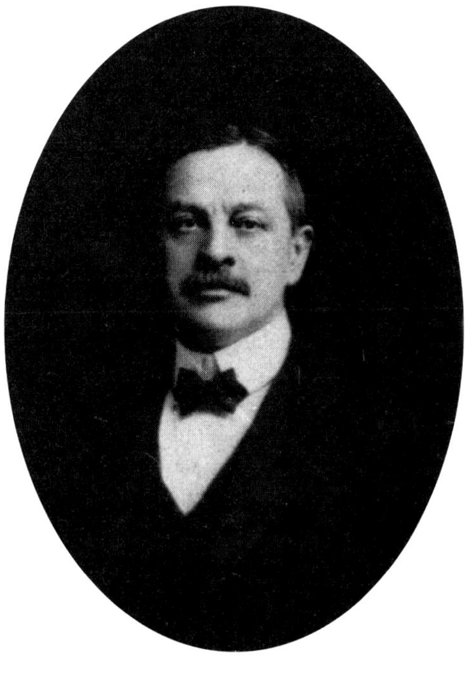

J. Chris Lange, M.D., professional associate of William H. Daly. (*Carnegie Library of Pittsburgh*)

General Nelson A. Miles (by special telegram from Washington, D.C.)—
"I am grieved," said General Miles, "yet when I recall that the attack of the grip left him in poor health and that the loss of his family, particularly his boy, depressed him greatly, it is not so surprising. Some time ago he told me that he intended giving up his practice altogether. His fortune was ample; he said particularly as he had no one to whom he could leave it. In Puerto Rico, he took exceedingly good care of the sick and wounded, and exercised a very close supervision of the hospice. His record in the Army was an exceedingly fine one. I do not think the embalmed beef investigation affected him. Dr. Daly proved his character, and those to cast doubt upon his professional standing had no effect upon him."

Dr. J. H. McClelland—
Dr. Daly was a man who occupied a very prominent place in the medical circles both at home and abroad. His reputation abroad was perhaps greater than here, as his articles on medical subjects were highly esteemed in Europe, where they were given wide circulation. The subjects dealt with were the air passages and the surgical treatment of the diseases of the nose, throat, and larynx. I think his articles won him honorary membership in several foreign medical societies. Socially he was very affable, and he made many friends where-ever he went. All that can be said of him in connection with the Army beef matter that he was elected by General Miles himself for his personal staff and the General would not be likely to select a man not fitted for that position.

U.S. Representative John Dalzell (by special telegram from Washington, D.C.)—
He was the last man of whom I expected to hear such news. His temperament was not such as would lead anyone to expect such an end. Oh, he must certainly have been mentally unbalanced. It couldn't have happened under any other circumstances. The doctor was so good to me in London last summer when I was ill for a while. The newspaper called special attention to the fact Mr. Dalzell's efforts enabled Dr. Daly to get the commission he held in the Army. He went to the President and Secretary of War for Daly and persuaded them to give him the commission.[17]

After his death, it was reported that Daly allegedly lost $75,000 in the Gottlieb-Bauernschmidt-Straus Brewing Company business venture. Remarkably, a personal check made payable to the brewing company, dated 10 June 1901 for the sum of $2,000, was found among his possessions at the time of his death.[18] The check supposedly represented a partial payment of the losses incurred. At least one newspaper surmised the loss was the cause of Daly's suicide.[19]

News reports of Daly's death and the testimonials offered by his friends attest to his prominence in professional medical circles and the community at large. Perhaps unintentionally, they also confirm the reality of Daly's fear that the "embalmed beef" matter would supplant all the things he set out to achieve in life. The fact that virtually all of the many obituaries and news reports covering his death prominently mentioned the beef controversy cannot be ignored.

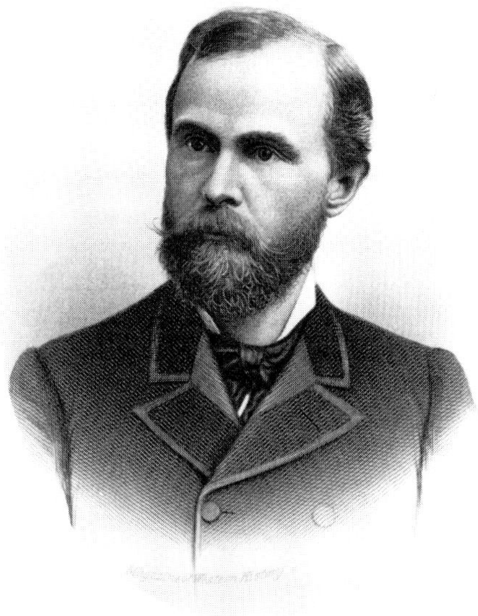

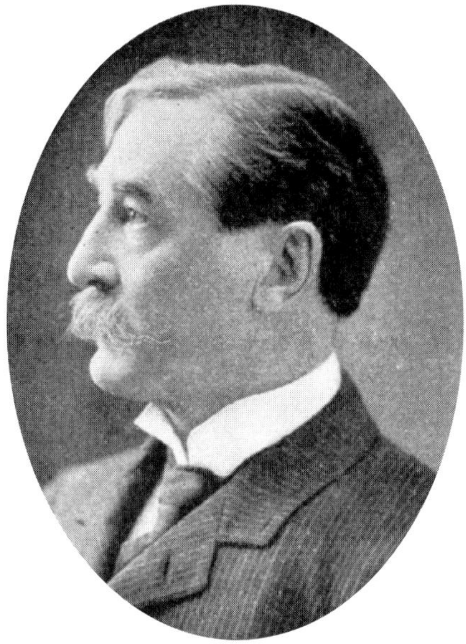

Above left: J. H. McClelland, M.D., professional associate of William H. Daly. (*Carnegie Library of Pittsburgh*)

Above right: U.S. Congressman John Dalzell, friend of William H. Daly. (*Carnegie Library of Pittsburgh*)

If Daly had lived another few years, he would have undoubtedly been delighted to realize the things he wrote on two pages about Army beef in a military report would change history. In this lone regard, Daly mastered Ben Franklin's precept—he wrote things worth reading and did things worth the writing. The country would soon come to learn the true impact of Daly's actions.

12

Legacy

On 10 June 1901, the day after Daly's death, General Miles offered perhaps the most poignant testimonial made about the doctor and the circumstance of his suicide: "Dr. Daly was no ordinary man, no ordinary physician. He was one of the best. His heart was broken when his little ones died of scarlet fever, and when his wife passed from him it broke his hold upon life."[1]

William H. Daly was buried close to his Howe Street home in Pittsburgh's Allegheny Cemetery. Located in the city's Lawrenceville area, the cemetery is one of the city's oldest burial grounds. He was laid to rest alongside his wife, Athalia, and children in Section 13, Lot 54. One of Daly's numerous obituaries contained a list of his friends and relatives. In a number of cases, it was the first time many of the family names appeared in association with the doctor. Besides listing the Daly children, James Cooper and William Theodore, other family members who were mentioned included Mrs. Agnes D. Johnstone, his sister from Pittsburgh, PA; Mrs. Jennie M. Dunaway, his sister from Virginia, IL; Mrs. Alexander McMahon, his sister from Monessen, PA; Thomas L. Daly, his brother from Gibsonton, PA; John M. Daly, his brother from Norfolk, VA; Hugh McMahon, a nephew from Pittsburgh, PA; Mrs. Joseph T. McKean, another relative from Gibsonton, PA; Dr. H. C. Daly and wife, his nephew and niece from Gibsonton, PA; Mr. and Mrs. Kerfoot W. Daly, his nephew and niece from Gibsonton, PA; Mr. and Mrs. W. H. R. Gass, his nephew and niece from Pittsburgh, PA; Mr. and Mrs. Harry D. Johnston, his nephew and niece from Pittsburgh, PA; Mr. and Mrs. Samuel Hubley, his nephew and niece from Pittsburgh, PA; John Cooper and wife, his nephew and niece from Baltimore, MD; and Mr. and Mrs. Mercer Cooper, his brother-in-law and sister-in-law from Garner, IA.[2]

The full extent of Daly's income, wealth, and alleged investment losses were a matter of wide conjecture while he was living. A much clearer picture emerged after his death. Only four months before his passing, he updated his last will and testament on 19 February 1901. It was a telling document that showed just how much he had loved and missed his wife. In part, it read:

> I, WILLIAM HUDSON DALY, of the City of Pittsburgh, the County of Allegheny and the State of Pennsylvania, being of sound mind, memory and understanding, do make this my last will and testament, hereby revoking and making void all former wills by me at any time heretofore made.
>
> *First.* I direct that all my just debts, funeral expenses and cost of granite cross similar to that I erected over my wife's grave, with date of my birth, September 14th, 1842, inscribed thereon, and the date of my death, be paid. I desire to be buried beside my children, so that they will lie between my deceased wife, Athalia, and myself.
>
> *Second.* There shall be no appraisement of my estate, and no sales made thereof unless deemed by its executors or trustees to be for its benefit, advantage and increase of income from same. They shall be the judges of this matter and have power to sell, build, improve or otherwise better the condition of my estate towards the end and uses for which I will it to be applied.
>
> *Third.* I direct, will and bequeath all my estate, both real, personal and mixed, and of all kinds wherever located, including life insurance, to the basic endowment, founding, establishment and maintenance of a home or homes for industrious girls and women, without respect to age or sect. The first to be established in the counties of Allegheny and Beaver.
>
> Others can be located elsewhere, as the fund shall grow adequately through the philanthropic generosity and consideration of others toward a worthy class of girls and women who have not received the attention and kindness they merit. If during my life, I shall have time and opportunity to establish the initial "Athalia Daly Home" in Pittsburgh, then my estate is to be applied to the further endowment, maintenance and purposes hereinbefore named. The bequest of my estate for the purpose hereinbefore indicated and named, being first subject to certain life annuities, to be paid in quarterly installments to the persons hereinafter named in equal sums during their natural lives, and to cease and determine at each of their respective deaths. The "Athalia Daly Home," or Homes, at once becoming the beneficiary of the sum or sums so determined, whether such respective deaths occur previous to or subsequent to my own death and the probating of this will.[3]

In his will, Daly thoughtfully suggested his properties in Baden, Beaver County, which included a farm, a mansion house, and associated farm buildings, might serve as a primary or secondary site for one of the homes. He surmised the rural settings and "invigorating influence" of such surroundings might be needed or preferred by some of the beneficiary women. He and Athalia had often used the properties in Baden for similar purposes and frequently rented them to others.

Besides making plans and creating an endowment for the Athalia Daly Home (or Homes), the document named a few personal beneficiaries. Those individuals included John M. Daly and his wife, Mary Daly, of VA; Thomas L. Daly and his wife, Carrie, of Gibsonton, Westmoreland County, PA; Jennie Mar Dunaway of Virginia, IL; Agnes D. Johnstone of Pittsburgh, PA; and Mary M. Short, his long-term housekeeper of Pittsburgh, PA. Each of these individuals was to receive $600 per year, paid in quarterly installments of $150 each during their natural lives. Daly's will also indicated he had held a mortgage on his brother's farm in Norfolk, VA. In his will, Daly specified: "The mortgage I hold against the farm of John M. Daly and his wife, Mary Daly, is not to be foreclosed nor payment demanded of interest or principal of same during the natural lives or ownership of either of them."

The value of Daly's estate at the time of his death was approximated at $250,000.[4] From that amount, about $220,000 was set aside for chartering the Athalia Daly Home or Homes.[5]

During Athalia's life, William was aware of and supportive of her interest in advancing the welfare of industrious women. Athalia's efforts in this regard were perhaps best expressed by the work she did among the Native American Indian tribes in the West while accompanying William on his hunting trips. As noted in an earlier chapter, she assisted in opening schools on reservations and in selling Indian-made lace to wealthy friends back in Pittsburgh. Anything she could do to help elevate the status of women was of paramount importance to her. Her interest in supporting unmarried, working women in Pittsburgh was an extension of her concern.

William took Athalia's interests in these matters to heart and crafted his will in a manner that would create a lasting tribute to the work she treasured. In the will, Daly described his intentions for the Home(s):

> The object, intent, aim and effect of the "Athalia Daly Home," or Homes, shall be to furnish home, shelter, protection, instruction and improvement to industrious girls and women, while either in or out of employment, at the lowest possible cost to them commensurate with maintaining the proper sense of self-respect and ambition on the part of the beneficiaries, who shall desire or require the shelter of plain, comfortable and cheerful home, surrounded by good influences, attended by proper and wholesome amusements, presided over by kind and friendly guardian officers, known to be interested in the happiness, prosperity, self-respect and welfare of the beneficiaries.[6]

The Athalia Daly Home was incorporated in March 1904. In preparing the Home's Articles of Incorporation, the trustees included William's "object and intent" language verbatim but broadened its aim by expanding it to another class of beneficiary. The home's beneficiaries would now include "girls who have strayed from the path of rectitude a helping hand toward restoration to the paths of usefulness, propriety, and industry, as set forth, contemplated, designed and specified in the will of William Hudson Daly."[7]

No further immediate action was taken after the incorporation due to a group of family members contesting Daly's will in local courts. The essence of the argument was based on the supposed impracticality of administering the home as devised in the will. Family members who challenged the will included John M. Daly, Thomas L. Daly, M. Maggie Gordley (administratrix for Jennie Mar Dunaway, deceased), M. Ella McMahon, and W. H. R. Gass (administrator of the estate of Agnes D. Johnstone, deceased). The primary point of contention was whether the corporation holding the home or the women who stayed in it were the true beneficiaries. In October 1904, after lengthy deliberations, the Supreme Court of Pennsylvania, Western Division, decided in favor of upholding Daly's will as written. The women who would stay in the home were determined to be the true beneficiaries. Thus, William's intentions were deemed practical and worthy of execution.

Once the matter was settled, planning for the Athalia Daly Home resumed. In restarting the planning, the executors made decisions seemingly at odds with William's expressed intentions. Rather than using one or more of Daly's real estate holdings, or other "plain dwellings," in Pittsburgh or Baden to serve as a site for the home, they decided otherwise. The executors opted instead to construct one large building in the city. The property they decided to build on was located at 366 Gross Street in the Bloomfield section of Pittsburgh not far from Daly's Howe Street home. Another change the executors made related to financing for the project. In his will, William expressly forbade selling his real estate, choosing instead to use the proceeds from the income generated from the holdings to finance the home's day-to-day operations. Once the decision was made to build a new structure on Gross Street, projected construction project costs far exceeded available liquid financial resources. Contrary to Daly's wishes, the executors sold the doctor's real estate, including his farm and mansion in Baden.[8]

Construction of the Athalia Daly Home began in 1905. The final cost of construction and related property improvements was $92,638. The home opened its doors on 20 November 1907, a little over six years after William's death and two days short of eight years since Athalia's passing. Once opened, the Athalia Daly Home fulfilled Daly's wishes, providing lodging and supportive services for "industrious girls and women."

The building was a magnificent three-story brick structure, containing fifty-four furnished rooms, visitor parlors, dining and laundry facilities, a sewing room, and recreational facilities including croquet lawns, tennis courts, a bowling alley, and a room with a pool table. Allowing for a number of double rooms and excluding rooms for staff, the facility could hold up to seventy women. Guest sleeping rooms faced the outside, each with a large window. The rooms contained a bed, washstand, dresser, chairs, wardrobe, and a table. Each floor contained four shared bathrooms fitted out with toilet rooms and washbasins with "running hot and cold water."

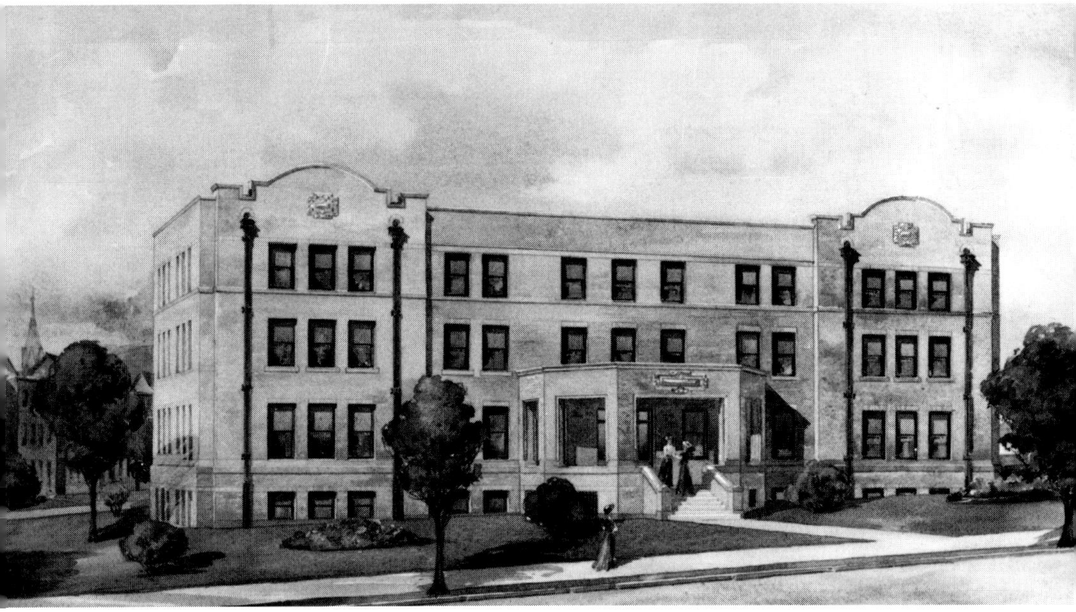

Athalia Daly Home architect's rendering, *c.* 1904.

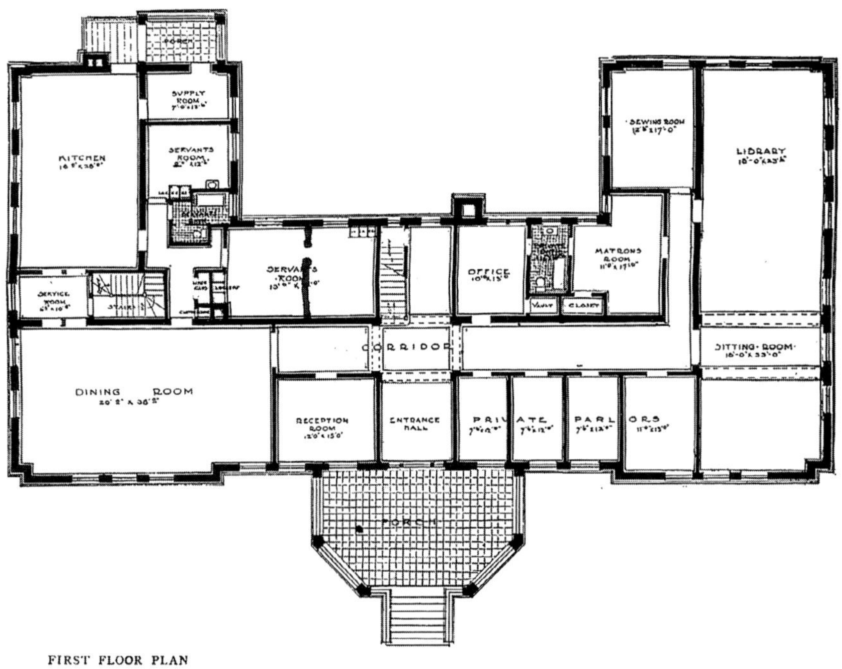

Athalia Daly Home first floor plan, 1913. (*Athalia Daly Home brochure*)

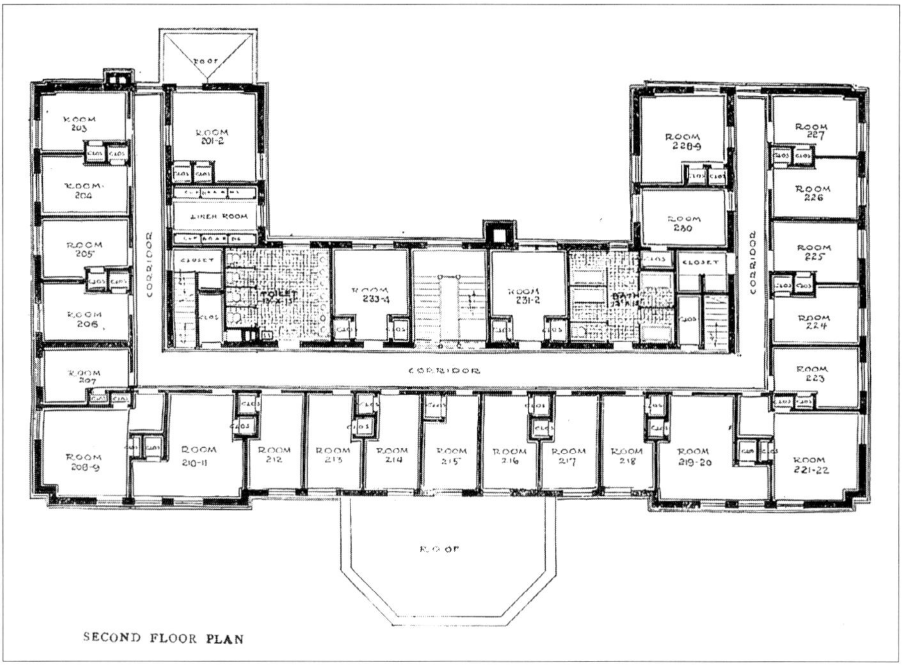

Athalia Daly Home second floor plan, 1913. (*Athalia Daly Home brochure*)

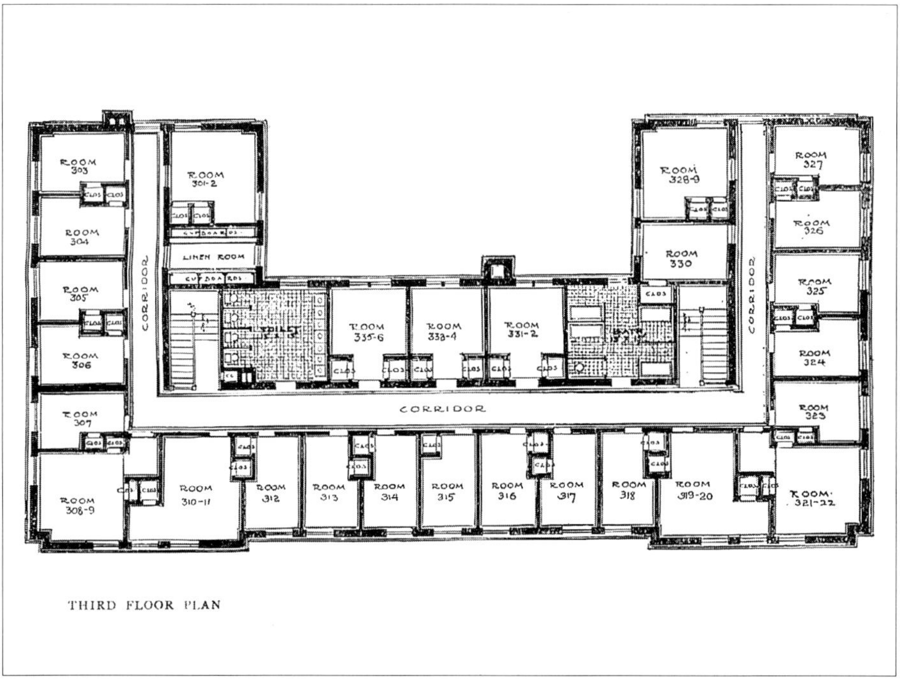

Athalia Daly Home third floor plan, 1913. (*Athalia Daly Home brochure*)

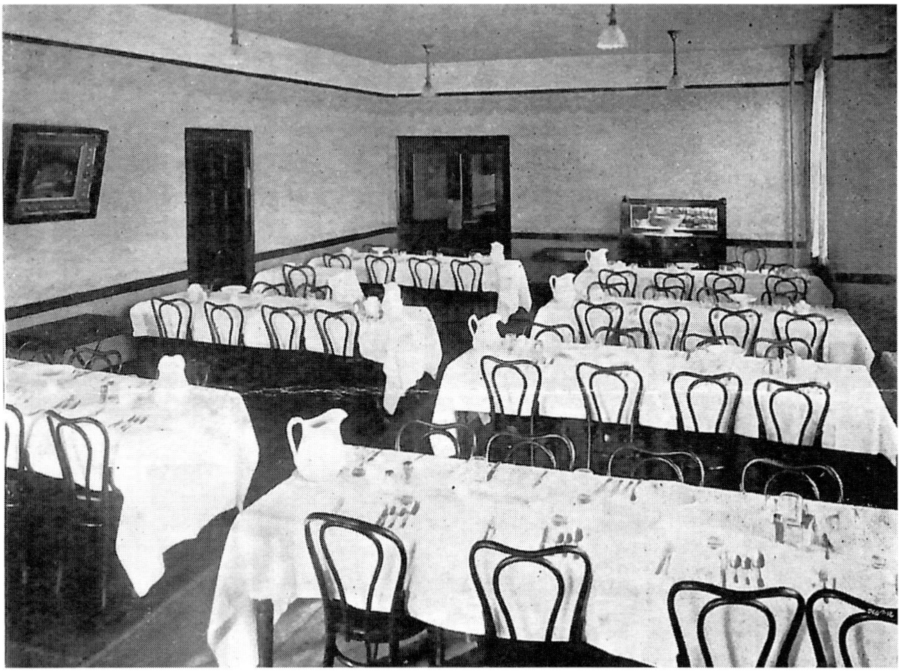

Above : Athalia Daly Home dining room plan, 1913. (*Athalia Daly Home brochure*)

Below: Athalia Daly Home bedroom plan, 1913. (*Athalia Daly Home brochure*)

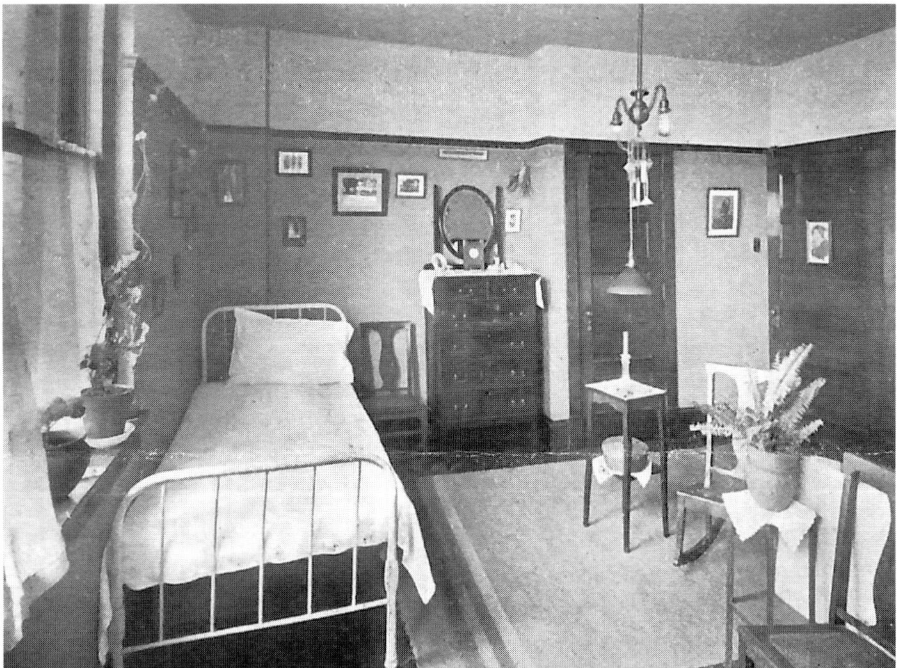

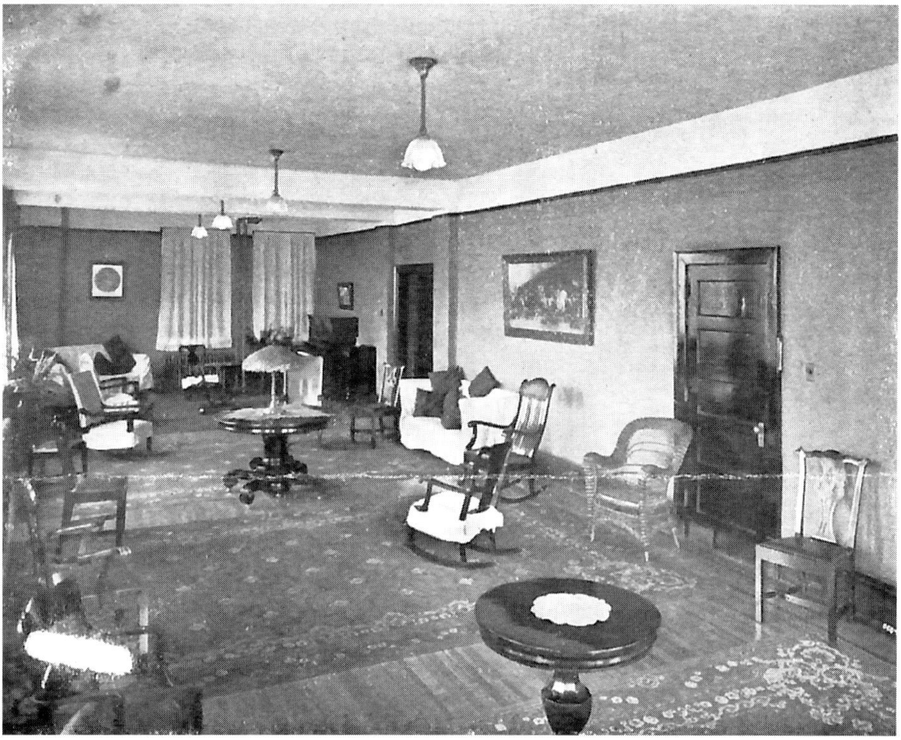

Above: Athalia Daly Home visitation room plan, 1913. (*Athalia Daly Home brochure*)

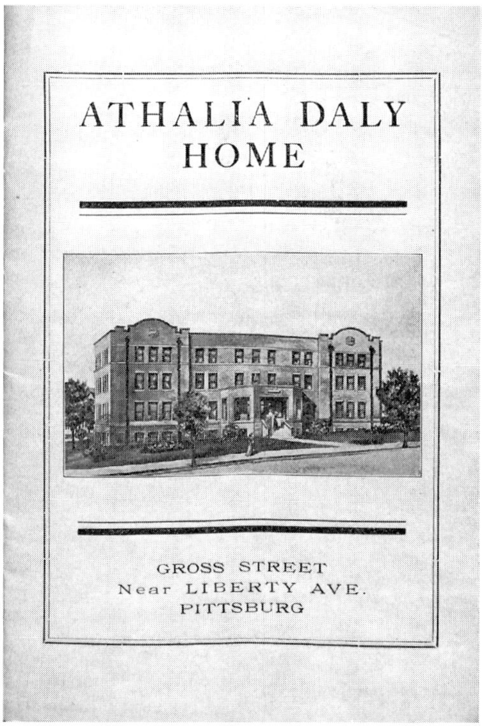

Right: Athalia Daly Home advertising brochure cover, 1913. (*Athalia Daly Home brochure*)

A brochure published several years after the home's opening addressed eligibility requirements for admittance. In defining which individuals were eligible, it explained:

> Not every girl, but any girl of good character who earns not more than $15.00 a week. This Home was not built to make money. It is not seeking to fill its rooms with anybody who can pay. It will not take girls not working for their living. It does not want a woman who is earning so much that she can pick and choose her home. It is looking for the respectable, self-supporting girl, tired of the lodging room and sick of the meager accommodations that her small salary compels her to accept. But while the Home is not run to make money, it must pay its own way. It is not a charity in the sense of giving something for nothing—the girl must pay her own way, thus she is wholly free and independent.[9]

Once admitted, the brochure noted residents would be served breakfast and dinner each day, including weekends and holidays. The food was described as "plentiful, good, wholesome, well cooked, and attractive in its variety." The cost of the meals was included in the weekly fee. The brochure also noted "lady friends" could be invited to stay overnight for a small fee, with the cost of their meals included.[10]

For more than seventy years, the home upheld the design of Daly's will. By the mid-1970s, however, social customs and improving economic circumstances for women began to reduce the number of individuals seeking the type of accommodations offered by the home. In 1975, under worsening financial circumstances, the Athalia Daly Home board of directors petitioned the Allegheny County Court of Common Pleas, Orphan's Court Division, for relief, with a recommendation "the operation of the Home should be discontinued, and that the real estate, all investments and all funds be transferred and delivered to the Western Pennsylvania Hospital."[11] In the petition, relative to its request to transfer its holdings to the hospital, the board noted: "Dr. Daly was associated as a member of the medical staff from the time he began practice in 1866 to the date of his death."[12] The board further noted the home had recently been appraised for insurance purposes. The structure was valued at $501,694, and the equipment in the building at $108,759. The group also informed the court they had operating funds on hand and owned $327,959 in investment securities.

The Athalia Daly Home and its financial assets were officially transferred to Western Pennsylvania Hospital on 31 March 1976. Before the transfer, it was reported that women who were living in the home were charged $30.50 per week for a shared room and $40.50 per week for a single room. The facility was staffed by a group of seventeen paid employees, including the board secretary, the directress (matron), her assistant, a bookkeeper, and thirteen cooks, maids, and helpers. Due to the irregular hours of operation, the directress and her assistant resided at the home.

A closing report on the operation of the home at the time of transfer offered interesting insights into the changes that had taken place since the home opened in 1907. Of particular interest:

> For many years the Home was fully occupied, and operating expenses were normally met by receipts from the guests so that it was not necessary to invade funds. For the last few years, the occupancy rate has been declining. On August 31, 1975, there were only 25 resident guests. Operating expenses for that month, $6,336.39, exceeded receipts from the residents by $2,864.78. This is a decline from 40 residents on January 1, 1975, and follows a trend with which the Board has been concerned for several years. Since January 1, 1975, 24 residents have moved into the Home; 40 have moved out, 20 to apartments and 20 returned to their homes.
>
> Current modes of living for single girls and women are increasingly liberal, and few will now accept for an extended period the dormitory-style living the Home provides. Wages of employed women now permit them to occupy small apartments of which there are many in the vicinity that have been created by subdivision of old single-family residences. Others, whose homes are in outlying districts and who formally would have been likely guests can now travel to work in Pittsburgh in their own automobiles. The monthly reports that the Trustees receive show clearly that the Home, instead of providing a more or less permanent residence, has become a way station on the route to apartment living.[13]

Before ending the Special Committee report, it was noted an attempt had been made in recent years to offer short-term accommodations to women whose husbands or other relatives were seriously ill in West Penn or St. Francis hospitals (West Penn was located one block away; St. Francis was located within easy walking distance).[14] Upon transfer of the home and in keeping with the above approach, the Western Pennsylvania Hospital board of directors decided to keep the facility open for this particular class of guests.

Between 1976 and 1990, West Penn retained the Athalia Daly Home's directress and maintained the facility using it primarily as overflow office space for hospital employees and as temporary lodging for relatives of out-of-town patients. After 1991, the facility was only used for office space and storage. Due to increasing maintenance costs and the outmoded layout of the facility, including the lack of elevators and an inability to otherwise meet federal standards under the Americans with Disabilities Act, the building was closed and demolished in early 2018.

One other item deserves mention relative to the final transfer of the Athalia Daly Home to West Penn Hospital. In harmony with Dr. Daly's intended purpose of assisting working girls and women, the hospital's board of directors offered to enter into an agreement that would have undoubtedly made William and Athalia happy. The agreement read: "The Western Pennsylvania Hospital agrees that if the Court awards to it the property and funds of Athalia Daly Home it will administer and apply the same for benefit and in aid of the instruction of girls and women as nurses, technical assistants, aides and such related matters as may be consistent with the wishes expressed in the Will of William Hudson Daly."[15] The trustees of the Athalia Daly Home were delighted to receive the offer and accepted it with gratitude.

At the time of his suicide, William H. Daly likely thought he could die in peace knowing what he had accomplished in life as a physician was well forged in writing and professional accomplishment. For him, that would serve as a sufficient legacy. Presumably, he likely surmised that Athalia's legacy would live on through the creation of the Athalia Daly Home and that it would serve as a lasting tribute to their love.

In contemplating death, Daly probably thought the "embalmed beef" controversy ended. He was wrong. He was simply not cognizant of how impactful his report of October 1898 and his testimony before the Dodge Commission and Wade Beef Board had been.

A few months before his death, Daly was aware that General Miles' nemesis in the War Department, Russell Alger, had resigned and Miles was planning a future in politics. Alger had been politically wounded by his highly criticized management of the War Department during the Spanish-American War, and more particularly by the actions and words of Commissary General Eagan during the "embalmed beef" controversy. Daly and General Miles most likely discussed the matter when Daly visited Washington to attend President McKinley's second inauguration in early March 1901. By then, it is also probable that Daly was already contemplating suicide based on the fact he updated his will only two weeks before leaving Pittsburgh for the inauguration. After returning to Pittsburgh, it would only be a matter of weeks before he shot himself.

Problems with food adulteration were known for many years before the "embalmed beef" scandal, but little had been done to resolve the issue. The matter may well have gone away after the Dodge Commission and Wade Beef Board completed their reports if not for Daly forcing the subject of tainted beef into full public attention by his suicide. His death and the great many newspaper reports that followed made certain the subject, and Daly's role in it, would not be forgotten.

Polish-American anarchist Leon Czolgosz unknowingly brought new attention to the matter on 06 September 1901 with his assassination of President McKinley. Theodore Roosevelt's ascent to the office after McKinley's death eight days later initiated some interesting coincidences that intersect with Daly's tainted meat investigations. From the date of Daly's death, a cascade of events would push Daly, President Theodore Roosevelt, author Upton Sinclair, U.S. Department of Agriculture chief chemist Harvey Washington Wiley, and others into convergence over the controversy. Within five years, the actions of these individuals would bring true focus to William H. Daly's most important legacy.

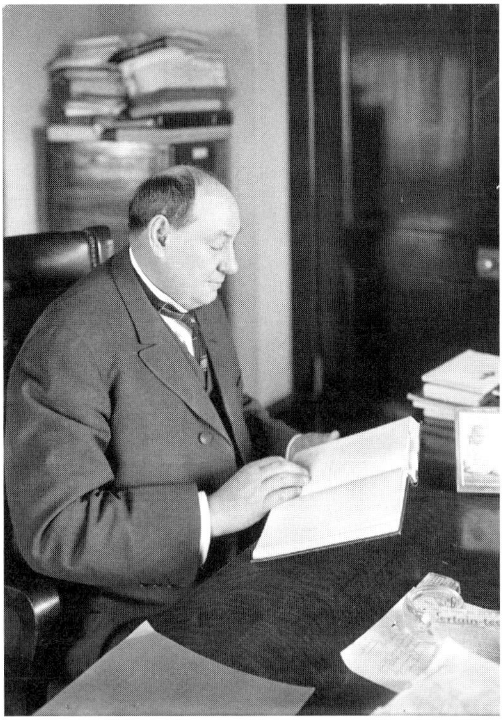

Dr. Harvey Washington Wiley, U.S. Department of Agriculture chief chemist, 1905. (*Library of Congress*)

In early 1904, while the executors of Daly's estate worked to incorporate the Athalia Daly Home and deal with court challenges seeking to stall or stop the project, Upton Sinclair began visiting meatpacking plants in Chicago. Sinclair's intent was to promote socialism and improve the condition of workers. He missed his target but managed to hit another that was not intended. The immediate product of his investigation was publication of serialized accounts printed in the socialist leaning *Appeal to Reason* newspaper between 25 February and 04 November 1905. His stories helped increase newspaper circulation, albeit not enough to ignite widespread sympathy for his cause. They did, however, create sufficient public indignation to suggest that publication of the columns in book form might prove more effective. Thus, Sinclair's novel *The Jungle* was conceived. It would be published in 1906. It was the same year that construction of the Athalia Daly Home was finished.

While Sinclair was investigating slaughterhouses in Chicago and writing the first installments for *Appeal to Reason*, Harvey Washington Wiley was busy investigating food adulteration and patent medicines on behalf of the government. Appointed under President Chester Arthur in the early 1880s, Wiley had long advocated for stronger controls on a range of industries, including meat packing. In March 1899, under instructions from the Agriculture Department, Wiley was one of the chemists assigned to test beef at six Chicago packinghouses.

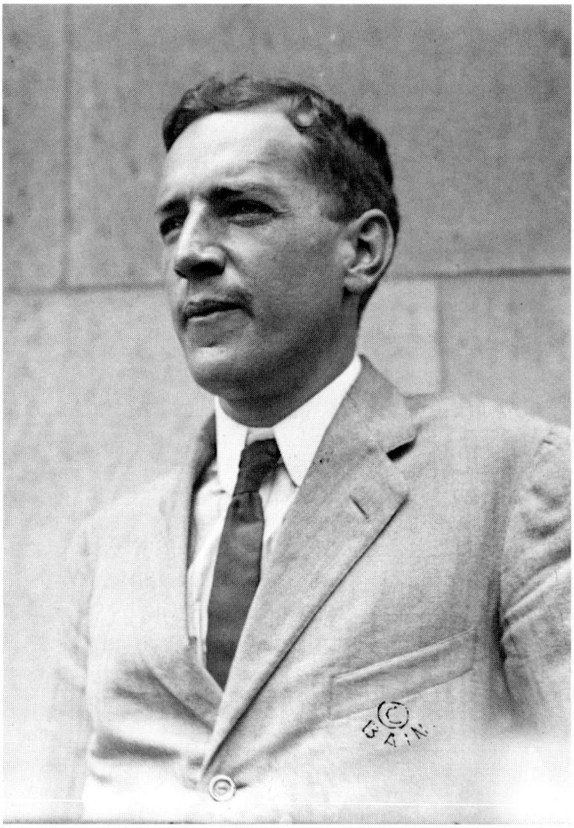

Upton Sinclair, 1900.
(*Library of Congress*)

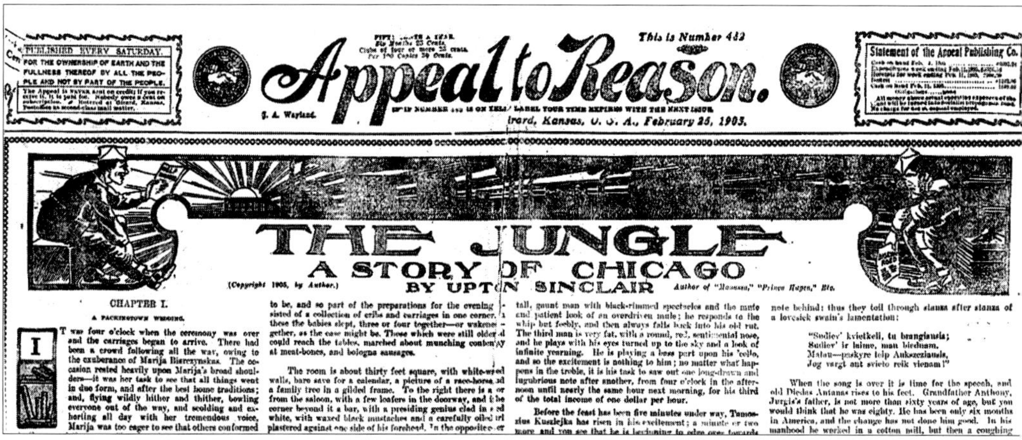

PUBLISHED EVERY SATURDAY.
FOR THE OWNERSHIP OF EARTH AND THE FULLNESS THEREOF BY ALL THE PEOPLE AND NOT BY PART OF THE PEOPLE.

Appeal to Reason.

J. A. Wayland.

This is Number 482

Girard, Kansas, U. S. A., February 25, 1905.

Statement of the Appeal Publishing Co.

THE JUNGLE
A STORY OF CHICAGO
BY UPTON SINCLAIR

(Copyright 1905, by Author.)

Author of "Manassas," "Prince Hagen," Etc.

CHAPTER I.

A PACKINGTOWN WEDDING.

IT was four o'clock when the ceremony was over and the carriages began to arrive. There had been a crowd following all the way, owing to the exuberance of Marija Berczynskas. The occasion rested heavily upon Marija's broad shoulders—it was her task to see that all things went in due form, and after the best home traditions; and, flying wildly hither and thither, bowling everyone out of the way, and scolding and exhorting all day with her tremendous voice, Marija was too eager to see that others conformed

to be, and so part of the preparations for the evening consisted of a collection of cribs and carriages in one corner, in these the babies slept, three or four together—or wakened together, as the case might be. Those which were still older and could reach the tables, marched about munching contentedly at meat-bones, and bologna sausages.

The room is about thirty feet square, with whitewashed walls, bare save for a calendar, a picture of a race-horse and a family tree in a gilded frame. To the right there is a door from the saloon, with a few loafers in the doorway, and in the corner beyond it a bar, with a presiding genius clad in soiled white, with waxed black mustaches and a carefully oiled curl plastered against one side of his forehead. In the opposite corner

tall, gaunt man with black-rimmed spectacles and the mute and patient look of an overdriven mule; he responds to the whip but feebly, and then always falls back into his old rut. The third man is very fat, with a round, red, sentimental nose, and he plays with his eyes turned up to the sky and a look of infinite yearning. He is playing a bass part upon his 'cello, and so the excitement is nothing to him; no matter what happens in the treble, it is his task to saw out one long-drawn and lugubrious note after another, from four o'clock in the afternoon until nearly the same hour next morning, for his third of the total income of one dollar per hour.

Before the feast has been five minutes under way, Tamoszius Kuszlejka has risen in his excitement; a minute or two more and you see that he is beginning to edge over towards

note behind: thus they toil through stanza after stanza of a lovesick swain's lamentation:

"Sudiev' kvietkeli, tu brangiausis;
Sudiev' ir laime, man biednam,
Matau—paskyre teip Aukszcziausis,
Jog vargt ant svieto reik vienam!"

When the song is over it is time for the speech, and old Diedas Antanas rises to his feet. Grandfather Anthony, Jurgis's father, is not more than sixty years of age, but you would think that he was eighty. He has been only six months in America, and the change has not done him good. In his manhood he worked in a cotton mill, but then a coughing

Appeal to Reason newspaper masthead and headline showing Upton Sinclair's first installment of *The Jungle*, 25 February 1905. (*Deception For Journalism's Sake: A Database dlib.nyu.edu/undercover/jungle-story-chicago-upton-sinclair-appeal-reason. Retrieved 25 February 2019*)

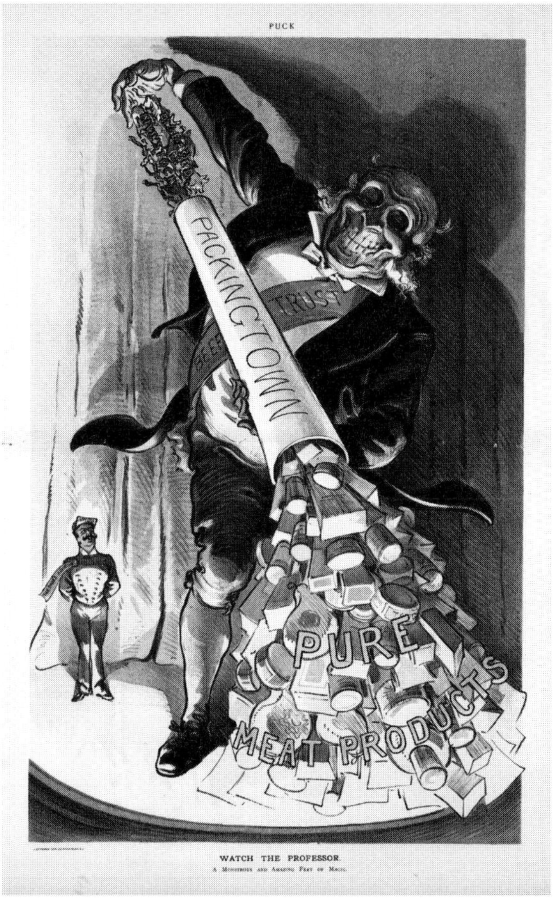

"Watch the Professor" cartoon illustration showing "Beef Trust" inserting diseased livestock through "Packingtown" cylinder to create "pure meat products" while government inspector watches. *Puck* magazine, Volume 50, Number 1525, 23 May 1906. (*Library of Congress*)

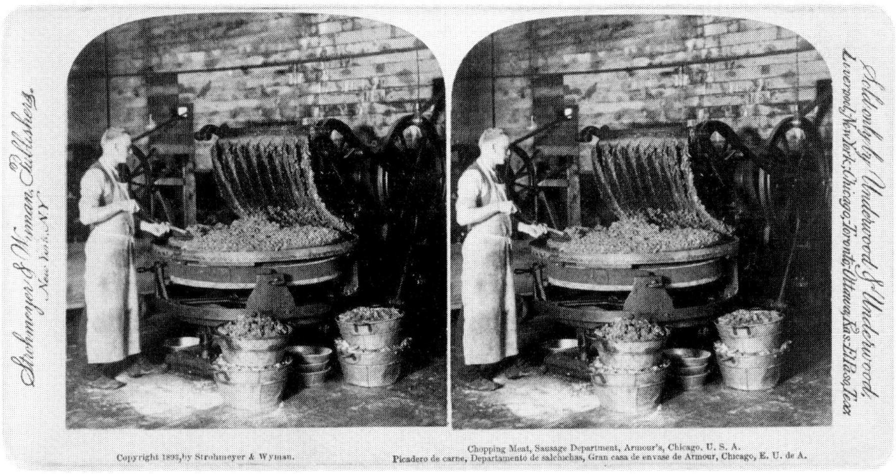

Chopping meat, sausage department at Armour's meat packing house, Chicago, IL, 1893. (*Library of Congress*)

His findings were presented to the Wade Beef Board on 14 April 1899. During his testimony, Wiley did not offer any opinion on refrigerated beef, as none of the beef from Cuba was available to him at the time. Much of his testimony concerned canned beef, the processes used in its canning and sterilization, and its nutritive value. While not entirely supportive of the issues Daly and Miles reported, Wiley's testimony nevertheless painted a very unflattering picture of inferior beef being fed to soldiers and sold to the public. Even though he provided solid research attesting to many abuses that were harmful to the public, Congress generally ignored his advocacy. That would soon change.

Shortly after publication, reports of Sinclair's *Appeal to Reason* articles reached President Roosevelt. The issues were not new to him. Roosevelt had written reports about the poor quality of beef while in the Army and offered testimony to the Dodge Commission. More recently, as Governor of New York, he had even testified in front of the Wade Beef Board. As President, he now also had to deal with the Beef Trust problem.

Having suspicions about Sinclair's reporting, however, and not wishing to act brashly, Roosevelt decided to send a pair of handpicked investigators to Chicago for further investigation. He chose Commissioner of Labor Charles Neill and social worker James Bronson Reynolds for the task. Neill and Reynolds were well-qualified and trustworthy investigators. Roosevelt felt he could rely on their report far more than Sinclair's. Upon conclusion of their investigation and after reading their report, Roosevelt found the problems were even worse than those Sinclair had uncovered. He decided to act.

On 05 May 1905, Roosevelt delivered his State of the Union Address to Congress. It set out a broad, aggressive agenda. In a follow-up to what he had just learned, he made certain to include a preview of his intentions regarding the beef matter. In his address, he stated: "I recommend that a law be enacted to regulate inter-State commerce in misbranded and adulterated foods, drinks, and drugs. Such law would protect legitimate manufacture and commerce and would tend to secure the health and welfare of the consuming public. Traffic in foodstuffs which have been debased or adulterated so as to injure health or to deceive purchasers should be forbidden."[16]

On a parallel track, others were sharpening their attacks on the patent medicine industry. Beginning in December 1905, *Collier's Weekly* magazine began publishing a series of articles by Samuel Hopkins Adams. Much like Sinclair's reports in *Appeal to Reason*, Adams' series exposed fraud among patent medicine purveyors. Abuses in the patent medicine industry were just as bad, if not worse than those happening in the beef industry.[17]

Upon its release on 26 February 1906, Sinclair's *The Jungle* became a bestseller. His story resonated with the public, but not for the reason Sinclair intended. Rather than gaining sympathy for the socialist cause or the plight of workers, the book managed to shine an even brighter light on the poor quality and frequently

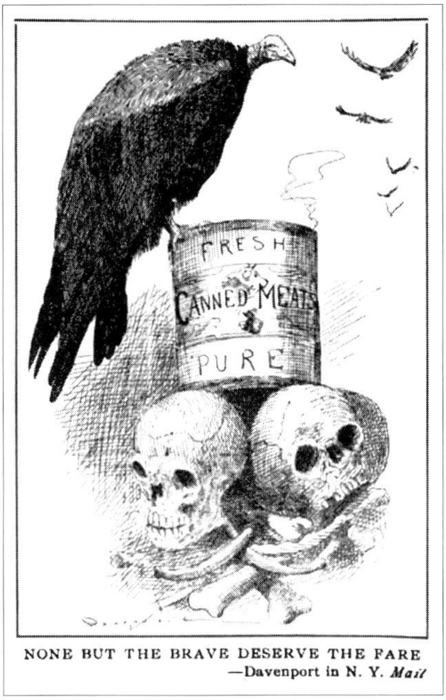

NONE BUT THE BRAVE DESERVE THE FARE
—Davenport in N. Y. *Mail*

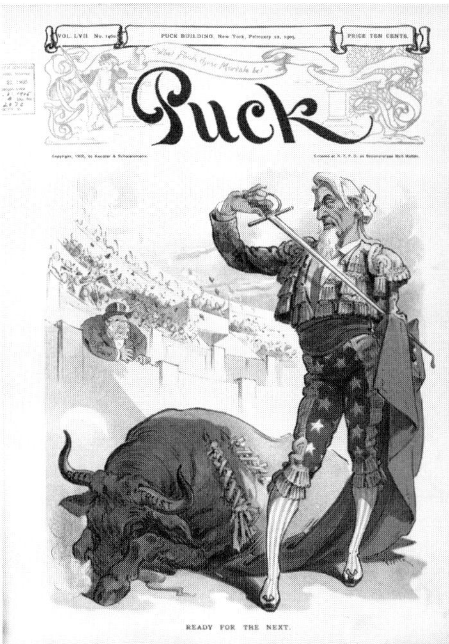

Above left: "None but the brave deserve the fare" cartoon illustration, *Current Literature*, Volume 41, Number 1, July 1906.

Above right: "Ready for the next" cartoon illustration showing Uncle Sam slaying "Beef Trust," *Puck* magazine, Volume 57, Number 1460, 22 February 1906. (*Library of Congress*)

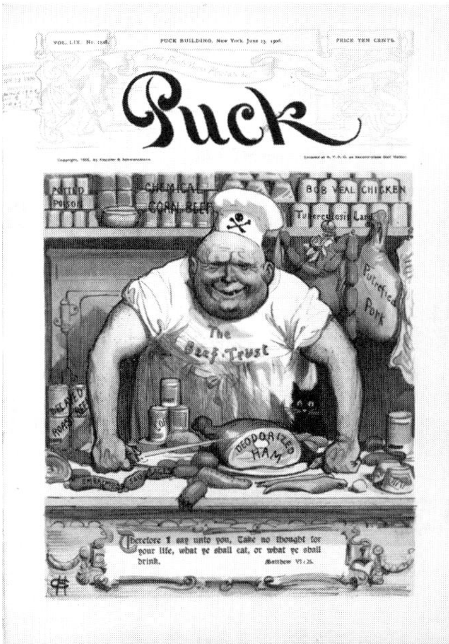

Cartoon illustration showing "The Beef Trust" at butcher shop counter surrounded by "Potted Poison, Chemical Corn Beef, Bob Veal Chicken, Tuberculosis Lard, Decayed Roast Beef, Deodorized Ham, Embalmed Sausages, and Putrefied Pork" meat products. Bible verse below reads: "Therefore I say unto you, Take no thought for your life, what ye shall eat, or what ye shall drink. Matthew VI:25." *Puck* magazine, Volume 59, Number 1528, 13 June 1906. (*Library of Congress*)

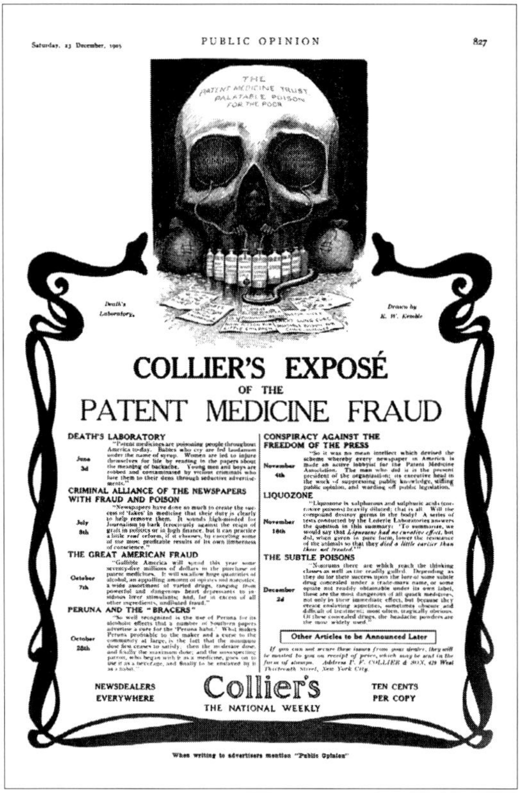

Saturday, 23 December, 1905 PUBLIC OPINION 827

THE PATENT MEDICINE TRUST PALATABLE POISON FOR THE POOR

Death's Laboratory. Drawn by E. W. Kemble

COLLIER'S EXPOSÉ
OF THE
PATENT MEDICINE FRAUD

DEATH'S LABORATORY

June 3d — "Patent medicines are poisoning people throughout America to-day. Babies who cry are fed laudanum under the name of syrup. Women are led to injure themselves for life by reading in the papers about the meaning of backache. Young men and boys are robbed and contaminated by vicious criminals who lure them to their dens through seductive advertisements."

CRIMINAL ALLIANCE OF THE NEWSPAPERS WITH FRAUD AND POISON

July 8th — "Newspapers have done so much to create the success of 'fakes' in medicine that their duty is clearly to help remove them. It sounds high-minded for Journalism to bark ferociously against the reign of graft in politics or in high finance, but it can practice a little *real* reform, if it chooses, by cancelling some of the most profitable results of its own limberness of conscience."

THE GREAT AMERICAN FRAUD

October 7th — "Gullible America will spend this year some seventy-five millions of dollars in the purchase of patent medicines. It will swallow huge quantities of alcohol, an appalling amount of opiates and narcotics, a wide assortment of varied drugs, ranging from powerful and dangerous heart depressants to insidious liver stimulants; and, far in excess of all other ingredients, undiluted fraud."

PERUNA AND THE "BRACERS"

October 28th — "So well recognized is the use of Peruna for its alcoholic effects that a number of Southern papers advertise a cure for the 'Peruna habit.' What makes Peruna profitable to the maker and a curse to the community at large, is the fact that the minimum dose first ceases to satisfy; then the moderate dose, and finally the maximum dose; and the unsuspecting patron, who began with it as a medicine, goes on to use it as a beverage, and finally to be enslaved by it as a habit."

CONSPIRACY AGAINST THE FREEDOM OF THE PRESS

November 4th — "So it was no mean intellect which devised the scheme whereby every newspaper in America is made an active lobbyist for the Patent Medicine Association. The man who did it is the present president of the organization; its executive head in the work of suppressing public knowledge, stifling public opinion, and warding off public legislation."

LIQUOZONE

November 18th — "Liquozone is sulphurous and sulphuric acids (corrosive poisons) heavily diluted; that is all. Will the compound destroy germs in the body? A series of tests conducted by the Lederle Laboratories answers the question in this summary: 'To summarize, we would say that *Liquozone had no curative effect*, but did, when given in pure form, lower the resistance of the animals so that they *died a little earlier than those not treated*.'"

THE SUBTLE POISONS

December 2d — "Nostrums there are which reach the thinking classes as well as the readily gulled. Depending as they do for their success upon the lure of some subtle drug concealed under a trade-mark name, or some opiate not readily obtainable under its own label, these are the most dangerous of all quack medicines, not only in their immediate effect, but because they create enslaving appetites, sometimes obscure and difficult of treatment; most often, tragically obvious. Of these concealed drugs, the headache powders are the most widely used."

Other Articles to be Announced Later

If you can not secure these issues from your dealer, they will be mailed to you on receipt of price, which may be sent in the form of stamps. Address P. F. COLLIER & SON, 420 West Thirteenth Street, New York City.

NEWSDEALERS EVERYWHERE — **Collier's** THE NATIONAL WEEKLY — TEN CENTS PER COPY

When writing to advertisers mention "Public Opinion"

Left: Public Opinion advertisement for "Patent Medicine Fraud" series by Samuel Hopkins Adams; *Collier's* magazine, Volume 39, Number 26, 23 December1905. (*Library of Congress*)

Below: Patent medicine advertisement for May's drug store, Pittsburg, Pennsylvania (*The Star Course magazine, Volume 1, Number 2, Carnegie, Pennsylvania 1895*)

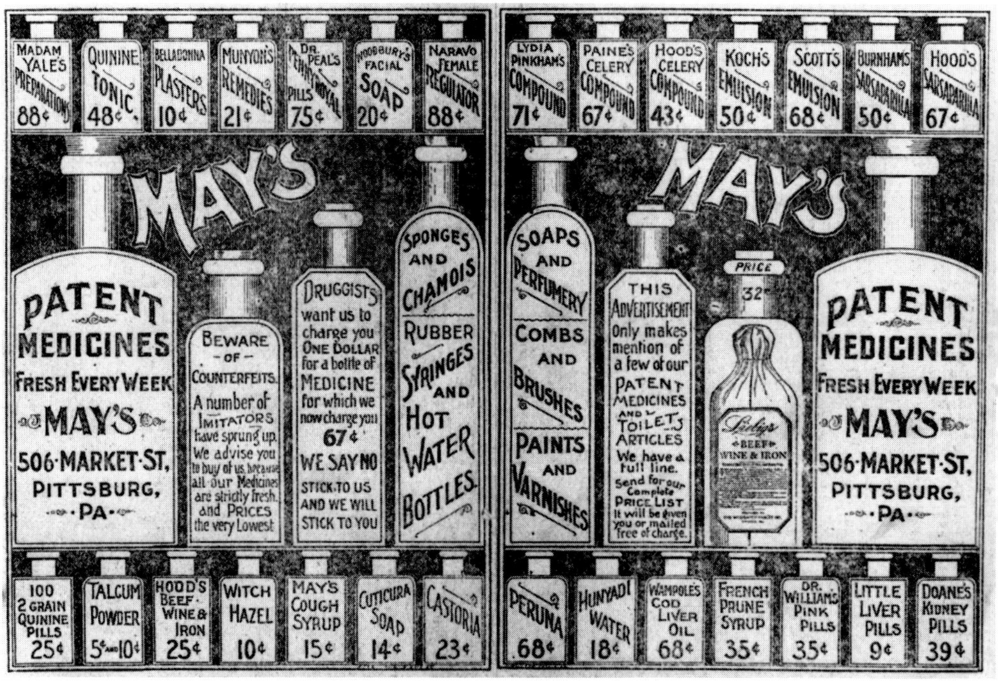

tainted beef being sold to the public and the government. Sinclair included a passage in his book about "embalmed beef," in which he wrote:

> It seemed that they must have agencies all over the country, to hunt out old and crippled and diseased cattle to be canned. There were cattle which had been fed on " whiskey-malt," the refuse of the breweries, and had become what the men called "steerly"—which means covered with boils. It was a nasty job killing these, for when you plunged your knife into them they would burst and splash foul-smelling stuff into your face; and when a man's sleeves were smeared with blood, and his hands steeped in it, how was he ever to wipe his face, or to clear his eyes so that he could see? It was stuff such as this that made the "embalmed beef" that had killed several times as many United States soldiers as all the bullets of the Spaniards; only the army beef, besides, was not fresh canned, it was old stuff that had been lying for years in the cellars.[18]

Sinclair also took the opportunity to include a section on canned beef:

> Jurgis spent his Christmas in this hospital, and it was the pleasantest Christmas he had had in America. Every year there were scandals and investigations in this institution, the newspapers charging that doctors were allowed to try fantastic experiments upon the patients; but Jurgis knew nothing of this—his only complaint was that they used to feed him upon tinned meat, which no man who had ever worked in Packingtown would feed to his dog. Jurgis had often wondered just who ate the canned corned beef and "roast beef" of the stockyards; now he began to understand—that it was what you might call "graftmeat," put up to be sold to public officials and contractors, and eaten by soldiers and sailors, prisoners and inmates of institutions, "shanty-men" and gangs of railroad laborers.[19]

Sinclair's exposé of the meatpacking industry's unsanitary practices and routine health code violations added another log on the fire that Daly had lit on board S.S. *Comal* in 1898. As sales of *The Jungle* increased, public outrage erupted anew, and they voiced their ire in the halls of Congress. Members of Congress who had long been unsuccessfully advancing legislation to deal with adulterated food and patent medicines now found new reason to stop talking and start acting. The more the public clamored for action and the louder the din became, the easier it became for congressional supporters to counter members who had supported the beef industry and blocked previous legislative attempts to intercede. With Roosevelt's support and arm-twisting, the Pure Food and Drug Act and the Meat Inspection Act were finally passed. On 30 June 1906, Theodore Roosevelt signed them into law. The safety of food and drugs was now assured.

William H. Daly's role in bringing attention to beef industry malfeasance at the turn of the twentieth century cannot be overstated. His reports and the

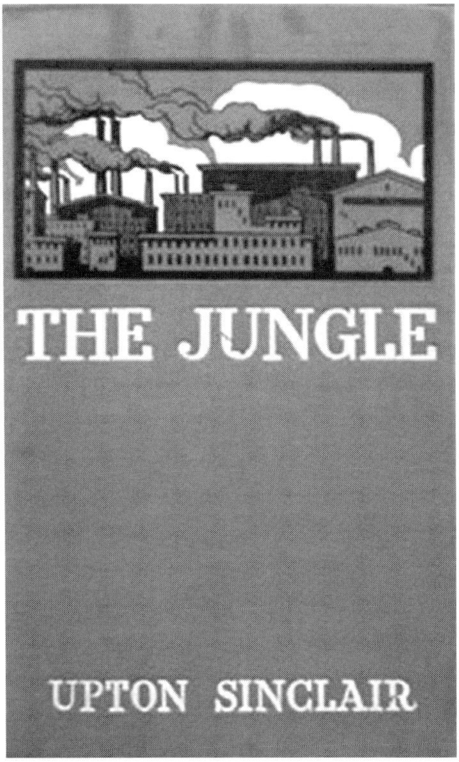

Cover of the first edition of *The Jungle* by Upton Sinclair, 1906. (*Wikimedia Commons*)

sensational outcome of his testimony at government hearings remained in the news for months and were etched in the public's memory. Despite the fact it took Roosevelt, Wiley, Sinclair, Adams, and many thousands of American citizens to sound the final clarion calls for government intervention, their involvement should not diminish Daly's exertions on behalf of Spanish-American War soldiers that ultimately resulted in passage of the landmark legislation. In many ways, we owe Daly gratitude for the consumer protections our country enjoys today.

William H. Daly deserves a place of honor in the history of the United States as a pioneering laryngologist, public health advocate, patriot, and soldier. As General Miles noted: "Dr. Daly was no ordinary man."

Endnotes

Introduction

1. Franklin, *Poor Richard's Almanac* (Philadelphia, 1738), spread 6.
2. *The Army Surgeon's Manual, for the use of Medical Officers, Cadets, Chaplains, and Hospital Stewards Regulations of the Medical Department, All General Orders from the War Department, and Circulars from the Surgeon-General's Office, From January 1st, 1861, to July 1st, 1864*, (1864), pp. 20-21.

Chapter 1

1. Daly Family Album (www.seltzerbooks.com/gen/daly/album.html).
2. Vivian, *Good Ol' Monongahela Rye and the Gibsonton Mills* (www.pre-pro.com/histories/gibson.htm).
3. Albert, *History of the County of Westmoreland, Pennsylvania* (1882), p. 565.
4. *Ibid.*, p. 566.

Chapter 2

1. "United States Census, 1860", Family Search (familysearch.org/ark:/61903/1:1:M418-TCP).
2. "President Abraham Lincoln's Union Blockade Proclamations" (1861), proclamations 82 and 86.
3. Evans, *Confederate military history; a library of Confederate States history, written by distinguished men of the south* (1899), p. 91.
4. *The Richmond Daily Dispatch,* 13 May 1861, p. 2.
5. Lain, *15th Virginia Infantry History, April 1861—Spring 1862*, pp. II-IV.
6. *Richmond Daily Dispatch* (15 May 1861), p. 1.
7. Schreier, "English Enfields In Confederate Service," *American Rifleman Journal* (1999).
8. Lain, *op. cit.*, pp. XII-XIII.
9. *Ibid.*, pp. IV-VII.
10. Lowe, "Magruder's Defense of the Peninsula," *Confederate Veteran* (1900), p. 105.

11. "Prince John" was the affectionate nickname that troops used to refer to Confederate General John B. Magruder. He was well educated, well-mannered, and at times somewhat flamboyant. His military exploits in outfoxing the Union Army were legendary. In particular, Magruder's use of "Quaker cannons," which were simply painted logs positioned amid regular cannons and mounted at the bastions to fool the enemy into thinking Confederate positions were better fortified than they actually were. When he used them early in war during the Peninsula Campaign they were sophisticated enough to help stop McClellan's advance on Richmond. Coupled with another of Magruder's tactics of having his men constantly beating drums and hooting and hollering, they made a small number of Confederate soldiers seem like a much larger and threatening enemy force. Colonel R. G. Lowe in his March 1900 article "Magruder's Defense of the Peninsula," in *Confederate Veteran,* wrote of Magruder's escapades stating, "McClellan, by his 'Own Story,' was about the worst fooled individual that ever came up the peninsula on a warlike mission." In relating his story, Lowe went on to add, "My purpose is not to belittle McClellan, who was deceived, but to magnify Magruder, the deceiver, for the relation of 53,000 to 7,000 men should have made the capture of Magruder and entire force a mere matter of military execution."
12. Day, *Down South; or, An Englishman's Experience at the seat of the American war, Volume 1*" (1862) p. 25.
13. *Ibid.*, pp. 36-37.
14. *Ibid.*, pp. 38-40.
15. *Richmond Daily Dispatch*, 13 June 1861, p. 4.
16. *The Union Army: a History of Military Affairs In the Loyal States, 1861–65—Records of the Regiments In the Union Army—Cyclopedia of Battles—Memoirs of Commanders And Soldiers* (1908), pp. 120-121.
17. Day, *op. cit.*, p. 41.
18. Douglas, "Reminiscences of the Peninsula," *Confederate Veteran* (1903), p. 554.
19. Lain, *op. cit.*, pp. XXXIII and XXXIV.
20. *Ibid.*, pp. XXXV and XXXVI.
21. *Ibid.*, pp. XXXVI.
22. *Ibid.*, pp. XXXVII and XXXVIII.
23. Douglas, *op. cit.*, p. 554.
24. *Ibid.*
25. Lain, *op. cit.*, p. XLVI.
26. *Ibid.*, p. XLVIII.
27. *Ibid.*, p. LVII.
28. Confederate Archives, Chapter 6, File No. 267, p. 5.
29. Confederate Archives, Manuscript No. 138.
30. Cunningham, "Confederate General Hospitals: Establishment and Organization," *The Journal of Southern History*, (1954) pp. 376-377' See also: Frank, *Women in the American Civil War* (2008), p. 339; and, "Daughters of our Presidents," *The Ladies Home Journal* (1897), p. 11.
31. Lain, *op. cit.*, p. LXV.
32. *Ibid.*, p. LXXI.
33. *The war of the rebellion: a compilation of the official records of the Union and Confederate armies.* Series 1, Volume II, Part III (1880–1901), p. 448.
34. *The Union Army: a History of Military Affairs In the Loyal States, 1861–65—Records of the Regiments In the Union Army—Cyclopedia of Battles—Memoirs of Commanders And Soldiers* (1908), p. 556.
35. *The war of the rebellion: a compilation of the official records of the Union and Confederate armies.* Series 1, Volume II, Part III. p. 437.

36. *The Union Army: a History of Military Affairs In the Loyal States, 1861–65,* Volume 6, pp. 556-557.
37. *The war of the rebellion: a compilation of the official records of the Union and Confederate armies.* Series 1, Volume II, Part III, pp. 448-449.
38. Douglas, *op. cit.*, p. 554.

Chapter 3

1. Company "B," 15th Regiment Va. Muster Roll (1862).
2. *Ibid.*
3. Netherton, *In the Path of History: Virginia Between the Rappahannock and the Potomac: An Historical Portrait* (2004).
4. Pickenpaugh, "Prisoner Exchange and Parole" (2018).
5. *Ibid.*
6. Wikisource contributors, "Dix-Hill Cartel."
7. *Ibid.*
8. Gesley, "The Lieber Code—the First Modern Codification of the Laws of War," (2018).
9. National Park Service, "Myth: Grant Stopped the Prisoner Exchange."
10. *Ibid.*
11. *Message of the President of the United States to the Two Houses of Congress at the Commencement of the Second Session of the Thirty-Seventh Congress,* Volume 2 (1861), p. 62.
12. The expression "galvanized Yankee" was a derisive term used to refer to captured Confederate soldiers who swore an oath of allegiance to the United States and volunteered in the Union army.
13. Hasegawa, "The Civil War's Medical Cadets: Medical Students Serving the Union," *Journal of the American College of Surgeons* (2001), p. 81.
14. *Ibid.*
15. *Ibid.*, p. 82.
16. *Ibid.*, p. 86. Note: Medical cadets did not have to complete a term before starting duty as a commissioned or contract surgeon.
17. Records of the Surgeon General, Record Group 112.12.3.
18. *Ibid.*
19. Record of Medical Officer Serving Department of the South for the Month of May 1865, William H. Daly Acting Assistant Surgeon, In Charge Provost Guards Hospital, S.C. to J. K. Barnes, Surgeon General USA (1865).
20. Letter from Acting Medical Director, Hilton Head S.C. to Surgeon General Joseph K. Barnes, 22 August 1865 (1865).

Chapter 4

1. Grom, *Physician Soldiers at the Forks* (2019), pp. 120-121.
2. "Students in Medicine," Department of Medicine and Surgery, University of Michigan *Catalogue of the Officers and Students for 1865–1866* (1866), p 27.
3. "Distinguished Alumni," *The Michigan Alumnus*, Volume VII, Number 8 (1901), p. 316.
4. "Students in Medicine," *op. cit.*, p. 27.
5. Shaw, "The University of Michigan, an Encyclopedic Survey" (1942), p. 792.
6. Holtz, "Bankrobbers, Burkers, and Bodysnatchers," *Michigan Quarterly Review* (1967), p. 92.

7. Medical Thesis Box 12, Michigan Historical Collections, Bentley Historical Library, University of Michigan, Ann Arbor.
8. "Degrees Conferred During the Year," *Catalogue of the Students for 1866–1867*, University of Michigan, Ann Arbor (1867), p. 7.
9. "Students in Medicine," *op. cit.*, p. 27.
10. *Annual Report of the Managers of the Western Pennsylvania Hospital for 1862*, p. 8.
11. *Ibid.*
12. "The United States Military Hospital," *The Daily Pittsburgh Gazette* (August 13, 1864), p. 1.
13. Grom, *op. cit.*, p. 207. Note: The Pittsburgh Sanitary Fair, held from 01 June to 18 June 1864, was a civilian philanthropic undertaking staged to raise funds for the relief and care of sick and wounded soldiers. Fair activities included numerous displays of machinery, model ships, weapons, livestock, floral arrangements, and art. Various entertainment and food venues were included, as were special areas where donated items were sold. Over its eighteen-day operation, more than $320,000 was raised.

Chapter 5

1. *Allegheny County Medical Society Membership History* (Pittsburgh, 1904).
2. Harris, "Minutes With Comments, The Allegheny County Medical Society 1865–1940 (16 April 1867 meeting)," *Pittsburgh Medical Bulletin* (1939), p 671.
3. *Ibid.* Note: The term "Irregular practitioners" included those who practiced homeopathy, phrenology, electrotherapy, botanical medicine, hydrotherapy, or other such movements that were considered outside mainstream (allopathic) medicine. Bleeders, cuppers, patent medicine purveyors, and galvanizers were likewise considered "irregular," or sometimes, simply as "quacks." Collectively, with the exception of the homeopaths, most of these practitioners were held to few or no professional or ethical standards. Until after the turn of the twentieth century when state and national laws and regulations were enacted, they openly competed with allopathic physicians as they peddled fraudulent cures to an unknowing public.
4. Officers of the Allegheny County Medical Society from 1865 to1904, Allegheny County Medical Society records (Pittsburgh, *c.* 1904).
5. The titles of Daly's contributions to Forest and Stream appear on the last page of the monograph: *A discussion of some questions relating to tonsillotomy: read before the State Medical Society of Pennsylvania, at its meeting in 1882, and published in The Medical Record of February, 1883; and, Clinical remarks upon deflections of the nasal septum, with a presentation of two cases made before the Allegheny County Medical Society, at its meeting, November, 1883*. From archive.org/details/b22454445/page/n1.
6. Daly, "Gunshot Wounds of the Larynx with the report of a case in which the vocal bands were involved." Monograph reprinted from the *New York Medical Journal* for July 12, 1884 (1884). Note: The two additional titles appear on the last page.
7. Thurston, *Directory of Pittsburgh and Allegheny Cities for 1868–69* (1868), p. 105; and *Directory of Pittsburgh and Allegheny Cities for 1869–70* (1868), p. 116.
8. Grom, "No Ordinary Man," *Pittsburgh History* (Spring 1991), p. 4.
9. "Distinguished Alumni, William Hudson Daly, '66 *m*" *The Michigan Alumnus* (1901), p. 317.
10. Cushing, "*History of Allegheny County Pennsylvania, Volume 1*" (1889), pp. 423-424.

11. Thurston, *Directory of Pittsburgh and Allegheny Cities for 1870; 1871–1872; 1872–1873, 1874, 1875, 1876, 1877*. Also see: Thurston and Diffenbacher, *Directory of Pittsburgh and Allegheny Cities for 1875 and 1876; and,* Diffenbacher, *Directory of Pittsburg(h) and Allegheny Cities*, 1878; 1880; 1882–1883; 1887; 1890–1891; 1892; 1894; 1896.
12. Diffenbacher, *Directory of Pittsburgh and Allegheny Cities, 1897–1898* (1897).
13. Thurston, *Directory of Pittsburg and Allegheny Cities for 1873–74* (1873), p. 43.
14. "Distinguished Alumni," *op. cit.*, pp. 316-317.
15. Brinton, (ed.), "Correspondence," *The Medical and Surgical Reporter: A Weekly Journal* (1878).
16. *Ibid.*, p. 368.
17. *Ibid.*, pp. 368-369.
18. Daly, "A Case of Stenosis of the Larynx, with Fibrous Adhesive Bands of the True Vocal Cords: Tracheotomy, Rupture of Bands, and Cure of Stenosis by General and Local Treatment," and "An Analysis of the Value of the Galvano-Cautery in the Treatment of Diseases and Growths of the Naso-Pharynx," *The Transactions of the American Medical Association*, (1880), pp. 647-656.
19. Daly, "Elongating Hyperthropy of the Femur and Tibia of Opposite Sides (The Osteitis Deformans of Paget)," *Medical Record*, Volume XVII, Number 9, February 28, 1880, pp. 225-227.
20. Elsberg, "A Case of Luxation of the Left Cornua of the Hyoid Bone," *Archives of Laryngology* (1881), pp. 162-163.
21. "Distinguished Alumni," *op. cit.*, p. 317.
22. "Letter from Dr. D. N. Rankin;" *The Journal of Laryngology and Rhinology*, (1887), p. 315-316; "Editors Reply," (1887), pp. 316-317.
23. "Editors Reply," *The Journal of Laryngology and Rhinology* (1887), pp. 316-317.
24. "Distinguished Alumni," *op. cit.*, p. 317.

Chapter 6

1. Gilmer, "Birth of the American Crucible Steel Industry," *The Western Pennsylvania Historical Magazine* (1953), pp. 27-28.
2. Durant, *History of Allegheny County Pennsylvania* (1876), p.76.
3. Hays, *City at the Point* (1989), p. 275.
4. Pennsylvania National Guard Veterans' Card File, 1867–1921 (series #13.36), Pennsylvania State Archives.
5. "Some Practical Observations On So-Called Malaria Being A Waterborne Disease," *Transactions of the American Climatological Association for the year 1893* (1893), p. 388.
6. *Pittsburg Bulletin* (1888), p.8.
7. "Making History," Pittsburgh Duquesne Club website, www.duquesne.org/about/history/ (2019).
8. Women were not admitted as members until 1980.
9. Grom, "No Ordinary Man," *Pittsburgh History* (Spring 1991), p. 5.
10. Grom, *Physician Soldiers at the Forks*, p. 209.
11. Daly, "Address in Medicine," *Transactions of the Medical Society of the State of Pennsylvania* (1884), p. 129.
12. *Journal of the American Medical Association* (1886), p. 551.
13. *Journal of the American Medical Association* (1887), p. 503.
14. *Pittsburg Bulletin*, (March 1890, p. 10. Note: In 1891, Pittsburgh's name was changed by dropping the final -h in response to a requirement of the U.S. Board on

Geographic Names. The -h was restored in 1911. During the period, both spellings were often used interchangeably.

15. *Pittsburg Dispatch*, 22 December 1891, p. 9.
16. *Pittsburg Bulletin*, 21 May 1892, p. 12.
17. Daly, "A Clinical Study of Glanders in the Horse," *Medical Record* (1893), p. 6.

Chapter 7

1. Jackson, *The Life of Chevalier Jackson: An Autobiography* (1938), p. 85.
2. *Ibid.*, p. 87.
3. *Ibid.*
4. Rankin, *The Journal of Laryngology and Rhinology* (August 1887), pp. 315-316 (London: 1887).
5. Wechsler, *Dr. Chevalier Jackson* (1994).
6. Grom, "No Ordinary Man", *Pittsburgh History* (Spring 1991), p. 5.
7. "Social Chatter," *Pittsburg Dispatch* (August 1892), p. 4.
8. "A Long Trip for Sport—Twelve Hundred Miles and Back Again for Prairie Chicken Shooting," *Pittsburg Dispatch* (09 October 1892), p. 15.
9. Miles, "Hunting Large Game," *North American Review* (October 1895), pp. 489-490.
10. *Ibid.,* p. 490.
11. *Ibid.*
12. *Ibid.*, p. 491.
13. *American Kennel Club Stud-Book, January 1–December 31, 1893* (1894), p. 353.
14. Morrill, *The Morrills and Reminiscences*, University Publishing Company (1918), p. 86.
15. *The Billings Gazette* (10 November 1899), p. 5.
16. Bonner, *William F. Cody's Wyoming Empire* (2007), p. 115.
17. Grom, *op. cit.,* p. 8.
18. Correspondence between U.S. Army Surgeon General George Miller Sternberg and Dr. William H. Daly (15 May 1894).
19. *Ibid.*

Chapter 8

1. "Transactions of the Fourth Annual Meeting of the American Laryngological, Rhinological, and Otological Society Held in Pittsburg, PA, May 11 and 12, 1898" (1899), pp. 1-2.
2. *Ibid.*, p. 201.
3. Miles, "The War with Spain—I", *North American Review* (1898) p. 523.
4. "Transactions of the Fourth Annual Meeting of the American Laryngological, Rhinological, and Otological Society Held in Pittsburg, PA, May 11 and 12, 1898" (1899), p. 201.
5. Koyle, "*I Shtart to free ould Cuba in the Mornin'*" (May 1898).
6. *Pennsylvania Medical Journal,* Volume 2, August 1898 (1898), p. 161.
7. Stewart, *Record of Pennsylvania volunteers in the Spanish-American War, 1898* (1900), p. 846.
8. "Miles Starts. General in Command of the U.S. Army, Departs from Washington for the Front," *Topeka State Journal*, 31 May 1898, p. 2. (Kansas: 1898).
9. United States. Surgeon General (Army) Office. Records relating to military personnel, Record Group 112.2.3 (Washington, D.C.: U.S. National Archives and

Records Administration). Note: Porto Rico and Puerto Rico are used in context throughout this work. Before the 1898 American invasion, the Spanish referred to the island as Puerto Rico. American government and military leaders, as well as the media, Americanized the name to Porto Rico during the Spanish-American War. At the end of hostilities and with the signing of the Treaty of Paris, Porto Rico was the official name. In 1931, the name was changed back to Puerto Rico by a joint resolution of Congress.

10. Miles, "The War with Spain—I," *North American Review* (1899), p. 528.
11. *Ibid.*, p. 523.
12. Miles, "The War with Spain—II," *North American Review* (1899), p. 755.
13. United States. Surgeon General (Army) Office. Records relating to military personnel, Record Group 112.2.3.
14. Cirillo, *Bullets and Bacilli: The Spanish–American War and Military Medicine*, (2004), p. 1.
15. *Ibid.*, p. 31.
16. United States. Adjutant-General's Office. "Correspondence Relating to the War With Spain: Including the Insurrection In the Philippine Islands And the China Relief Expedition, April 15, 1898, to July 30, 1902, Volume 1" (1993), p. 381.
17. "Official Dispatches," *United States Army and Navy Journal and Gazette* (10 September 1898), p.43.
18. "The Sick on the Panama," *The Sun* (18 September 1898), p. 4.
19. Surgeon General (Army) Office. "Records relating to military personnel," Record Group 112.2.3
20. W. H. Daly, Major and Chief Surgeon U.S. Volunteers, to Assistant Adjutant-General, Headquarters of the Army, Washington, D.C. "Spanish American War, 1898, government documents: pamphlet collection," (1897–1900), pp. 51-52. See also: *Report of the Commission Appointed by the President to Investigate the Conduct of the War Department In the War With Spain*, p. 3,397.
21. Halstead, *The Life of Theodore Roosevelt* (1903), pp. 118-119.
22. *Ibid.*, p. 119.
23. "The Bombardment of the War Department," *The Literary Digest* (1898) p. 302.
24. "Criticism of Army Administration," *The Literary Digest* (1898), p. 212.

Chapter 9

1. "Gen. Miles Repeats His Charges and Lays the Facts Bare," *New York Journal and Advertiser* (08 September 1898), p. 1.
2. United States. "Reports to President—Secretary R. A. Alger's letter to President." *Report of the Commission Appointed to Investigate the Conduct of the War Department in the War with Spain, Minutes of Meetings, Volume 1, Appendix A* (1899).
3. United States. Commission Appointed by the President to Investigate the Conduct of the War Department in the War with Spain. *Report of the Commission Appointed to Investigate the Conduct of the War Department in the War with Spain, Volume 1*, (1899), Title Page.
4. Testimony was taken in Washington, D.C.; Jacksonville, Florida; Fort McPherson, Georgia; Anniston, Alabama; Huntsville, Alabama; Chattanooga, Tennessee; Knoxville, Tennessee; Lexington, Kentucky; Chicago, Illinois; Cincinnati, Ohio; Detroit, Michigan; Harrisburg, Pennsylvania; New York City; Boston, Massachusetts; Burlington, Vermont; Tampa, Florida, and Fernandina, Florida. Indeed, Commission members traveled extensively during the course of their

deliberations. Besides holding formal hearings, they also inspected and took testimony at a number of military bases around the country, including: Camp Cuba Libre, Jacksonville, Florida; Camp Tampa, Tampa, Florida; Camp Amelia, Fernandina, Florida; Camp Thomas, Chickamauga, Georgia; Camp Shipp, Anniston, Alabama; Camp Forse, Huntsville, Tennessee; Camp Poland, Knoxville, Tennessee; Camp Bradley, Lexington, Kentucky; and Camp Meade, Middletown, Pennsylvania. While at the camps, Commission members also inspected troops and supplies, which allowed them an opportunity to communicate directly with officers and enlisted men. For further details see: United States. *Report of the Commission Appointed by the President to Investigate the Conduct of the War Department In the War With Spain*" (1899), p. 6.

5. United States. "Reports to President—President William McKinley's letter to Commission" *Report of the Commission Appointed to Investigate the Conduct of the War Department in the War with Spain, Minutes of Meetings, Volume 1, Appendix B* (1899).
6. Ranson, "The Investigation of the War Department, 1898–1899", *The Historian*, (November 1971), pp. 78, 89. Also see: "Army Beef Scandal," *The Literary Digest*, (February 1899), p. 151.
7. United States. "Statement of Major General Nelson A. Miles," *Report of the Commission Appointed by the President to Investigate the Conduct of the War Department in the War with Spain*, *Volume 7* (1899), p. 3,241.
8. *Ibid.*
9. *Ibid.*
10. *Ibid.*, p. 3,242.
11. *Ibid.*, p. 3,258.
12. United States. "Testimony of William H. Daly," *Report of the Commission Appointed by the President to Investigate the Conduct of the War Department In the War With Spain*, *Volume 7 (1899)*, p. 3,710.
13. *Ibid.*, pp. 3,715-3,716
14. *Ibid.*, p. 3,716.
15. *Ibid.*
16. Early in the Spanish American War there was consensus in Washington that fighting a war on tropical islands could potentially be disastrous for troops who were not conditioned, by lifestyle or prior illness—particularly with malaria and yellow fever—to service in such climates. In May 1898, Congress approved plans for recruitment of a volunteer force to be composed of troops thought to be immune to tropical diseases. The reality was many of those possessing such qualities were citizens of the South and most were African-American. A number of regiments were subsequently raised, deployed, and fought with valor. Collectively, they became known as "immune regiments," or more popularly, as the "Immunes."
17. United States. Surgeon General (Army) Office. Records relating to military personnel, Record Group 112.2.3.
18. *Ibid.* Daly's reports were dated 05 November 1898, 03 December 1898, and 01 January 1899.
19. United States, "Testimony of William H. Daly," *op. cit.*, p. 3,724.
20. *Ibid.*, p. 3,725.
21. *Ibid.*
22. *Ibid.*, pp. 3,725-3,726
23. "The Progress of the World," *The American Monthly Review of Reviews*, (1898), p. 500.
24. Camp Alger was created in May 1898 for specific use as an assembly base for troops from several states during the Spanish American War. Shortly after opening,

it was determined there were serious flaws with the location due to poor water supply and inherent sanitary control problems due to its remote location some six miles from the Potomac River. A major outbreak of typhoid fever began ravaging troops between July and November 1898. The outbreak was so bad that in late August troops were being relocated to other camps. By September the site was abandoned and the property put up for sale.

25. United States. "Statement of Major Gen. Nelson A. Miles," *Report of the Commission Appointed by the President to Investigate the Conduct of the War Department In the War With Spain,*" *Volume 7,* (1899), p. 3,256.
26. In conducting a Google search of the term "embalmed beef," more than 100,000 results are reported.
27. United States. "Statement of Major Gen. Nelson A. Miles," *Report of the Commission Appointed by the President to Investigate the Conduct of the War Department In the War With Spain, Volume 7* (1899), pp. 3,257-3,258.
28. United States. "Extracts from letters, reports, etc., from officers, enlisted men, etc., Theodore Roosevelt, 09 January 1899," *Report of the Commission Appointed by the President to Investigate the Conduct of the War Department In the War With Spain*, Volume 8, p. 417 (Washington, D.C.: Government Printing Office, 1899).
29. *Ibid.*
30. United States. "Canned and Refrigerated Beef—Correspondence, Documents, Papers, Affidavits, etc., Relating to the Amount of Beef Supplied to the Army, its Character, etc., Correspondence from Charles P. Eagan, Commissary-General of Subsistence." *Report of the Commission Appointed by the President to Investigate the Conduct of the War Department In the War With Spain, Volume 8*, (1899), p. 408.
31. United States. "Brigadier General Charles P. Eagan—Recalled" *Report of the Commission Appointed by the President to Investigate the Conduct of the War Department In the War With Spain, Volume 7* (1899), p. 3,564.
32. *Ibid.*, p. 3,572.
33. *Ibid.*, p. 3,574.
34. *Ibid.*, pp. 3,574-3,575.
35. *Ibid.*, p. 3,576.
36. United States. "Food Furnished By Subsistence Department to Troops in the Field, Letter from The Secretary Of War, Transmitting in Response to Resolution of the Senate of March 30, 1900," *The Original Record of the Court of Inquiry Relative to the Unfitness for Issue of Certain Articles of Food Furnished by the Subsistence Department to Troops in the Field During the Recent Operations in Cuba and Porto Rico, Part III,* (1899), pp. 2,509-2,510.
37. United States. "Brigadier General Charles P. Eagan—Recalled" *Report of the Commission Appointed by the President to Investigate the Conduct of the War Department In the War With Spain, Volume 7,*" (1899), p. 3,577.
38. *Ibid.*, pp. 3,577-3,578.
39. *Ibid.*, p. 3,578.
40. "Calls Gen. Miles a Liar," *New York Sun* (13 January 1899), p. 1.
41. "The President's Commission—General Eagan's Testimony," *The United States Army and Navy Journal and Gazette of the Regular and Volunteer Forces* (14 January 1899), pp. 470-471.
42. "General Eagan's Outbreak," *The United States Army and Navy Journal and Gazette of the Regular and Volunteer Forces* (14 January 1899), p. 458.
43. *Ibid.*
44. U.S. Government, "General Order No. 24," *General Orders and Circulars Adjutant General's Office, 1899* (1900), pp. 1-3.

45. *Ibid.*, p. 3.
46. *Ibid.*
47. "Papers of the Estate of Dr. W. H. Daly, Pittsburg, Pa, Nov. 10th, 1902" (1902).
48. United States. "Testimony of William H. Daly," *Report of the Commission Appointed by the President to Investigate the Conduct of the War Department In the War With Spain, Volume 7*, (1899), pp. 3,733-3,734.
49. United States. "Testimony of Prof. Frank W. Clarke," *Report of the Commission Appointed by the President to Investigate the Conduct of the War Department In the War With Spain, Volume 7*, (1899), p. 3,749.
50. United States, "Refrigerated Beef," *Report of the Commission Appointed to Investigate the Conduct of the War Department in the War with Spain, Minutes of Meetings, Volume 1*, (1899), p. 163.
51. United States, "Canned Meats," *Report of the Commission Appointed to Investigate the Conduct of the War Department in the War with Spain, Minutes of Meetings, Volume 1,* (1899), pp. 166-167.
52. United States. War Department. "Letter of Transmittal," *Food Furnished by Subsistence Department to troops in the field: letter from the Secretary of War, Part I,* (1890), p. 5.

Chapter 10

1. United States War Department. "Letter from the Secretary of War, Transmitting, in response to resolution of the Senate of March 30, 1900, the Original Record of the Court of Inquiry relative to the Unfitness for Issue of Certain Articles of Food Furnished by the Subsistence Department to Troops in the Field During the Recent Operations in Cuba and Porto Rico," *Food Furnished by Subsistence Department to the Troops in the Field, Part 2,* (1900), p. 1,855.
2. United States War Department. "Record of a Court of Inquiry," *Food Furnished by Subsistence Department to the Troops in the Field, Part 1*, (1900), p. 5.
3. United States War Department. "Letter from the Secretary of War, Transmitting, in response to resolution of the Senate of March 30, 1900, the Original Record of the Court of Inquiry relative to the Unfitness for Issue of Certain Articles of Food Furnished by the Subsistence Department to Troops in the Field During the Recent Operations in Cuba and Porto Rico," *Food Furnished by Subsistence Department to the Troops in the Field, Part 3,* (1900), p. 1,921.
4. United States War Department. "Record of a Court of Inquiry," *Food Furnished by Subsistence Department to the Troops in the Field, Part 2,* (1900), p. 1,849.
5. "Investigation of the Army Administration," *Harper's Weekly*, (12 November 1898), p. 1,098.
6. "M'Dougall Investigates," *New York Journal* (14 October 1898), p. 6. Note: The Crédit Mobilier reference referred to General Dodge's involvement in the scandal of 1872–1873 when the Union Railroad created Crédit Mobilier to hold and finance lucrative construction contracts. Shares of company stock were either sold at a discount or given free of charge to members of Congress. Congress, in turn, awarded generous federal subsidies to the company. After his military career, Grenville M. Dodge became chief engineer of the Union Pacific Railroad and was subsequently elected to Congress. As such, he was allegedly involved on both sides of the scandal.
7. "General Miles Sustained," *The Evening Times* (21 March 1899), p. 4. Note: The pejorative term "Alger Relief Commission" was coined shortly after the Dodge Commission was formed in September 1898. Its original connotation suggested

President McKinley had selected General Dodge and the other members of the Commission for the express purpose of whitewashing Secretary Alger's handling of the Spanish-American War.

8. "The Army Beef Inquiry," *New York Times* (23 February 1899), p. 1.
9. United States War Department. "Record of a Court of Inquiry," *Food Furnished by Subsistence Department to the Troops in the Field, Part 2,* (1900), p. 1,361.
10. *Ibid.*
11. *Ibid.*, p. 1,362.
12. *Ibid.*, p. 1,847.
13. *Ibid.*, p. 1,343.
14. *Ibid.*, p. 1,844.
15. United States War Department. "Conclusion," *Food Furnished by Subsistence Department to the Troops in the Field, Part 2*, (1900), pp. 1,893-1,894.
16. "Report of Army Beef Commission," *Literary Digest* (13 May 1899), p. 537.
17. *Ibid.*, p. 538.
18. "Whitewash for Beef and Boodle," *New York Journal and Advertiser* (08 May 1899), p. 1.

Chapter 11

1. "Miles' Pittsburg Visit," *Scranton Tribune* (21 June 1899), p. 1.
2. "General Miles at Pittsburg—A Busy Time As Guest Of All Organized Labor," *Scranton Tribune*, (01 July 1900), p. 1.
3. *The National Cyclopedia of American Biography, Volume 10*, (1900), pp. 268-269; Correspondence between Daly, James T. White & Co., and Harry L. Christy (1900).
4. *Ibid.*, p. 268.
5. *Journal of the American Medical Association* (1899), p. 384.
6. Correspondence—"Letter of Good Standing" dated 28 June 1900 from Surgeon General Sternberg addressed 'To Whom it may concern;' Correspondence between Nelson A. Miles and William H. Daly dated 09 July 1900 regarding letter of introduction to U.S. Military Attaches in care of London Bankers, Brown, Shipley & Co.; Letter from Nelson A. Miles addressed to Military Attaches to United States Embassies and Legations, dated 07 July 1900 containing letter introducing William H. Daly requesting assistance for Daly to visit military facilities and maneuvers of foreign troops; sanitary facilities and food supplies (1900).
7. William H. Daly passport application dated 03 July 1901.
8. Alger, *The Spanish-American War* (1901).
9. Alger, "The Food of the Army during the Spanish War," *North American Review* (January 1901), pp. 39-58.
10. "Roast Beef for Alger," *Daily Inter Mountain* (09 January 1901), p. 3.
11. "List of Fire Insurance Policies with Date of Expiration," Estate of William H. Daly (1901).
12. "Brookston Beer Bulletin," www.brookstonbeerbulletin.com/tag/maryland/.
13. "William H. Daly Coroner's Report, 10 June 1901" Allegheny County Coroner's Case Files (1901).
14. "W. S. Foster, M.D. Coroner's Affidavit," Allegheny County Coroner's Case Files (1901).
15. "Revolver Shot Ends The Life Of Dr. W.H. Daly," *Pittsburg Dispatch* (10 June 1901), p. l.
16. *Ibid.*

17. *Ibid.*
18. William H. Daly personal bank check No. 20, T. Mellon & Sons' Bank, dated 10 June 1901 (1901).
19. "Dr. Daly's Suicide," *The Forest Republican* (19 June 1901), p. 1.

Chapter 12

1. "Maj. W. H. Daly Shoots Himself," *Pittsburgh Commercial* (10 June 1901) p. 1.
2. "Revolver Shot Ends The Life Of Dr. W.H. Daly," *Pittsburg Dispatch* (10 June 1901), p. l.
3. "Will of William H. Daly," Registered in Register's office June 12, 1901, Will Book, Volume 66, p. 450.
4. "The Estate of Dr. William H. Daly," *Journal of the American Medical Association* (13 July 1901), p. 121.
5. Athalia Daly Home Corporation, Court Order, 1975, Allegheny County Court of Common Pleas, Orphan's Court Division (1975). Note: In his will, Daly thought his properties, in Baden, Beaver County, including a farm, a farm mansion house, and associated farm buildings, might serve as a primary or secondary site for one of the Homes. He surmised the rural settings and "invigorating influence" of such surroundings might be needed or preferred by some of the beneficiary women.
6. "Paper Book of Appellees," *Supreme Court of Pennsylvania, Western District*, Numbers 8, 9, 10, 11 and 12, October term, 1904, in Re: Estate of Dr. W. H. Daly, Deceased (1904).
7. Articles of Incorporation of the Athalia Daly Home, Court of Common Pleas No. 1 of Allegheny County, April Term, 1904 (1904).
8. Swetnam, "Dr. Daly's Dream Home," *Pittsburgh Press* (27, August 1972), p. 3.
9. Athalia Daly Home brochure (15 January 1913).
10. *Ibid.*
11. Athalia Daly Home Corporation, Petition for Distribution of Assets, No. 5152 of 1975, Allegheny County Court of Common Pleas, Orphans' Court Division (1975), p. 3.
12. *Ibid.*, pp. 3-4.
13. Athalia Daly Home Report of Special Committee on Operation of the Home, 20 October 1975 (1975).
14. *Ibid.*
15. Athalia Daly Home Sale to Western Pennsylvania Hospital, Agreement Undertaking, Exhibit "C" (1975).
16. "Theodore Roosevelt State of the Union Address 05 December 1905," Teaching American History.org. teachingamericanhistory.org/library/document/state-of-the-union-address-part-ii-10/. Retrieved 21 February 2019,
17. Adams, *The Great American Fraud*, 4th edition, Reprinted from *Collier's Weekly* (1905–1907).
18. Sinclair, *The Jungle* (1906), p. 114.
19. *Ibid.*, p. 267.

Bibliography

Books

Adams, S. H., *The Great American Fraud*, 4th edition. Reprinted from *Collier's Weekly*, (Chicago: P. F. Collier & Son, 1905–1907).
Albert, G. D., *History of the County of Westmoreland, Pennsylvania* (Philadelphia: L. H. Everts & Co., 1882).
Alger, R. A., *The Spanish-American War* (New York: Harper & Brothers, 1901).
American Kennel Club Stud-Book, Volume X, January 1–December 31, 1893 (Philadelphia, PA: S. M. Larzelere, 1894).
Anderson, O. E., *The Health of a Nation: Harvey W. Wiley and the Fight for Pure Food* (Chicago, IL: University of Chicago Press, 1958).
Annual Report of the Managers of the Western Pennsylvania Hospital for 1862 (Pittsburgh, PA: W. S. Haven & Co., 1863).
Blum, D., *The Poison Squad* (New York: Penguin Press, 2018).
Brown, D. A., *The Galvanized Yankees* (Urbana, IL: University of Illinois Press, 1963).
Cirillo, V. J., *Bullets and Bacilli: The Spanish–American War and Military Medicine*, (New Brunswick, NJ: Rutgers University Press, 2004).
Cosmas, G. A., *An Army for Empire* (Columbia, MO: The Curators of the University of Missouri, 1971).
Cushing, T., *History of Allegheny County Pennsylvania*, Volume 1 (Chicago, IL: A. Warner & Co., 1889).
Day, S. P., *Down South; or, An Englishman's Experience at the Seat of the American War*, Volume 1 (London: Hurst and Blackett, 1862).
"Degrees Conferred During the Year," *Catalogue of the Students for 1866–1867* (Ann Arbor: University of Michigan, 1867).
DeMontravel, P. R., *A Hero to His Fighting Men* (Kent, Ohio: Kent State University Press, 1998).
Diffenbacher, J. F., *Directory of Pittsburgh and Allegheny Cities*, 1878; 1880; 1882–1883; 1887; 1890–1891; 1892; 1894; 1896, 1897–1898 (Pittsburgh, PA: G. H. Thurston).
"Distinguished Alumni," *The Michigan Alumnus*, Volume VII, Number 8, May 1901 (Ann Arbor, MI: University of Michigan Alumni Association, 1901).
Durant, S. W., *History of Allegheny County Pennsylvania* (Philadelphia, PA: L. H. Everts & Co., 1876).
Evans, C. A., (ed.), *Confederate military history; a library of Confederate States history, written by distinguished men of the south* (Atlanta: Confederate Publishing Company, 1899).
Frank, L. T., *Women in the American Civil War* (Santa Barbara, CA: ABC-CLIO, 2008)
Grom, R. M., *Physician-Soldiers at the Forks* (Mount Pleasant, SC: Arcadia Publishing, 2019).
Halstead, Murat, *The Life of Theodore Roosevelt* (London: Grant Richards, 1903).

Hays, S., *City at the Point*, (Pittsburgh, PA: University of Pittsburgh Press, 1989).
Jackson, C. (Chevalier), *The Life of Chevalier Jackson: An Autobiography*, (New York: Macmillan Company, 1938).
Message of the President of the United States to the Two Houses of Congress at the Commencement of the Second Session of the Thirty-Seventh Congress, Volume 2 (Washington, D.C.: Government Printing Office, 1861).
Miles, N. A., "Hunting Large Game," *North American Review*, Volume 161, Number 467 (Boston, MA: October 1895); *Personal Recollections & Observations of General Nelson A. Miles* (Chicago, IL: The Werner Company, 1896); *Serving the Republic: Memoirs of the Civil and Military Life of Nelson A. Miles* (New York: Harper & Brothers, 1911).
Roosevelt, Theodore and Greene, Vinton, *The Works of Theodore Roosevelt: The Rough Riders* (New York: P. F. Collier & Son, 1899).
Shaw, W. B., (ed.), *The University of Michigan, an Encyclopedic Survey* (Ann Arbor, MI: University of Michigan Press, 1942).
Sifakis, S., *Compendium of the Confederate Armies: Virginia* (Westminster, Maryland: Heritage Books, Inc. 1992).
Stewart, T. J., *Record of Pennsylvania Volunteers in the Spanish-American War, 1898* (Pennsylvania: William Stanley Ray, 1900).
"Students in Medicine," *Catalogue of the Students for 1865–1866* (Ann Arbor: University of Michigan, 1866).
"The Army Surgeon's Manual, for the use of Medical Officers, Cadets, Chaplains, and Hospital Stewards Regulations of the Medical Department, All General Orders from the War Department, and Circulars from the Surgeon-General's Office, From January 1st, 1861, to July 1st, 1864," (New York: Bailliere Brothers, 1864).
"The National Cyclopedia of American Biography, Volume 10" (New York: James T. White & Company, 1900).
"The Union Army: A History of Military Affairs in the Loyal States, 1861–65, Records of the Regiments In the Union Army, Cyclopedia of Battles, Memoirs of Commanders And Soldiers," (Madison, WI: Federal Publishing Co., 1908).
The war of the rebellion: a compilation of the official records of the Union and Confederate armies. Series 1, Volume II, Part III (Washington, D.C.: Government Printing Office 1880–1901).
Thurston, G. H., *Directory of Pittsburgh and Allegheny Cities for 1868–69; 1869–70; 1870; 1871–1872; 1872–1873; 1873–74, 1874* (Pittsburgh, PA: A. A. Anderson & Sons).
Thurston, G. H., and Diffenbacher, J. F., *Directory of Pittsburgh and Allegheny Cities for 1875, 1876, 1877* (Pittsburgh, PA: G. H. Thurston).
Transactions of the Fourth Annual Meeting of the American Laryngological, Rhinological, and Otological Society Held in Pittsburg, PA, May 11 and 12, 1898, (New York, NY: American Laryngological, Rhinological, and Otological Society, 1899).
United States Adjutant-General's Office. Correspondence Relating to the War With Spain: Including the Insurrection In the Philippine Islands And the China Relief Expedition, April 15, 1898, to July 30, 1902, Volume 1 (Washington, D.C.: Center of Military History, U.S. Army, 1993).
United States Adjutant General's Office, "General Order No. 24," *General Orders and Circulars Adjutant General's Office, 1899* (Washington, D.C.: Government Printing Office 1900).
United States War Department, *Report of the Commission Appointed by the President to Investigate the Conduct of the War Department in the War With Spain, Volumes 1–8* (Washington, D.C.: Government Printing Office, 1899).
Wallace, L. A., *A Guide to Virginia Military Organizations, 1861–1865* (Richmond, VA: Civil War Commission, 1964).

Wechsler, H. (Harry) L., *Dr. Chevalier Jackson* (Pittsburgh, PA: The West Penn Hospital Foundation, 1994).

"Women and the Trades," *The Pittsburgh Survey* (New York: Russell Sage Foundation, 1909).

Young, J. H., *Pure Food: Securing the Federal Food and Drug Act of 1906* (Princeton: Princeton University Press, 1989).

ARTICLES

Alger, R. A., "The Food of the Army during the Spanish War," *North American Review*, Vol. 172, No. 530, January 1901 (Boston, 1901).

"A Long Trip for Sport—Twelve Hundred Miles and Back Again for Prairie Chicken Shooting," *Pittsburg Dispatch*, 09 October 1892 (Pittsburg, PA, 1892).

"Army Beef Scandal," *The Literary Digest*, Volume XVIII, Number 6 (New York, NY: 11 February 1899).

Brinton, D. G., (ed.), "Correspondence," *The Medical and Surgical Reporter: A Weekly Journal*," Volume 39 (Philadelphia, PA: 1878).

"Calls Gen. Miles a Liar," *New York Sun*, 13 January 1899, p. 1 (New York, NY: 1899)

"Criticism of Army Administration," *The Literary Digest*, Volume XVII, Number 8, 20 August 1898 (New York, NY: 1898).

Cunningham, H. H., "Confederate General Hospitals: Establishment and Organization," *The Journal of Southern History*, Volume 20, Number 3, August 1954 (Houston, TX: 1954).

Daly, W. H., "Address in Medicine," *Transactions of the Medical Society of the State of Pennsylvania*, Volume 16 (Philadelphia, PA: Collins, 1884); "A Case of Luxation of the Left Cornua of the Hyoid Bone," *Archives of Laryngology*, Volume 1, Number 2, 1880 (New York, NY: G. P. Putnam's Sons, 1881); "A Case of Stenosis of the Larynx, with Fibrous Adhesive Bands of the True Vocal Cords: Tracheotomy, Rupture of Bands, and Cure of Stenosis by General and Local Treatment," *The Transactions of the American Medical Association*, Volume 31 (Chicago, IL: American Medical Association, 1880); "A Clinical Study of Glanders in the Horse," *Medical Record*, Volume 43, 07 January 1893 (New York, NY: *New York Medical Journal*, 1893); "An Analysis of the Value of the Galvano-Cautery in the Treatment of Diseases and Growths of the Naso-Pharynx," *The Transactions of the American Medical Association*, Volume 31 (Chicago, IL: American Medical Association, 1880); "Elongating Hyperthropy of the Femur and Tibia of Opposite Sides (The Osteitis Deformans of Paget)," *Medical Record*, Volume XVII, Number 9, February 28, 1880, (New York, NY: 1880); "Extensive Burn Involving the Cavity of the Knee-Joint," *British Medical Journal*, Volume 2, Number 1250, 13 December 1884, (London: 1884); "Gunshot Wounds of the Larynx with the report of a case in which the vocal bands were involved." Monograph reprinted from the *New York Medical Journal* for July 12, 1884, (New York: D. Appleton and Company, 1884); "Some Practical Observations On So-Called Malaria Being A Waterborne Disease," *Transactions of the American Climatological Association for the year 1893*, Volume 10, 1893 (New York, NY: American Climatological Association, 1893).

"Daughters of our Presidents," *The Ladies Home Journal*, Vol. 14, No. 3, 1897 (Philadelphia: 1897).

Douglas, H. T., "Reminiscences of the Peninsula," *Confederate Veteran*, Vol. XI, No. 12 (Nashville, TN: December 1903).

"Dr. Daly's Suicide," *The Forest Republican*, Volume XXXIV, Number 11, 19 June 1901 (Tionesta, PA: 1901).

"Dr. W. H. Daly Kills Himself," *Pittsburgh Times*, 10 June 1901 (Pittsburgh, PA: 1901)

"General Eagan's Outbreak," *The United States Army and Navy Journal and Gazette of the Regular and Volunteer Forces,* 14 January 1899, Volume 36 (New York, NY: Army and Navy Journal, Inc., 1899).

"General Miles at Pittsburg—A Busy Time As Guest Of All Organized Labor," *Scranton Tribune*, 01 July 1900 (Scranton, PA: 1900).

"Gen. Miles Repeats His Charges and Lays the Facts Bare," *New York Journal and Advertiser*, 08 September 1898 (New York, NY: 1898).

"General Miles Sustained," *The Evening Times*, 21 March 1899 (Washington, D.C.: 1899).

Gilmer, H., "Birth of the American Crucible Steel Industry," *The Western Pennsylvania Historical Magazine,* Volume 36, Number 1, March 1953 (Pittsburgh, PA: Historical Society of Western Pennsylvania, 1953).

Grom, R. M., "No Ordinary Man," *Pittsburgh History*, Spring 1991(Pittsburgh, PA: Historical Society of Western Pennsylvania, 1991).

Harris, G. R., "Minutes With Comments, The Allegheny County Medical Society 1865–1940 (16 April 1867 meeting)," *Pittsburgh Medical Bulletin*, 23 September 1939 (Pittsburgh, PA: Allegheny County Medical Society, 1939).

Hasegawa, G. R., "The Civil War's Medical Cadets: Medical Students Serving the Union," *Journal of the American College of Surgeons,* Volume 193, Issue 1 (Chicago, IL: American College of Surgeons, 2001).

Holtz, W., "Bankrobbers, Burkers, and Bodysnatchers," *Michigan Quarterly Review*, Vol. 6, No. 2, Spring 1967 (Ann Arbor, MI: University of Michigan, 1967).

"Investigation of the Army Administration," *Harper's Weekly*, Volume XLII, Number 2186, 12 November 1898 (New York, NY: 1898).

Keuchel, E. F., "Chemicals and Meat: The Embalmed Beef Scandal of the Spanish-American War," *Bulletin of the History of Medicine*, Volume 48, Number 2, Summer 1974 (Baltimore, MD: Johns Hopkins University Press, 1974).

Lowe, R. G., "Magruder's Defense of the Peninsula," *Confederate Veteran*, Vol. VIII, No. 3, March 1900 (Nashville, TN: 1900).

"Maj. W. H. Daly Shoots Himself," *Pittsburgh Commercial*, 10 June 1901 (Pittsburgh, PA, 1901).

"M'Dougall Investigates," *New York Journal*, 14 October 1898 (New York, NY, 1898)

Miles, N. A., "The War with Spain—I", *North American Review*, Volume 168, Number 510 (Boston, MA: May 1899); "The War with Spain—II", *North American Review*, Volume 168, Number 511 (Boston, MA: June 1899).

"Miles' Pittsburg Visit," *Scranton Tribune*, 21 June 1899 (Scranton, PA, 1899).

"Miles Starts. General in Command of the U.S. Army, Departs from Washington for the Front," *Topeka State Journal*, 31 May 1898 (Topeka, KS: 1898).

"Official Dispatches," *United States Army and Navy Journal and Gazette*, Volume 36, 1898–99 (Washington, D.C.: 10 September 1898).

Rankin, D. N., "Letter from Dr. D. N. Rankin—Editor's Reply," *The Journal of Laryngology and Rhinology*, Volume 1, Number 8, August 1887, (London, 1887).

Ranson, E., "The Investigation of the War Department, 1898–1899," *The Historian*, Volume 34, Number 1, November 1971 (New Jersey: 1971).

"Report of Army Beef Commission," *Literary Digest*, Volume XVIII, Number 19, 13 May 1899 (New York, NY: 1899).

"Revolver Shot Ends the Life of Dr. W. H. Daly," *Pittsburg Dispatch*, 10 June 1901 (Pittsburgh, PA: 1901).

"Roast Beef for Alger," *Daily Inter Mountain,* 09 January 1901 (Butte, MT, 1901)

Sinclair, U., "The Condemned-Meat Industry," *Everybody's Magazine*, Volume XIV, Number 5, May 1906 (New York, NY: 1906); *The Jungle*, (New York: Doubleday, Page & Company, 1906).

"Social Chatter," *Pittsburg Dispatch*, 24 August 1892 (Pittsburgh, PA: 1892).
Swetnam, G., "Dr. Daly's Dream Home," *Pittsburgh Press,* 27 August 1972 (Pittsburgh, PA: 1972).
"The Army Beef Inquiry," *New York Times*, 23 February 1899 (New York, NY: 1899).
"The Bombardment of the War Department," *The Literary Digest*, Volume XVII, Number 11, 10 September 1898 (New York, NY: 1898).
"The Estate of Dr. William H. Daly," *Journal of the American Medical Association*, Volume 37, Number 2, 13 July 1901 (Chicago, IL: 1901).
"The President's Commission—General Eagan's Testimony," *The United States Army and Navy Journal and Gazette of the Regular and Volunteer Forces,* 14 January 1899, Volume 36 (New York, NY: Army and Navy Journal, Inc., 1899).
"The Progress of the World," *The American Monthly Review of Reviews*, Volume 18, No 5 (New York, NY: November 1898).
"The Sick on the Panama," *The Sun* (New York, NY: 18 September 1898).
"Whitewash for Beef and Boodle," *New York Journal and Advertiser*, 08 May 1899 (New York, NY: 1899).
Young, J. H., "The Pig that Fell Unto the Privy: Upton Sinclair's 'The Jungle' and the Meat Inspection Amendments of 1906," *Bulletin of the History of Medicine*, Volume 59, Number 04, Winter 1985 (Baltimore, MD: Johns Hopkins University Press, 1985).

Brochures and Pamphlets

Allegheny County Medical Society Membership History, 1904 (Pittsburgh, PA: Allegheny County Medical Society, *c.* 1904).
Athalia Daly Home brochure (Pittsburgh, PA: Archives of Western Pennsylvania Hospital, 15 January 1913).

Correspondence

Daly, William H., Acting Medical Director, Hilton Head S.C, to Surgeon General Joseph K. Barnes, 22 August 1865" (Washington, D.C.: Records of the Surgeon General, Record Group 112.12.3, U.S. National Archives and Record Administration).
General Nelson A. Miles to Military Attaches to United States Embassies and Legations, introducing William H. Daly and requesting assistance for Daly in visiting military facilities and maneuvers of foreign troop; sanitary facilities and food supplies, 07 July 1900 (Pittsburgh: Archives of Western Pennsylvania Hospital, 1900).
General Nelson A. Miles to William H. Daly, 09 July 1900 (Pittsburgh, PA: Archives of Western Pennsylvania Hospital, 1900).
General Nelson A. Miles to William H. Daly regarding letter of introduction to U.S. Military Attaches in care of London Bankers, Brown, Shipley & Co.; 09 July 1900 (Pittsburgh, PA: Archives of Western Pennsylvania Hospital, 1900).
Surgeon General Sternberg to whom it may concern, "Letter of Good Standing," 28 June 1900 (Pittsburgh, PA: Archives of Western Pennsylvania Hospital, 1900).

Legal Documents and Related Materials

Articles of Incorporation of the Athalia Daly Home, Court of Common Pleas No. 1 of Allegheny County, April Term, 1904 (Pittsburgh, PA: Archives of Western Pennsylvania Hospital).
Athalia Daly Home Corporation, Court Order, 1975, Allegheny County Court of Common Pleas, Orphan's Court Division (Pittsburgh, PA: Archives of Western

Pennsylvania Hospital, 1975).

Athalia Daly Home Corporation, Petition for Distribution of Assets, Number 5152 of 1975, Allegheny County Court of Common Pleas, Orphan's Court Division (Pittsburgh, PA: Archives of Western Pennsylvania Hospital, 1975).

Athalia Daly Home Report of Special Committee on Operation of the Home (Pittsburgh, PA: Archives of Western Pennsylvania Hospital, 20 October 1975).

Athalia Daly Home sale to Western Pennsylvania Hospital, Agreement Undertaking, Exhibit "C" (Pittsburgh, PA: Archives of Western Pennsylvania Hospital, 1975).

Bill of Sale, Athalia Daly Home to the Western Pennsylvania Hospital (Pittsburgh, PA: Archives of Western Pennsylvania Hospital, 31 March 1976).

Daly, W. H., Acting Assistant Surgeon Contract, Records of the Surgeon General, Record Group 112.12.3 (Washington, D.C.: U.S. National Archives and Record Administration).

Fire Insurance Policies with Date of Expiration, Estate of William H. Daly (Pittsburgh, PA: Archives of Western Pennsylvania Hospital, 1901).

"Paper Book of Appellees," Supreme Court of Pennsylvania, Western District, Numbers 8, 9, 10, 11 and 12, October term, 1904, in Re Estate of Dr. W. H. Daly, Deceased. (Pittsburgh, PA: Archives of the Western Pennsylvania Hospital, 1904).

"Papers of the Estate of Dr. W. H. Daly, Pittsburgh, Pennsylvania" (Pittsburgh, PA: Archives of the Western Pennsylvania Hospital, 10 November 1902).

"William H. Daly Coroner's Report, 10 June 1901" Allegheny County Coroner's Case Files, (Pittsburgh, PA: Archives of Industrial Society, University of Pittsburgh).

William H. Daly passport application (Pittsburg, PA: Archives of Western Pennsylvania Hospital, 03 July 1901).

"Will of William H. Daly," Registered in Register's office June 12, 1901, Will Book, Volume 66 (Pittsburgh, PA: Archives of Western Pennsylvania Hospital).

"W. S. Foster, M.D. Coroner's Affidavit," Allegheny County Coroner's Case Files, Archives of Industrial Society, University of Pittsburgh (Pittsburgh, PA).

Manuscripts and Archival Materials

Company "B," 15th Regiment Va. Muster Rolls, 26 April 1862 and 31 December 1862, Manuscript No. 1038, (Washington, D.C.: U.S. National Archives and Records Administration).

Confederate Archives, Chapter 6, File No. 267, Page 5 (Washington, D.C.: National Archives and Record Administration).

Confederate Archives, Manuscript No. 138 (Washington, D.C.: National Archives and Record Administration).

Daly, W. H., *Report to Assistant Adjutant-General, Headquarters of the Army, Washington, D. C.,* Spanish American War, 1898, government documents: pamphlet collection (Washington, D.C.: Government Printing Office, 1897–1900).

Koyle, F. H., *"I Shtart to free ould Cuba in the Mornin',"* (Pittsburgh, PA: Archives of Western Pennsylvania Hospital, May 1898).

Lain, C. Y., *15th Virginia Infantry History, April 1861–Spring 1862* (Blacksburg, Virginia: Ms2009-111, Special Collections, Virginia Polytechnic and State University, 1862).

William Hudson Daly, "Sympathetic Pruritus with More Special Reference to that Form Affecting the Scrotum of the Male," Medical Thesis Box 12, Michigan Historical Collections, Bentley Historical Library (Ann Arbor: University of Michigan).

Officers of the Allegheny County Medical Society from 1865 to 1904 (Pittsburgh, PA: Allegheny County Medical Society, *c.* 1904).

Pennsylvania National Guard Veterans' Card File, 1867–1921, series #13.36 (Harrisburg, PA: Pennsylvania State Archives).

"President Abraham Lincoln's Union Blockade Proclamations (Proclamations 82 and 86), 4/27/1861–8/16/1861," Record Group 21: Records of District Courts of the United States. (Washington, D.C.: U.S. National Archives and Records Administration).

Record of Medical Officers Serving Department of the South for the Month of May 1865, William H. Daly Acting Assistant Surgeon, In Charge Provost Guards Hospital, S.C. to J. K. Barnes, Surgeon General USA, Records of the Surgeon General, Record Group 112.12.3 (Washington, D.C., U.S. National Archives and Record Administration).

United States Surgeon General's (Army) Office. "Records relating to military personnel," Record Group 112.2.3 (Washington, D.C.: National Archives and Records Administration).

William H. Daly personal bank check No. 20, T. Mellon & Sons' Bank (Pittsburg, PA: Archives of Western Pennsylvania Hospital, 10 June 1901).

Newspapers

Audubon County Journal (Exira, IA)
Cameron County Press (Emporium, PA)
Custer County Republican (Broken Bow, NE)
Daily Inter Mountain (Butte, MO)
Daily Pittsburgh Gazette (Pittsburgh, PA)
Evening Times-Republican (Marshalltown, IA)
Forest Republican (Tionesta, PA)
Houston Daily Post (Houston, TX)
Journal Courier (New Haven (CT)
Keowee Courier (Walhalla, SC)
Lincoln County Record (Pioche, NV)
Little Falls Weekly (Little Fall, MN)
McCook Tribune (McCook, NE)
New York Daily Tribune (New York, NY)
New York Journal and Advertiser (New York, NY)
New York Sun (New York, NY)
New York Times (New York, NY)
Omaha Daily Bee (Omaha, NE)
Pittsburg Bulletin (Pittsburgh, PA)
Pittsburgh Chronicle Telegraph (Pittsburgh, PA)
Pittsburgh Commercial (Pittsburgh, PA)
Pittsburg Dispatch (Pittsburgh, PA)
Pittsburgh Gazette (Pittsburgh, PA)
Pittsburgh Press (Pittsburgh, PA)
Pittsburg Times (Pittsburgh, PA)
Rock Island Argus (Rock Island, IL)
Richmond Daily Dispatch (Richmond, VA)
St. John's Herald (St. John's Apache County, Arizona Territory)
Scranton Tribune (Scranton, PA)
Spirit of the Age (Woodstock, VT)
The Abbeville Press and Banner (Abbeville, SC)
The Anaconda Standard (Anaconda MT)
The Arizona Republican (Phoenix, AZ)
The Billings Gazette (Billings, MO)
The Chronicle (Camden, NJ)
The Citizen (Frederick City MD)

The Columbian (Bloomsburg, PA)
The Daily Sentinel (Grand Junction, CO)
The Dalles Daily Chronicle (The Dalles, OR)
The Denison Review (Denison, IA)
The Dickinson Press (Dickinson, ND)
The Evening Bulletin (Nashville, KY)
The Evening Star (Washington, D.C.)
The Evening Times (Washington, D.C.)
The Farmers Leader (Canton, SD)
The Globe Republican (Dodge City, KS)
The Herald (Shenandoah, PA)
The Kansas City Journal (Kansas City, MO)
The Lehi Banner (Lehi, UT)
The Madison Daily Leader (Madison, SD)
The Nebraska Independent (Lincoln, NE)
The Oregon Mist (St. Helens, OR)
The Philipsburg Mail (Philipsburg, MO)
The Record-Union (Sacramento, CA)
The St. Paul Globe (St. Paul, MN)
The Salt Lake Herald (Salt Lake City, UT)
The San Francisco Call (San Francisco, CA)
The Seattle Post-Intelligencer (Seattle, WA)
The Semi-Weekly Messenger (Wilmington, NC)
The Sun (New York, NY)
The Times (Washington, D.C.)
The Topeka State Journal (Topeka, KS)
The Watchman and Southron (Sumter, SC)
The Wheeling Intelligencer (Wheeling, WV)
Virginian-Pilot (Norfolk, VA)
Waterbury Evening Democrat (Waterbury, CT)
Wichita Daily Eagle (Wichita, KS)

Periodicals

Archives of Laryngology
Confederate Veteran
Forest and Stream
Harper's Weekly
Journal of the American College of Surgeons
Journal of the American Medical Association
Literary Digest
Medical Record
Michigan Quarterly Review
New York Medical Journal
North American Review
Pennsylvania Medical Journal
Pittsburgh History
Pittsburgh Medical Bulletin
Timely Topics
The American Monthly Review of Reviews
The Conservative

The Journal of Laryngology and Rhinology
The Ladies Home Journal
The Laryngoscope
The Literary Digest
The Medical and Surgical Reporter
The Medical Times and Register
The Michigan Alumnus
Transactions of the American Climatological Association
Transactions of the Medical Society of the State of Pennsylvania
United States Army and Navy Journal and Gazette

Web Pages

Brookston Beer Bulletin, brookstonbeerbulletin.com/tag/maryland/. Retrieved 19 February 2019.

Daly Family Album (Daly Family Genealogy), www.seltzerbooks.com/gen/daly/album.html. Retrieved 25 October 2018.

Daly, W. H., "A discussion of some questions relating to tonsillotomy: read before the State Medical Society of Pennsylvania, at its meeting in 1882, and published in the *Medical Record* of February, 1883 and Clinical remarks upon deflections of the nasal septum, with a presentation of two cases made before the Allegheny County Medical Society, at its meeting, November, 1883" (London: Royal College of Surgeons, 1883). Retrieved from archive.org/details/b22454445/page/n1 on 01 January 2019.

Descendants of Hugh Daly, www.genealogy.com/ftm/w/h/i/David-E-Whitby/GENE4-0003.html. Retrieved 25 October 2018.

"Dix-Hill Cartel," Wikisource contributors, en.wikisource.org/wiki/Dix-Hill_Cartel. Retrieved 10 December 2018.

Franklin, B., *Poor Richard's Almanac* (Philadelphia, PA: 1738), Historical Society of Pennsylvania. Spread 6, www.rarebookroom.org/Control/frapou/index.html?page=6. Retrieved 22 October 2018.

Gesley, J., "The Lieber Code—the First Modern Codification of the Laws of War," Library of Congress, April 24, 2018, blogs.loc.gov/law/2018/04/the-lieber-code-the-first-modern-codification-of-the-laws-of-war/. Retrieved 11 December 2018.

"John Daly, United States Census, 1860," Family Search (familysearch.org/ark:/61903/1:1:M418-TCP). Retrieved 04 November 2018.

"Making History," Pittsburgh Duquesne Club from www.duquesne.org/about/history/. Retrieved 10 January 2019.

"Myth: Grant Stopped the Prisoner Exchange," National Park Service, www.nps.gov/ande/learn/historyculture/grant-and-the-prisoner-exchange.htm. Retrieved 09 December 2018.

Netherton, R., *In the Path of History: Virginia Between the Rappahannock and the Potomac: An Historical Portrait* (Falls Church, VA: Higher Education Publications, 2004).

alexlibraryva.org/custom/web/lhsc/genealogyresources/oath/oath1.html. Retrieved 11 September 2018.

Pickenpaugh, R., "Prisoner Exchange and Parole," Essential Civil War Curriculum," www.essentialcivilwarcurriculum.com/prisoner-exchange-and-parole.html. Retrieved 09 December 2018.

Schreier, Philip, "English Enfields In Confederate Service," *American Rifleman Journal*, Thursday, July 7, 2016 (Virginia: National Rifle Association of America, 2016). From www.americanrifleman.org/articles/2016/7/7/english-enfields-in-confederate-service/. Retrieved 06 November 2018.

"Theodore Roosevelt State of the Union Address 05 December 1905," From Teaching American History.org, teachingamericanhistory.org/library/document/state-of-the-union-address-part-ii-10/. Retrieved 26 February 2019.

"United States Census, 1860", Family Search (familysearch.org/ark:/61903/1:1:M418-TCP). Retrieved 04 November 2018.

Vivian, C., *Good Ol' Monongahela Rye and the Gibsonton Mills*. www.pre-pro.com/histories/gibson.htm. Retrieved 26 October 2018.

Index